INTERNATIONAL UNION OF THEORETICAL AND
APPLIED MECHANICS (IUTAM)

# COLLOQUIUM ON FATIGUE
STOCKHOLM MAY 25-27, 1955 PROCEEDINGS

# COLLOQUE DE FATIGUE
STOCKHOLM 25-27 MAI 1955 COMPTES RENDUS

# KOLLOQUIUM ÜBER ERMÜDUNGSFESTIGKEIT
STOCKHOLM 25.-27. MAI 1955 VERHANDLUNGEN

EDITORS

WALODDI WEIBULL
DR. PHIL. PROFESSOR EMERITUS
KUNGL. TEKNISKA HÖGSKOLAN
(ROYAL INSTITUTE OF TECHNOLOGY)
STOCKHOLM

FOLKE K. G. ODQVIST
DR. PHIL. PROFESSOR
KUNGL. TEKNISKA HÖGSKOLAN
(ROYAL INSTITUTE OF TECHNOLOGY)
STOCKHOLM

WITH 194 FIGURES

1956

SPRINGER-VERLAG/BERLIN·GÖTTINGEN·HEIDELBERG

ISBN-13: 978-3-642-99856-0     e-ISBN-13: 978-3-642-99854-6
DOI: 10.1007/978-3-642-99854-6

# Preface

Upon the request of the International Union of Theoretical and Applied Mechanics (IUTAM) the Swedish National Committee for Mechanics organized a colloquium on fatigue, which was held at the Royal Institute of Technology (Kungl. Tekniska Högskolan) in Stockholm, May 25—27, 1955.

35 lectures were delivered, principally dealing with problems of statistical and basic nature. Among the topics were to be found statistical theory of fatigue, cumulative damage, mechanism of fatigue, metallurgical aspects on fatigue, velocity of fatigue cracks, fatigue at elevated temperature, and fatigue at combined stresses.

Lectures were going on simultaneously in two sections. Each lecturer had 15 minutes for presentation of his communication, and afterwards 15 minutes were reserved for discussion. Abstracts of the lectures were distributed about a month before the colloquium.

The colloquium was attended by 149 participants from the following countries: Denmark (1), Finland (2), France (5), Germany (6), Italy (2), Netherlands (2), Norway (2), Poland (2), Saar (1), Spain (3), Sweden (100), Switzerland (1), United Kingdom (10), USA (8), USSR (3), and Yugoslavia (1). A complete list of the participants will be found below.

The languages of the Colloquium were English, French, German and Italian. No lectures were delivered in Italian. Also, all contributions to the discussions have been translated to one of the first three languages.

Statements and opinions advanced are always those of the individual authors or participants in the discussions.

The present volume contains the papers presented at the Colloquium in full. Reference to bibliographies at the end of each paper will be made with numbers in brackets of the type [2], [5].

The units employed in this volume are usually left with the individual author. In order to help the reader the notation of units has been somewhat standardized, so that:

1 psi = 1 pound per square inch
1 tsi = 1 ton per square inch
1 ksi = 1000 psi
1 kg/mm² = 1 kilogramme per square millimetre.

The following relations will facilitate the conversion of units:
1 kg/mm² = 1422 psi = 0.6350 tsi.

If not otherwise indicated, the following frequency unit will be used
1 Hz = 1 period per second.

The editors regret that limitations of space have necessitated certain
reductions of the original manuscripts and particularly omitting of a
number of figures.

At the end of the meeting some participants expressed the view that
the picture of fatigue research as conveyed by the colloquium as a whole
was a rather confusing one. It is believed that the reading of the complete papers does not contradict this view. It was also suggested that
before closing the meeting, someone should have undertaken to summa-
rize the papers so as to let different opinions and points of view stand
out clearly. Of course such summary would have been highly desirable.
Anyhow it would have exceeded the powers of the Organizing Committee. If a subsequently prepared summary had been included in this
volume this would have meant a not inessential exceeding of the originally allotted space. In printing the discussions comparatively complete, and certainly not free from truisms, we have tried to form as true
a picture of the proceedings as has been possible. As a substitute for
a conclusive summary a comparatively complete Subject index in three
languages has been included. In preparing the manuscript for this
index the editors were faced with partly unsurmountable difficulties
of translation. Errors in translation of many index words must be tolerated, due to lack of equivalence in the different languages. Inconsis-
tency and vagueness of terms have called for uniting of similar or nearly
equivalent words to larger groups.

To cover part of the travelling expenses and subsistance of participants the IUTAM Bureau had granted an amount of $3500. To this
the Swedish government and industry added the equivalent of about
$1500 for publications and administration purposes and for entertain-
ments.

The editors want to express their gratitude to the publisher, Springer
Verlag, for having complied with all wishes regarding the presentation
of this volume.

Finally, the editors would like to express their high appreciation of
the unselfish work, laid down by Mr. ÅKE ISAKSSON, secretary of the
Colloquium on Fatigue, in preparation of the manuscript and reading
the proofs.

Stockholm and Bockamöllan.

**Folke K. G. Odqvist**          **Waloddi Weibull**

# Organizing committee

*President*:

Prof. W. WEIBULL, Bockamöllan, *Brösarp Station*.

*v. President*:

Prof. F. ODQVIST, Kungl. Tekniska Högskolan, *Stockholm 70*.

*Secretaries*:

Civ. ing. Å. ISAKSSON, Kungl. Tekniska Högskolan, *Stockholm 70*.
Civ. ing. G. WÅLLGREN, Flygtekniska Försöksanstalten, *Ulvsunda 1*.

Övering. S. FORNANDER, Jernkontoret, Kungsträdgårdsgatan 6, *Stockholm C*.
Överdir. O. FORSMAN, Statens Provningsanstalt, *Stockholm 26*.
Civ. ing. C. SCHAUB, Fagersta Bruks AB, *Fagersta*.

# List of authors

*Denmark*:

Øveringeniør P. E. WIENE, A/S Burmeister & Wain's Maskin- og Skibsbyggeri,
*Copenhagen*.

*Finland*:

Fil. mag. J. SALOKANGAS, Statens Tekniska Forskningsanstalt, Lönnrotsgatan
37, *Helsingfors*.

*France*:

M. F. BASTENAIRE, Docteur-ès-Sciences, Institut de Recherches de la Siderurgie,
185, Rue Président Roosevelt, *St. Germain-en-Laye* (S.-&-O.).
M. R. CAZAUD, Docteur-ès-Sciences, Institut de Recherches de la Siderurgie,
185, Rue Président Roosevelt, *St. Germain-en-Laye* (S.-&-O.).
M. R. JAQCUESSON, Docteur-ès-Sciences, Ecole Nationale Supérieure de
Mécanique et d'Aérotechnique, Place Montierneuf, *Poitiers*.
M. A. KAMMERER, Docteur-ès-Sciences, Ecole Centrale des Arts & Manu-
factures, 1 Rue Montgolfier, *Paris* (IIIe).
M. M. WEISZ, Institut de Recherches de la Siderurgie, 185, Rue Président
Roosevelt, *St. Germain-en-Laye* (S.-&-O.).

*Germany*:

Dr.-Ing. E. GASSNER, Laboratorium für Betriebsfestigkeit, *Darmstadt*,
Jahnstraße 107.
Dr.-Ing. M. HEMPEL, Max-Planck-Institut für Eisenforschung, *Düsseldorf*,
August-Thyssen-Straße 1.
Prof. F. WEVER, Max-Planck-Institut für Eisenforschung, *Düsseldorf*, August-
Thyssen-Straße 1.

*Netherlands*:

Dr. Ir. F. J. PLANTEMA, National Luchtvaartlaboratorium, Sloterweg 145,
*Amsterdam W*.

*Italy*:

Ing. A. FERRO, Laboratori FIAT, *Torino*.
Dr. Ing. F. GATTO, Istituto Sperimentale dei Metalli Leggeri, Divisione Ricerche, Casella Postale N. 169, *Novara*.
Dr. Ing. L. LOCATI, FIAT, Laboratorio Ricerche e Controlli, Auto-Avio, *Torino*.
Ing. U. ROSSETTI, Consiglio Nazionale delle Ricerche, Centro di Studio Sugli Stati di Coazione Elastica, Castello del Valentino, *Torino*.

*Saar*:

M. le Directeur P. LAURENT, Institut de Recherches Métallurgiques, *Sarrebruck 15*.

*Sweden*:

Flygdirektör A. FRANSSON, Centrala Flygverkstäderna, *Malmslätt*.
Chefsingenjör A. JOHANSSON, STAL, *Finspång*.
Ingenjör W. LIEDTKE, Fagersta Bruks AB, *Fagersta*.
Dr.-Ing. O. LISSNER, ASEA, *Västerås*.
Civilingenjör C. SCHAUB, Centrallaboratoriet, Fagersta Bruks AB, *Fagersta*.
Prof. W. WEIBULL, Bockamöllan, *Brösarp Station*.

*Switzerland*:

Dipl.-Ing. L. MARTINAGLIA, c/o Gebrüder Sulzer A.G., *Winterthur*.

*United Kingdom*:

Dr. R. B. HEYWOOD, F. Hangar, Structures Department, R.A.E., *Farnborough, Hants, England*.
Mr. C. E. PHILLIPS, Mechanical Engineering Research Laboratory, East Kilbride, *Glasgow, Scotland*.
Dr. D. G. SOPWITH, Mechanical Engineering Research Laboratory, East Kilbride, *Glasgow, Scotland*.
Mr. R. J. TAYLOR, British Iron and Steel Research Association, 11 Park Lane, *London, W 1*.
Dr. E. W. C. WILKINS, Royal Aeronautical Society, 4 Hamilton Place, *London W 1*.

*USA*:

Prof. W. N. FINDLEY, Brown University, *Providence 12, R.I.*
Prof. A. M. FREUDENTHAL, Department of Civil Engineering, Columbia University, *New York 27, N.Y.*
Mr. P. KUHN, Structures Research Division, NACA, *Langley Field, Virginia*.
Dr. F. A. McCLINTOCK, Room 1—321, M.I.T., *Cambridge 39, Mass.*
Mr. R. E. PETERSON, Research Laboratories, Westinghouse Electric Corporation, *East Pittsburg, Pa.*
Dr. J. T. RANSOM, Engineering Research Laboratory, E.I. du Pont de Nemours and Comp. Inc., *Wilmington 98, Delaware*.
Prof. F. R. SHANLEY, The RAND Corporation, 1700 Main St., *Santa Monica, Calif.*

*USSR*:

Prof. I. A. ODING, Corr. Memb. Akademia NAUK USSR, *Moscow*.
Prof. A. I. PETRUSSEWITSCH, Akademia NAUK USSR, *Moscow*.
Prof. G. V. UZHIK, Akademia NAUK USSR, *Moscow*.

# List of other participants

*Finland:*

Prof. A. YLINEN, Tekniska Högskolan, *Helsingfors.*

*Germany:*

Dir. L. BÜCHNER, C. Schenck Maschinen-Fabrik, *Darmstadt.*
Prof. Dr.-Ing. H. EBNER, *Hamburg-Fu.*, Flughafen, Haus 15.
Dipl.-Ing. B. JACOBY, Losenhausenwerk, *Düsseldorf-Grafenberg*, Schlüterstr. 19.

*Netherlands:*

Mr. K. SCHIJVE, Nationaal Luchtvaartlaboratorium, Sloterweg 145, *Amsterdam W.*

*Norway:*

Prof. A. MARKESTAD, Norges Tekniske Høgskole, Materialprøvningsanstalten, *Trondheim.*
Ingenjör K. ØDEGÅRD, Norges Tekniske Høgskole, Materialprøvningsanstalten, *Trondheim.*

*Poland:*

Prof. MACHAL LUNC.
Mr. JAROSLAV NALESZKIEVICZ.

*Spain:*

Prof. G. MILLÁN, Instituto Nacional de Técnica Aeronáutica, Claudio Cuello St. -88, *Madrid.*
Prof. A. PÉREZ-MARÍN, Instituto Nacional de Técnica Aeronáutica, Esteban Terradas, Serrano 43, *Madrid.*
Mr. SARDINERO, Instituto Nacional de Técnica Aeronáutica, Esteban Terradas, Serrano 43, *Madrid.*

*Sweden:*

Civ. ing. B. ÅBERG, AB Scania-Vabis, *Södertälje.*
Ing. T. ÅKERSTRÖM, AB Volvo, *Göteborg.*
Ing. S. ALFREDSON, Flygtekniska Försöksanstalten, *Ulvsunda 1.*
Tekn. lic. O. ANDERSSON, Sv. Träforskningsinstitutet, Drottning Kristinas väg 61, *Stockholm Ö.*
Bergsing. T. ANGEL, Sandvikens Jernverk AB, *Sandviken.*
Civ. ing. L. B. ARONSSON, Carl Gustafs Stads gevärsfaktori, *Eskilstuna.*
Ing. I. ÅSLUND, AB Bofors, *Bofors.*
Civ. ing. N. BERGNER, AB Separator, Fleminggatan 8, *Stockholm K.*
Civ. ing. J. BERGSTRÖM, Sv. Träforskningsinstitutet, Drottning Kristinas väg 61, *Stockholm Ö.*
Bergsing. P. BJÖRKMAN, AB Kanthal, *Hallstahammar.*
Byråing. A. BJÖRKLUND, Kungl. Vattenfallsstyrelsen, Postfack, *Stockholm 1.*
Prof. G. BOESTAD, Kungl. Tekniska Högskolan, *Stockholm 70.*
Teknolog M. BROMAN, Stockholms Hamnstyrelses Materialprovn. laboratorium, Götgatan 139, *Stockholm.*
Ing. C. BRÖNN, SAAB, *Linköping.*

*Sweden:*

Ing. B. CARLSSON, AB de Lavals Ångturbin, Box 15 025, *Stockholm 15.*

Teknolog K. CEDERWALL, Eriksbergsgatan 34 IV, *Stockholm.*

Ing. S. CURIC, Jugoslaviska Handelsavdelningen, Drottninggatan 30, *Stockholm.*

Tekn. lic. S. EGGWERTZ, Valkyrievägen 3, *Djursholm 1.*

Ing. G. EKSTRAND, AB Garphytte Bruk, *Garphyttan.*

Civ. ing. R. ENG, Atlas Diesel AB, *Stockholm 1.*

Ing. L. ENGSTRÖM, Kungl. Armétygförvaltningen, *Stockholm 80.*

Ing. E. ERIKSSON, Kungl. Tekniska Högskolan, *Stockholm 70.*

Bergsing. S.-E. ERIKSON, Elektriska Svetsnings AB, *Göteborg.*

Prof. O. H. FAXÉN, Kungl. Tekniska Högskolan, *Stockholm 70.*

Civ. ing. H. C. FISCHER, Atlas Diesel AB, *Stockholm 1.*

Byråing. N. FOGHAGEN, Kungl. Flygförvaltningen, *Stockholm 80.*

Ing. G. FOLKESTAD, Berzeliigatan 4, *Linköping.*

Ing. L. FORSBERG, AB Garphytte Bruk, *Garphyttan.*

Ing. G. FREDRIKSSON, S.A.S., Bromma Flygplats, *Stockholm 40.*

Civ. ing. S. FRÖDERSTRÖM, AB Contram, Lagman Linds väg 12, *Stocksund.*

Tekn. lic. R. GUNNERT, AGA, *Lidingö.*

Fil. lic. G. GUSTAFSSON, Flygtekniska försöksanstalten, *Ulvsunda 1.*

Övering. J. GÖTZLINGER, ASEA, *Västerås.*

Ing. K. HEDSTRÖM, SAAB, *Linköping.*

Civ. ing. H. HELLSTRÖM, Sv. Träforskningsinstitutet, Drottning Kristinas väg 61, *Stockholm Ö.*

Doc. R. HILTSCHER, Kungl. Tekniska Högskolan, *Stockholm 70.*

Tekn. lic. J. HULT, Kungl. Tekniska Högskolan, *Stockholm 70.*

Civ. ing. E. HULTMARK, Sandhamnsgatan 62, *Stockholm Ö.*

Civ. ing. C. T. INGWALL, Sandgatan 12 A, *Norrköping*

Doc. A. JOHNSSON, Kungl. Tekniska Högskolan, *Stockholm 70.*

Civ. ing. L.-E. JONSSON, Kungl. Tekniska Högskolan, *Stockholm 70.*

Ing. L. JOHANSSON, AB Svenska Metallverken, *Västerås.*

Bergsing. T. KREY, AB Bofors, *Bofors.*

Ing. E. KOBBERNAGEL, AB de Lavals Ångturbin, *Stockholm 15.*

Civ. ing. J. LARSÉN, Atlas Diesel AB, *Stockholm 1.*

Civ. ing. N. G. LEIDE, Kockums Mek. Verkstad AB, *Malmö.*

Dir. R. LILJEBLAD, ASEA, *Västerås.*

Civ. ing. O. LJUNGSTRÖM, SAAB, *Linköping.*

Överdir. B. LUNDBERG, Flygtekniska Försöksanstalten, *Ulvsunda 1.*

Bergsing. B. LUNDGREN, S.K.F., *Göteborg.*

Byråing. B. LÖNNSTEDT, Kungl. Vattenfallsstyrelsen, Postfack, *Stockholm 1.*

Ing. E. MATTSSON, Kungl. Vattenfallsstyrelsen, Postfack, *Stockholm 1.*

Civ. ing. J. MUNCK, Atlas Diesel AB, *Stockholm 1.*

Civ. ing. L. E. NELSON, Kungl. Tekniska Högskolan, *Stockholm 70.*

Civ. ing. K. E. NIELSEN, Cement- o. Betonginstitutet, Kungl. Tekniska Högskolan, *Stockholm 26.*

Civ. ing. R. NILSON, Råsundavägen 70 V, *Solna.*

Dr. phil. F. NIORDSON, Backvägen 9, *Solna.*

Bergsing. T. NORÉN, Elektriska Svetsnings AB, *Göteborg.*

Civ. ing. R. NORBECK, Atlas Diesel AB, *Stockholm 1.*

Civ. ing. A. NORR, Strålgatan 23, *Stockholm K.*

Mr. B. R. NOTON, Ängkärrsgatan 10 II, *Solna 4.*

Prof. H. NYLANDER, Kungl. Tekniska Högskolan, *Stockholm 70.*

Ing. K. G. OLSSON, Statens Provningsanstalt, *Stockholm 26.*

*Sweden:*

Civ. ing. L. Östlund, Kungl. Tekniska Högskolan, *Stockholm 70.*
Civ. ing. S. Petrelius, Enspännargatan 10, *Stockholm-Vällingby.*
Doc. O. Pettersson, Kungl. Tekniska Högskolan, *Stockholm 70.*
Prof. T. Rand, Kungl. Tekniska Högskolan, *Stockholm 70.*
Ing. Å. Romander, S.A.S., Bromma Flygplats, *Stockholm 40.*
Prof. J. O. Roos af Hjelmsäter, Karlavägen 21, *Stockholm Ö.*
Civ. ing. S. Sabelström, Petterbergsvägen 41, *Hägersten.*
Civ. ing. S. Sahlin, Kungl. Tekniska Högskolan, *Stockholm 70.*
Civ. ing. N. J. Sandström, Carl Gustafs Stads gevärsfaktori, *Eskilstuna.*
Dr.-Ing. F. Schücker, AB Svenska Metallverken, *Västerås.*
Civ. ing. N. E. Sjöholm, Carl Gustafs Stads gevärsfaktori, *Eskilstuna.*
Tekn. lic. S. Sjöström, AB Scania-Vabis, *Södertälje.*
Tekn. lic. E. Steneroth, Rederi-AB Nordstjernan, Box 7196, *Stockholm 7.*
Ing. B. Ström, AB Svenska Metallverken, *Finspång.*
Ing. F. Svensson, Flygtekniska Försöksanstalten, *Ulvsunda 1.*
Ing. N. Sylvén, Kungl. Flygförvaltningen, *Stockholm 80.*
Ing. L. Söderberg, AB Svenska Metallverken, *Finspång.*
Civ. ing. T. Tarandi, Kungl. Marinförvaltningen, *Stockholm 80.*
Byrådir. J. U. Thran, Kungl. Vattenfallsstyrelsen, Postfack, *Stockholm 1.*
Ing. F. Turner, SAAB, *Linköping.*
Dr. H. Unckel, AB Svenska Metallverken, *Finspång.*
Ing. B. Wadell, Atlas Diesel AB, *Stockholm 1.*
Ing. S. Wallmark, de Lavals Ångturbin AB, *Stockholm 15.*
Byrådir. B. Wesslén, Kungl. Flygförvaltningen, *Stockholm 80.*
Ing. B. Wirgelius, Rindögatan 44 II, *Stockholm Ö.*
Laborator L. E. Zachrisson, Försvarets Forskningsanstalt, *Stockholm 80.*

*United Kingdom:*

Mr. P. P. Benham, Imperial College, *London, S.W.*
Mr. A. Binns, W. & T. Avery Limited, Soho Foundry, *Birmingham 40.*
Dipl.-Ing. T. Haas, Fatigue Section, Engineering Development Laboratory, The Bristol Aeroplane Company, Ltd., Filton House, *Bristol.*
Mr. G. P. Kennedy, Brettenham House, Strand, *London, W.C. 2.*
Prof. G. Temple (Treasurer IUTAM), Mathematical Institute, 10 Parks Road, *Oxford.*

*USA:*

Dr. H. L. Dryden, (President IUTAM), NACA, 1724 F.Str. N.W., *Washington 25, D.C.*
Mr. L. Himmel, Scientific Liaison Officer, Office of Naval Research, Keysign House, 429 Oxford Street, *London, W. 1.*

*Yugoslavia:*

Prof. A. Kuhelj, Faculty of Engineering, *Ljubljana,* Cojzova 5.

# Contents    Sommaire    Inhalt

# Étude critique de la notion de dommage appliquée à une classe étendue d'essais de fatigue

Par

**F. Bastenaire**

Avec 3 figures

## 1. Préambule

Le comportement des matériaux dans des essais de fatigue où l'amplitude de la contrainte est variable est ordinairement apprécié par comparaison à des critères qui varient selon les types d'essais et selon les auteurs.

Le concept de dommage a le grand avantage de s'appliquer à une classe d'essais très étendue mais son existence même dépend de plusieurs conditions.

Nous avons d'abord procédé à l'inventaire et à la critique de ces conditions, puis, ne conservant que les plus essentielles, nous avons défini et caractérisé des généralisations de ce concept en insistant particulièrement sur celles qui utilisent la notion de probabilité.

Dans l'espace qui nous est accordé ici, il ne nous a pas été possible de donner les démonstrations mathématiques de tous nos résultats. Nous nous sommes parfois limité à énoncer les hypothèses et leurs conséquences et ce mémoire n'est que le résumé d'un travail qui sera publié ultérieurement in extenso.

## 2. Introduction

En matière de résistance à la fatigue, les premiers chercheurs se sont limités, pour simplifier, à des essais pour lesquels l'amplitude de variation de la contrainte restait constante. On a admis qu'ils représentaient plus ou moins bien les conditions ordinaires d'utilisation où l'amplitude est en réalité aléatoire mais oscille autour d'une moyenne.

Des expérimentateurs ont essayé de faire subir à des éprouvettes un certain nombre de cycles sous chacune de plusieurs valeurs distinctes de la contrainte maximum (que nous appellerons désormais plus brièvement la contrainte). Ces essais, qui peuvent varier à l'infini, n'appartiennent en pratique qu'à un petit nombre de types. Les plus fréquents sont:

a) Les essais où la contrainte ne prend que deux valeurs différentes: l'understressing et l'overstressing.

b) Les essais où elle croît par paliers étagés en progression arithmétique (coaxing).

c) Les essais où elle varie par paliers croissants ou décroissants une ou plusieurs fois.

Weibull/Odqvist, Ermüdungsfestigkeit

d) La méthode de M. Prot dans laquelle elle croît en fonction linéaire du nombre des cycles effectués, la contrainte initiale étant inférieure à la limite d'endurance.

Ces types d'essais peuvent être envisagés comme des cas particuliers de la famille plus générale des essais où la contrainte $S$ est définie en fonction du nombre de cycles par une fonction arbitraire à une variable : $S = f(N)$. On est alors surpris de leur trouver des explications théoriques différentes ; l'understressing, peut-être à cause de l'apparente simplicité de l'essai, a bénéficié de l'attention des chercheurs mais il ne semble pas que l'on ait vu que les explications proposées doivent être généralisables à des essais plus complexes. Le concept de dommage sur lequel nous reviendrons est l'idée la plus hardie par sa généralité puisqu'elle s'applique à tous les types d'essais mais, bien que des formes mathématiques très différentes en aient été proposées, il semble qu'aucune d'elles ne donne entièrement satisfaction.

### 3. Définition des effets de l'understressing

a) **Première définition.** Le fait de soumettre une éprouvette à $N_1$ cycles sous la contrainte $S_1$ et de la porter ensuite sous la contrainte $S_2$ ne constitue évidemment pas, à notre point de vue, une préparation suivie d'un essai mais un essai unique défini par une fonction $f(N)$ ($N$ désigne le nombre total de cycles) possédant simplement une discontinuité en $N_1$ (Fig. 1).

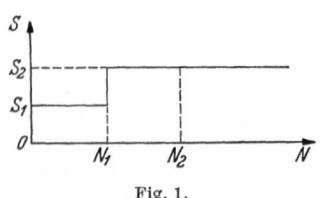

Fig. 1.

Le sort d'une éprouvette doit être, en effet, relié à la totalité de son histoire.

Ceci dit, on a souvent considéré que la proportion des éprouvettes rompues après $N_2$ cycles parmi celles qui ont survécu aux $N_1$ premiers devrait être égale à la proportion normale de rompues sous $S_2$ après $(N_2 - N_1)$ cycles[1]. Lorsque les observations n'ont pas justifié cette égalité, on a attribué la différence aux effets de l'understressing.

Il est normal d'étudier d'abord les conséquences logiques d'une telle

---

[1] C'est la méthode dans laquelle on commence par soumettre une série d'éprouvettes à $N_1$ cycles sous la contrainte $S_1$. Les éprouvettes non rompues sont alors reportées en $S_2$ et leurs durées de vie directement comparées à celles d'éprouvettes n'ayant pas travaillé. Au point de vue statistique, l'égalité des durées de vie doit être comprise comme l'identité des distributions, c'est-à-dire comme l'égalité des probabilités de rupture pour un même nombre donné arbitraire de cycles sous la contrainte $S_2$. Cependant, comme nous nous repérons ici au moyen du nombre total des cycles parcourus, les probabilités de rupture à comparer sont celles qui correspondent à $N_2$ cycles pour les éprouvettes ayant travaillé en $S_1$ et à $(N_2 - N_1)$ cycles pour les autres.

définition quand on suppose l'absence de tout effet car un comportement de référence n'a de sens que s'il est possible.

Les valeurs $N_1$, $N_2$, $S_1$, $S_2$ étant arbitraires, nous prendrons $N_2 = 2\,N_1$ et ferons tendre $S_2$ vers $S_1$ jusqu'à ce que $S_2 = S_1$. Soit $p$ la proportion de ruptures de 0 à $N_1$ cycles sous $S_1$ et $p'$ cette proportion sous $S_2$ pour un même nombre de cycles. Il résulte de la définition précédente qu'en l'absence de tout effet, la proportion totale d'éprouvettes non rompues rapportée à *l'effectif initial* devrait, au bout de $N_2$ cycles, être égale à $(1-p)\,(1-p')$.

Lorsque $S_2$ tend vers $S_1$, $p'$ tend vers $p$ et la proportion d'éprouvettes non rompues tend vers $(1-p)^2$. Il est facile d'étendre le raisonnement à une succession de $k$ phases de $N_1$ cycles chacune à des contraintes $S_1$, $S_2$, $S_3$ .... et de faire tendre ensuite $S_2$, $S_3$ ..... $S_k$ vers $S_1$ (Fig. 2).

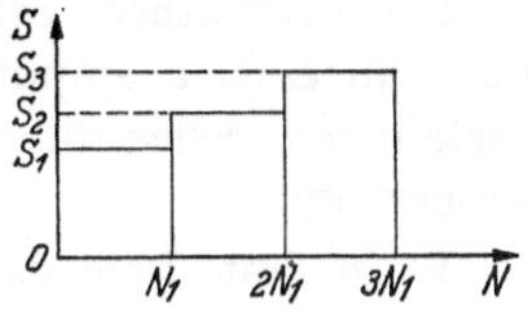

Fig. 2.

Au bout de $kN_1$ cycles, la proportion d'éprouvettes non rompues devrait donc être $(1-p)^k$, cette formules s'étendant d'ailleurs par un raisonnement simple aux valeurs fractionnaires de $k$ et, si l'on admet la continuité, à $k$ quelconque.

En désignant par $p_0$ la proportion de ruptures après $N_0$ cycles, la proportion de survies après $N = kN_0$ est donnée par:

$$(1 - p_0)^k = (1 - p_0)^{N/N_0}$$

En posant:

$$(1 - p_0)^{1/N_0} = e^{-1/a}$$

on peut mettre cette loi sous la forme exponentielle:

$$\text{Probab. de non rupture} = e^{-N/a}$$

L'expérience ne confirme pas cette forme de distribution. Il semble d'ailleurs maladroit de choisir une définition qui implique quelque chose quant à la distribution des durées de vie, déjà mal connue. Elle fera conclure à la présence d'understressing toutes les fois que la distribution n'aura pas la forme exponentielle.

**b) Seconde définition.** La première définition a été critiquée par E. Epremian et R. F. Mehl ([1] p. 58) qui ont fait remarquer que les éprouvettes restant après les $N_1$ premiers cycles étant les plus résistantes, il était logique de les voir durer plus longtemps en moyenne dans un nouvel essai que les éprouvettes neuves d'un échantillon représentatif de la population d'origine contenant toutes les catégories.

Ils considèrent que le résultat de la première phase de l'essai est une sélection et que la proportion $(1-p)$ des éprouvettes non rompues devrait naturellement se comporter par la suite de la même façon que la proportion $(1-p)$ des éprouvettes neuves *dont les durées de vie sont les plus longues*.

1*

Dans la terminologie du calcul des probabilités, leur distribution devrait être la distribution conditionnelle des durées supérieures au quantile $p$.

Si l'on applique cette hypothèse quel que soit le passé des éprouvettes, on peut démontrer la possibilité de faire survivre une proportion arbitraire d'éprouvettes à des essais de durée indéfinie pratiqués à une contrainte arbitraire.

Il est clair qu'Epremian et Mehl attribuent aux éprouvettes non rompues des qualités identiques à celles qu'elles avaient avant l'essai puisqu'ils supposent qu'elles doivent se comporter ultérieurement comme elles se comporteraient si elles n'avaient pas subi une «préparation».

Cette hypothèse est peut-être admissible pour les éprouvettes qui, dans un essai à amplitude constante, ne rompront jamais mais il est certain que celles qui doivent se rompre subissent une transformation progressive.

Il ne faut donc pas confondre les éprouvettes qui *ne doivent pas rompre* avec celles qui finiront par le faire. Ces dernières ne sont plus dans leur état initial. C'est de cette fausse supposition que nous tirons l'absurdité énoncée plus haut.

Pour appliquer le critère d'Epremian et Mehl, il faut admettre que les éprouvettes non rompues ne doivent pas rompre, c'est-à-dire que $N_1 = \infty$, $N_2 = \infty$, etc. . . .; nous n'avons pas le droit de nous arrêter en chemin comme nous l'avons admis dans notre raisonnement. Ce critère ne peut donc être appliqué qu'à des essais d'un type particulier.

Nous n'irons pas plus loin dans l'étude des définitions directes qui conduisent souvent à des impasses pour le traitement du problème général.

## 4. Le concept de dommage

Les essais à deux niveaux ne sont que des cas particuliers d'essais plus généraux dans lesquels la contrainte peut varier plusieurs fois et que l'on a tenté d'interpréter au moyen du concept de dommage.

L'idée de base est, en fait, d'associer un certain état physique à chaque moment de l'histoire de l'éprouvette et, dans la conception classique, à supposer que cet état est, du point de vue fatigue tout au moins, caractérisable par un paramètre unique.

a) **Conceptions classiques du dommage.** Elles font toutes intervenir, dans l'expression du dommage la durée de vie $N_i$ sous la contrainte $S_i$ (par exemple $\delta = \sum \dfrac{n_i}{N_i}$ ). Or, $N_i$ est une grandeur statistique dont la tendance centrale peut s'exprimer aussi bien par le mode, la médiane ou la moyenne. Ce choix pose un premier problème.

En supposant s'être arrêté à une définition arbitraire de $N_i$, on peut toutefois définir le nombre de cycles $\nu_1$ qui, sous une contrainte $S_1$ donnée, est équivalent à un nombre $\nu_0$ de cycles sous la contrainte $S_0$ de référence (Fig. 3) de la façon suivante:

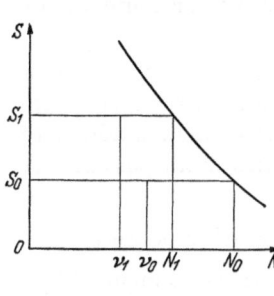

Fig. 3.

Nous dirons que $(S_1, \nu_1)^1$ est *équivalent* à $(S_0, \nu_0)$ que nous noterons $(S_1, \nu_1) \to (S_0, \nu_0)$ si des éprouvettes ayant subi $(S_1, \nu_1)$ étant reportées à la contrainte $S_0$, leur durée de vie comptée à partir de cet instant y est égale à celle des éprouvettes qui ont subi $(S_0, \nu_0)$, c'est-à-dire à la différence $(N_0 - \nu_0)$ entre la durée de vie totale $N_0$ sous $S_0$ et le nombre $\nu_0$, ref. [2].

Il faut distinguer la relation:

$$(S_1, \nu_1) \to (S_0, \nu_0)$$

de la relation:

$$(S_0, \nu_0) \to (S_1, \nu_1)$$

car il n'est pas dit qu'en reportant en $S_1$ les éprouvettes ayant subi $(S_0, \nu_0)$, celles-ci se trouveront dans un état équivalent à $(S_1, \nu_1)$ et que leur durée de vie y sera $(N_1 - \nu_1)$ à partir de de cet instant. En d'autres termes, rien ne permet d'affirmer que l'equivalence est une relation réciproque.

En l'admettant, soit maintenant $S_2$ un troisième niveau de $S$ et $\nu_2$ le nombre de cycles tel que:

$$(S_2, \nu_2) \rightleftarrows (S_0, \nu_0)$$

Supposons également satisfaite la relation:

$$(S_1, \nu_1) \rightleftarrows (S_0, \nu_0)$$

Rien ne permet de démontrer que:

$$(S_1, \nu_1) \rightleftarrows (S_2, \nu_2)$$

qui, si elle a lieu, exprime la transitivité de l'équivalence. C'est un postulat qu'il reste à prouver par l'expérience.

Ou peut démontrer que la condition nécessaire et suffisante pour qu'il existe un «dommage» caractérisable par une valeur numérique $\delta$ est précisément qu'il y ait à la fois réciprocité et transitivité pour tout système de deux et de trois contraintes respectivement.

Mais ces conditions d'existence ne suffisent encore pas à faire du dommage un concept utilisable s'il ne peut pas être appliqué à des essais plus généraux que ceux où $S$ est constant. C'est pourquoi on a toujours admis l'hypothèse:

1. Tout traitement défini par un parcours $S = f(N)$ *quelconque* possède au moins un équivalent à contrainte constante.

---

[1] Nous représenterons désormais par la notation $(S, \nu)$ un essai consistant en $\nu$ cycles sous la contrainte $S$.

Elle revient à admettre que les parcours $S = f(N)$ quelconques ne peuvent conduire à des états différents de ceux que l'on peut atteindre au moyen des essais du type $S = $ Constante.

Lorsque l'on ajoute à 1. les conditions de réciprocité et de transitivité précédentes, on voit que l'équivalence existe de plus pour toute valeur de $S$.

Or, $S$ étant déterminé, on ne peut parvenir en faisant varier $N$ qu'à une simple infinité d'états; l'ensemble de 1. et des conditions de réciprocité et de transitivité dans les essais $S = $ Constante revient donc à admettre une correspondance biunivoque entre la totalité des états possibles et la valeur d'un paramètre unique.

Il va sans dire que l'on ne peut non plus se passer de l'hypothèse:

2. Deux traitements équivalents suivis de deux traitements identiques *quelconques* donnent des résultats finaux équivalents.

Il faut encore faire une hypothèse de dérivabilité qui n'a aucune nécessité logique mais dont on accepte mal de se passer. On admettra, qu'à l'instant où le dommage est $\delta$, son accroissement le long du parcours $S = f(N)$ sera:

$$d\delta = A(\delta, S) \, dN + B(\delta, S) \, dS$$

car il dépend en effet de la contrainte présente et du dommage existant mais pas directement du nombre de cycles parcourus dont l'effet s'exprime entièrement, d'après l'hypothèse 2. par $\delta$.

D'autre part, dans la catégorie des expériences de fatigue, les seuls effets possibles sont dûs, par définition, aux sollicitations répétées; dans le cas où quelques cycles suffisent à produire une modification irréversible de la matière, on peut dire que l'on sort de cette catégorie.

On peut donc admettre:

3. Qu'une variation de $dS$ qui a lieu à $N$ constant ($dN = 0$) ne produit aucun dommage et que $B(\delta, S)$ est identiquement nul.

En définitive, on admettra que:

$$d\delta = A(\delta, S) \, dN$$

Cette formule résume les hypothèses précédentes; elle permettrait si $A(\delta, S)$ était connue de calculer la variation de $\delta$ le long d'un parcours $S = f(N)$ quelconque.

Voilà le résultat auquel on parvient après avoir posé des hypothèses dont il ne semble pas possible de se passer quand on part de la notion d'équivalence entre des traitements du type $S = $ Constante.

On notera que $d\delta$ dépend à priori à la fois de $S$ et de $\delta$ lui-même, ce que les formules proposées actuellement pour $\delta$ ne font pas ressortir.

Elles donnent de $\delta$ une valeur indépendante de l'ordre dans lequel on fait subir à l'éprouvette les traitements $(S_i, n_i)$.

**b) Conception probabiliste du dommage.** La dispersion des résultats d'essais de fatigue est due, en majeure partie, à l'hétérogénéité du matériau lui-même et une description adéquate du phénomène peut être donnée par des statistiques de ces résultats sans s'occuper des valeurs individuelles.

La distinction entre les caractéristiques des populations et celles des individus s'applique aussi à *leurs histoires.*

On peut admettre que la population passe elle aussi par une succession d'états qui peuvent être décrits en termes statistiques et que son évolution peut être caractérisée en fonction du nombre de cycles par celle des paramètres statistiques définissant ces états.

Deux états de la population seront dits équivalents et correspondront par définition à des dommages égaux si ces populations ne se distinguent pas dans des expériences de fatigue ultérieures.

La notion d'équivalence introduite dans la conception déterministe va seulement se trouver définie de manière différente dans la conception probabiliste: en fait, il suffira de remplacer le terme «durée de vie» par le terme «distribution de la durée de vie».

Pour que $(S_1, \nu_1)$ soit équivalent à $(S_0, \nu_0)$, il faut qu'en reportant les éprouvettes qui restent après $(S_1, \nu_1)$ en $S_0$, la distribution statistique de leurs durées de vie soit *identique* à celle des éprouvettes qui restent de $(S_0, \nu_0)$ *comptée à partir* de $\nu_0$, les secondes phases des essais ayant lieu toutes deux sous $S_0$.

**c) Existence d'équivalences plus générales.** Si l'on recherche les valeurs du nombre de cycles qui, sous des contraintes $S$ variées, produisent des effets équivalents à $(S_0, \nu_0)$ de telle sorte qu'il y ait en même temps réciprocité et transitivité, il ne faut pas oublier que, ce faisant, on cherche un dommage à un paramètre. En effet, quel que soit $S$ et $\nu$, on recherche la valeur du paramètre unique $\nu_0$ qui, sous la contrainte $S_0$ de référence, est tel que $(S, \nu) \rightleftarrows (S_0, \nu_0)$.

Il est assez rationnel d'admettre qu'il existe des états équivalents. Pour qu'il n'y en ait pas, il faudrait qu'il y ait autant d'états possibles de la population qu'il y a de traitements c'est-à-dire de fonctions d'une variable. On tente généralement en physique de représenter l'état d'un système par un nombre fini de paramètres (en thermo-dynamique par exemple). L'ensemble des fonctions étant, on le sait, beaucoup plus «riche» que n'importe quel espace euclidien à $n$ dimensions, il est vraisemblable qu'il existe des états équivalents mais il n'est par sûr qu'un seul paramètre suffise à les décrire.

## 5. Étude théorique du concept statistique de dommage supposé défini par un paramètre unique

L'hypothèse la plus simple sur le nombre des paramètres représentant une famille d'états équivalents est de supposer qu'il se réduit à l'unité. Elle sera maintenue dans toute cette partie et ses subdivisions.

Bien qu'elle paraisse difficile à vérifier sous cette forme abstraite on peut en déduire des conséquences qui seront, elles, susceptibles de donner lieu aux vérifications qui s'imposent (et qui peuvent très bien l'infirmer).

**a) Le dommage et la probabilité de rupture.** Lorsque nous avons recherché une définition directe de l'équivalence dans la conception probabiliste, il nous est immédiatement venu à l'esprit d'exiger l'identité des distributions des *éprouvettes restantes* au cours d'un nouvel essai. Mais nous n'avons rien dit des éprouvettes rompues tant par suite de $(S_1, v_1)$ que de $(S_0, v_0)$ qui n'ont pourtant aucune raison de ne pas entrer en ligne de compte dans l'évaluation du dommage.

On ressent même intuitivement que *les proportions d'éprouvettes rompues devraient être égales dans les deux cas.*

D'ailleurs, si l'état de la population *toute entière* peut être à tout moment représenté par un seul paramètre, la proportion des éprouvettes rompues à un instant donné, qui en est une caractéristique essentielle, ne doit dépendre comme tous les autres que de celui-là.

Le paramètre qu'il convient de choisir pour repérer l'état de la population est d'ailleurs, indifférent puisque tous varient simultanément et il est tout indiqué de choisir la probabilité de rupture elle-même qui est une quantité susceptible d'être estimée statistiquement.

Ainsi, chaque fois que deux essais quelconques produiront des proportions égales de rupture, on pourra en déduire que les populations seront, à la fin de l'essai, dans des états équivalents et que, dans tout nouvel essai, elles se comporteront (ou ce qu'il en reste) de façon *statistiquement* identiques.

**b) Équations fondamentales du dommage à un paramètre.** Il est possible d'établir des équations dont la résolution fournit les distributions des durées de vie et des contraintes de rupture pour des essais quelconques.

L'hypothèse 1. du paragraphe 4a) équivaut, avec les conditions de transitivité et de réciprocité, à admettre, nous l'avons vu, que les états possibles d'une éprouvette sont représentables par un paramètre. Il suffit de remplacer le mot «éprouvette» par «population» pour retrouver l'hypothèse fondamentale de la cinquième partie.

En renouvelant les autres hypothèses de 4a) mais en les appliquant au paramètre descriptif de l'évolution de la population, on aboutit évidemment encore à l'équation:

$$\mathrm{d}\,\delta = A\,(\delta,\,S)\,\mathrm{d}N$$

applicable en particulier à la probabilité de rupture $p$:

$$\mathrm{d}\,p = A\,(p,\,S)\,\mathrm{d}N$$

On pourrait aussi caractériser le dommage par le nombre $\nu_0$ de cycles qui, sous une contrainte $S_0$ de référence engendrerait le même dommage.

En désignant par $F(S,\,\nu)$ la fonction donnant la probabilité de rupture avant $\nu$ cycles sous l'amplitude $S$ supposée constante, $\nu_0$ sera obtenu en écrivant que la probabilité du rupture $p$ résultant du traitement considéré est égale à celle qui est associée à $(S_0,\,\nu_0)$:

$$p = F\,(S_0,\,\nu_0)$$

Il est plus intéressant d'introduire le nombre $\nu$ de cycles qui, sous la contrainte actuelle $S$, aurait produit (si $S$ avait été maintenu constant depuis le début) un dommage égal au dommage actuel; $\nu$ est déterminé par l'équation

$$p = F\,(S,\,\nu) \tag{1}$$

Tandis que $\nu_0$ est le nombre équivalent de cycles (en abrégé n.e.c.) rapporté à la contrainte *fixe* $S_0$; $\nu$ est le n.e.c. rapporté à *la valeur actuelle* $S$.

La dérivation de l'équation $p = F(S,\,N)$ donne la variation du dommage qui résulte d'une augmentation $\mathrm{d}N$ du nombre réel de cycles dans un essai à $S$ constant:

$$\mathrm{d}\,p = \frac{\partial F\,(S,\,N)}{\partial N}\,\mathrm{d}N$$

mais si cet accroissement réel $\mathrm{d}N$ a lieu à un instant où le n.e.c. est égal à $\nu$ (en général différent de $N$ quand le trajet antérieur n'a pas été effectué à $S$ constant), alors:

$$\mathrm{d}\,p = \frac{\partial F\,(S,\,\nu)}{\partial \nu}\,\mathrm{d}N \tag{2}$$

On en déduit que la fonction $A\,(p,\,S)$ est telle que

$$A\,(p,\,s) = \frac{\partial F\,(S,\,\nu)}{\partial \nu}$$

et que (2) s'applique aussi au cas où $S$ n'est pas constant vu que $\mathrm{d}p$ ne dépend d'après l'équation:

$$\mathrm{d}\,p = A\,(p,\,S)\,\mathrm{d}N$$

que de $p$, $S$ et $\mathrm{d}N$ ou, ce qui revient au même, de $\nu$, $S$ et $\mathrm{d}N$ mais pas de $\mathrm{d}S$. D'autre part,

$$\mathrm{d}\,p = \frac{\partial F}{\partial S}\,\mathrm{d}S + \frac{\partial F}{\partial \nu}\,\mathrm{d}\nu$$

et par élimination de d$p$ avec (2), il vient:

$$\frac{\partial F}{\partial \nu}(d\nu - dN) + \frac{\partial F}{\partial S}\,dS = 0 \qquad (3)$$

Si l'on tient compte de la relation $S = f(N)$ définissant le chemin suivi, on peut dans (3) se débarrasser de $N$ ou de $S$ indifféremment par substitution. Si l'on a éliminé $S$ par exemple, (3) se réduit à une équation différentielle dont l'intégration fournit la relation entre le *nombre réel N de cycles et le nombre équivalent de cycles* $\nu$.

Lorsque $\nu$ exprimé en fonction de $N$ est introduit dans (1) on obtient *la loi de probabilité* de la rupture en fonction du nombre réel de cycles parcourus.

**c) Application de ces équations.** De nombreuses recherches ont été entreprises sur la distribution des durées de vie et l'équation de la courbe de Wöhler.

La description complète de résultats d'essais à amplitude constante n'est possible que par une fonction à deux variables $F(S, N)$ donnant la probabilité de rupture avant $N$ cycles sous la contrainte $S$ mais cette fonction n'est pas encore bien connue.

Dans le seul but de montrer une application des formules précédentes nous ferons sur $F(S, N)$ deux hypothèses assez larges:

1. Nous supposerons que les lois de distribution de $S$ définies par la fonction $F(S, N)$ à $N$ constant, ont même forme quel que soit $N$ et se déduisent les unes des autres par translation parallèlement à l'axe des $S$ sans toutefois supposer quoi que ce soit sur la nature de ces distributions.

2. Nous adopterons pour équation de la courbe de Wöhler définie ici comme la courbe médiane:

$$F(\widetilde{S}, N) = 0,5$$

une équation proposée par W. Weibull [3]:

$$\nu\,(\widetilde{S} - E)^m = k$$

que nous simplifierons en faisant $m = 1$ à la manière de M. Prot [4]. On démontre alors aisément que (3) s'écrit dans ce cas:

$$\frac{k}{\nu^2}(d\nu - dN) + dS = 0 \qquad (4)$$

et, en tenant compte de la relation linéaire

$$S = S_0 + \alpha N \qquad (5)$$

on obtient:

$$dS = \alpha\,dN$$

d'où l'équation différentielle:

$$\frac{k}{\nu^2} \cdot (d\nu - dN) + \alpha\,dN = 0$$

Son intégration en tenant compte de la condition initiale $N = 0$ pour $v = 0$ donne :

$$N = \frac{1}{2} \sqrt{\frac{k}{\alpha}} \log \left( \frac{1 + v \sqrt{\alpha/k}}{1 - v \sqrt{\alpha/k}} \right) \qquad (6)$$

Il ne faut pas oublier que l'on doit y joindre (5) et l'équation :

$$p = F(S, v)$$

Si l'on se propose par exemple de rechercher la valeur de $S$ correspondant à $50\%$ de ruptures dans *l'essai Prot*, on écrira :

$$F(S, v) = 0,50$$

qui se réduit ici à :

$$v = \frac{k}{S - E} \qquad (7)$$

Par substitution dans (6) de $v$ donné par (7) et de $N$ tiré de (5), on en déduit l'equation :

$$\frac{S - S_0}{\alpha} = \frac{1}{2} \sqrt{\frac{k}{\alpha}} \log \left( \frac{S - E + \sqrt{\alpha k}}{S - E - \sqrt{\alpha k}} \right) \qquad (8)$$

dont la racine $S_R$ est la contrainte de rupture médiane dans l'essai Prot. Elle dépend évidemment de la vitesse de mise en charge $\alpha$.

· Bien que (8) soit transcendante, on peut en étudier les propriétés. On démontre que :

$$\lim_{\alpha \to 0} \frac{S_R - E}{\sqrt{\alpha k}} = 1$$

ce que l'on peut encore écrire :

$$S_R = E + \sqrt{\alpha k} + \varepsilon \sqrt{\alpha k}$$

où $\varepsilon$ tend vers zéro quand $\alpha$ tend lui-même vers zéro.

D'après cette équation, la contrainte $S_R$ de rupture n'est linéaire en fonction de la racine carrée de la vitesse de mise en charge que de façon approchée et d'autant mieux que $\alpha$ est plus petit ; d'autre part, la limite de $S_R$ pour $\alpha$ tendant vers zéro est égale à la limite d'endurance $E$, en accord avec les intentions de la méthode de charge progressive.

**d) Vérifications expérimentales.** On doit naturellement se demander comment il est possible de soumettre la théorie probabiliste du dommage à un paramètre à des vérifications. On peut, d'après ses conséquences, le faire de bien des manières. Par exemple :

Ayant selon des trajets quelconques, mais différents, rompu une même proportion d'éprouvettes dans deux échantillons, ceux-ci devraient par la suite avoir les mêmes caractéristiques dans un essai unique arbitraire.

En particulier, en désignant par $S_1$ et $S_2$ ($S_1 < S_2$) deux contraintes
du domaine d'endurance et par $p_1$ et $p_2$ ($p_1 < p_2$) les proportions *limites*
d'éprouvettes rompues en $S_1$ et $S_2$ respectivement, portons les éprouvettes non rompues du fait d'un essai ($S_1$, $\infty$) à la contrainte $S_2$.

Puisque $p_1 < p_2$, il existe sous $S_2$ un nombre $\nu_2$ tel que:

$$F (S_2, \nu_2) = p_1$$

C'est dire que ($S_2$, $\nu_2$) est équivalent à ($S_1$, $\infty$) et que tout devrait
se passer comme si l'on avait accompli $\nu_2$ cycles sous la contrainte $S_2$
quand on en a, en fait, accompli un très grand nombre (théoriquement $\infty$)
sous $S_1$.

En poursuivant à partir de là l'essai sous $S_2$ jusqu'à $\nu = \infty$, la proportion limite de ruptures (rapportée comme toujours à l'effectif *total
initial*) doit évidemment tendre, d'après la théorie, vers $p_2$.

Si un matériau suivait ces lois, le procédé de coaxing ne devrait
donc avoir aucune influence sur ses fréquences limites de ruptures. Ce
sont les résultats expérimentaux que STULEN ([*5*] p. 36) a obtenu sur
un acier SAE 4330.

Nous ne prétendons pas qu'il doit en être ainsi dans tous les cas
mais au lieu de définir les effets de l'understressing par des méthodes
directes (voir paragraphe 3), il nous semble plus simple (quoique cela
n'ait de nécessité qu'avec nos hypothèses) de considérer par définition
que ses effets sont nuls lorsqu'un seul paramètre suffit à représenter le
dommage, ce qui peut être vrai de certains matériaux. Il n'y aurait
d'understressing que sur des matériaux dont les états équivalents ne
pourraient être définis que par deux ou plus de deux paramètres.

## 6. Conceptions possibles d'un dommage à plusieurs paramètres

Si l'on renonce à admettre que le dommage s'exprime par un seul
paramètre, il ne devient guère possible de rechercher des définitions du
dommage par la méthode directe (4) car il n'existe en général aucun
$\nu_1$ tel que ($S_1$, $\nu_1$) $\rightleftarrows$ ($S_0$, $\nu_0$) lorsque $S_0$, $S_1$ et $\nu_0$ sont arbitraires.

Il est préférable d'aborder le problème sous l'angle très général du
paragraphe 4c) et de rechercher les hypothèses qu'il est rationnel de
garder.

Il est raisonnable de maintenir toutes celles de 4a) à l'exception
de 1., de la réciprocité et de la transitivité qui équivalent à supposer
que le dommage est à un paramètre.

Si $u$ et $v$ désignaient par exemple les deux paramètres caractéristiques du dommage, leurs accroissements ne dépendraient, d'après ces
seules hypothèses, que de leurs valeurs actuelles, de l'accroissement $dN$
du nombre réel de cycles et de la contrainte sous laquelle il aurait lieu.

Les équations d'évolution de $u$ et $v$ auraient la forme générale suivante

$$d\,u = \varphi\,(u,\,v,\,S)\,d\,N$$
$$d\,v = \psi\,(u,\,v,\,S)\,d\,N$$

la probabilité de rupture se trouvant, comme toutes les autres caractéristiques de la population, entièrement spécifiée par une fonction de $u$ et de $v$:

$$p = p\,(u,\,v)$$

On peut aussi imaginer qu'il en faut plus de deux et leur nombre est peut-être égal au nombre d'effets distincts se produisant dans le métal: écrouissage, vieillissement, etc . . .

Il semble d'ailleurs que dans ce cas, l'observation d'une seule grandeur telle que la durée de vie ne nous renseigne que partiellement sur l'état physique atteint par une population et qu'il y aurait intérêt à en observer simultanément plusieurs autres.

### Bibliographie

[1] EPREMIAN, E. et MEHL, F. R.: ASTM Spec. Techn. Publ., Nr. 137 (1952).

[2] NEWMARK, N. M. dans W. M. MURRAY (Edit.): Fatigue and Fracture of Metals, New York 1952.

[3] WEIBULL, W.: KTH Handl. (Trans. Roy. Inst. Tech.). (Stockholm) Nr. 27 (1949).

[4] PROT, M.: Rev. Métall., 45, 481 (1948).

[5] STULEN: ASTM Spec. Techn. Publ., Nr. 121 (1951).

# Essais de fatigue statistiques suivant la méthode de charge progressive

Par

**F. Bastenaire, R. Cazaud et M. Weisz**

Avec 2 figures

Les essais ont comporté trois parties dont les résultats ont été analysés par les méthodes statistiques:

1. Détermination de la courbe de Wöhler (15 éprouvettes dont 12 rompues).
2. Etude de la zone d'endurance par la méthode à charge constante (80 éprouvettes).
3. Essais en charges progressives (71 éprouvettes).

Ces essais ont été effectués sur des éprouvettes toriques (fig. 1) prélevées dans une seule barre d'un acier demi-dur recuit, de caractéristiques mécaniques suivantes:

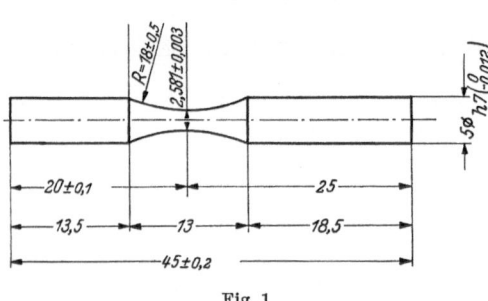

Fig. 1.

$$R = 57,3 \text{ kg/mm}^2$$
$$A\% = 26,5$$
$$E_{0,2} = 36,5 \text{ kg/mm}^2$$
$$S\% = 55$$

et d'analyse:

| | |
|---|---|
| C % = 0,38 | Si % = 0,13 |
| Mn % = 0,5 | S % = 0,022 |
| P % = 0,017 | |

Les caractéristiques essentielles de cet acier du point de vue fatigue ont été déterminées d'après les résultats des deux premières parties puis comparées à celles qui peuvent être déduites des essais en charge progressive.

## 1. Courbe de Wöhler

Une première série d'éprouvettes a servi à tracer la courbe de Wöhler entre 32 et 40 kg/mm². À 30, 31 et 32 kg/mm², les essais ont été arrêtés après trente millions de cycles sans observer la rupture, ce qui situait donc la limite d'endurance aux environs de 32 kg/mm².

A cette première série de 12 observations, nous avons ajusté une courbe d'équation[1]:
$$N (S - E)^\mu = K \qquad (1)$$

---

[1] Voir la liste des notations.

d'un type proposé par W. WEIBULL [*1*], en déterminant la régression du logarithme du nombre de cycles à la rupture par rapport au logarithme de $(S-E)$; (1) s'écrit en effet:

$$\log N = k - \mu \log (S - E)$$

Un tel ajustement est difficile à cause du paramètre inconnu $E$ figurant sous le signe du logarithme mais nos essais à charge constante nous donnaient de $E$ une estimation beaucoup plus précise que celle que l'on pouvait obtenir à partir de la première série d'observations et nous avons préféré l'introduire directement dans (1) de façon à n'estimer que $K$ et $\mu$ par les méthodes classiques. Nous avons ainsi obtenu l'équation de régression:

$$\log N = 6{,}4261 - 1{,}075 \log (S - E) \qquad (2)$$

La décomposition de la variance totale est indiquée dans le tableau 1. Grâce à quelques observations en double et en triple à certains niveaux, on a pu estimer la variance d'erreur et lui comparer la variance des moyennes autour de la droite de régression.

Tableau 1. *Régression de* $\log N$ *par rapport à* $\log (S - E)$

| | Somme des carés | Degrès de liberté | Carré moyen | Rapport des variances | Seuil de signif. de $F$ [1]) |
|---|---|---|---|---|---|
| Régression linéaire | $b^2 \Sigma (x-\bar{x})^2$   0,6803 | 1 | $s_1^2 = 0{,}6803$ | $\dfrac{s_1^2}{s_3^2} = 18{,}09$ | $F_{0{,}01} = 16{,}26$ |
| Variation non linéaire | $\Sigma n_i (\bar{y}_i - y_i)^2$   0,4927 | 5 | $s_2^2 = 0{,}0985$ | $\dfrac{s_2^2}{s_3^2} = 2{,}61$ | $F_{0{,}05} = 5{,}05$ |
| Variance intraclasse | $\Sigma_{i,j}(y_{ij}-\bar{y}_i)^2$   0,1882 | 5 | $s_3^2 = 0{,}0376$ | | |
| Total | $\Sigma_{i,j}(y_{ij}-\bar{y})^2$   1,3612 | 11 | | | |

Nouvelle estimation de la variance d'erreur: $\dfrac{0{,}4927 + 0{,}1882}{10} = 0{,}06809$

---

[1] Test de comparaison des variances de SNÉDÉCOR [*4*].

Le rapport de ces variances n'excédant pas le seuil de signification, on peut admettre la validité de l'ajustement linéaire en se souvenant toutefois qu'il n'est basé que sur 12 points.

Les estimations de $\mu$ et de $\log K$:

$$\mu = - 1{,}075$$
$$k = 6{,}4261$$

ont les intervalles de confiance à 95% suivants:

$$0{,}315 < \mu < 1{,}835$$
$$5{,}872 < \log K < 6{,}980$$

## 2. Limite d'endurance par la méthode à charge constante

La limite d'endurance à trente millions de cycles a été déterminée de façon directe par la méthode à charge constante.

D'après les résultats de la première série d'observations, quatre valeurs de la contrainte maximum ont été choisies régulièrement espacées les unes des autres de 0,750 kg/mm² et vingt éprouvettes essayées pour chacune de ces quatre valeurs.

Les nombres d'éprouvettes rompues sont indiqués dans le tableau 2.

Tableau 2. *Résultats des essais à charge constante*

| Charge en kg/mm² | Nombre d'éprouvettes | | Total |
|---|---|---|---|
| | Rompues | Non rompues | |
| 30,500 | 1 | 19 | 20 |
| 31,250 | 6 | 14 | 20 |
| 32,000 | 7 | 13 | 20 |
| 32,750 | 17 | 3 | 20 |

L'ajustement d'une courbe sigmoïde (intégrale de la loi de Laplace-Gauss) à ces résultats peut être effectué de diverses manières. La méthode du maximum de vraisemblance nous a conduit pour les paramètres de cette courbe aux estimations suivantes:

$$e = 31,93 \text{ kg/mm}^2$$
$$s = 1,21 \text{ kg/mm}^2$$

$e$ désignant l'estimation de la contrainte pour laquelle il y a 50% de ruptures avant trente millions de cycles et $s$ l'estimation de l'écart-type de la courbe sigmoïde.

Ces estimations sont elles-mêmes des variables aléatoires, approximativement normales, d'écart-type:

$$\sigma_e = 0,209 \text{ kg/mm}^2$$
$$\sigma_s = 0,402 \text{ kg/mm}^2$$

On en déduit les intervalles de confiance à 95% de $E$ et de $\sigma$ en leur ajoutant et en leur retranchant 1,96 fois leurs écarts-types:

$$31,52 \text{ kg/mm}^2 < E < 32,34 \text{ kg/mm}^2$$
$$0,42 \text{ kg/mm}^2 < \sigma < 2 \quad \text{ kg/mm}^2$$

Ajoutons que les résultats ne sont pas en désaccord avec l'hypothèse que la proportion des ruptures observées avant trente millions de cycles varie en fonction de la contrainte selon l'intégrale d'une loi de Laplace-Gauss.

## 3. Essais en charge progressive

a) **Conditions générales des essais.** Ils ont été effectués sur des machines réalisant automatiquement de petites augmentations discontinues de la contrainte au moyen d'un dispositif laissant tomber des billes dans un seau suspendu à l'éprouvette.

Ces augmentations périodiques de $0,1\ kg/mm^2$ peuvent avoir lieu tous les 1.000 cycles au minimum jusqu'à 631.000 au maximum; les vitesses extrêmes de mise en charge sont donc:

minimum: $1,585 \cdot 10^{-7}\ kg/mm^2/cycle$
maximum: $10^{-4}\ kg/mm^2/cycle$

et les essais ont été effectués en couvrant la totalité de cet intervalle (Tableau 3).

*Tableau 3*

| $\alpha$ | $S_R$ |
|---|---|
| $10^{-4}$ | 46,53 |
| $1,585 \cdot 10^{-5}$ | 40,35 |
| $2,630 \cdot 10^{-6}$ | 36,63 |
| $0,631 \cdot 10^{-6}$ | 35,87 |
| $1,585 \cdot 10^{-7}$ | 37,52 |

**b) Interprétation des résultats d'ensemble.** Environ quinze éprouvettes réparties sur trois machines ont été essayées à chaque vitesse et l'essai PROT a porté sur 71 éprouvettes au total. Les moyennes des contraintes de rupture $S_R$ (Tableau 3) ont été reportées fig. 2 à des abscisses proportionnelles aux racines carrées des vitesses.

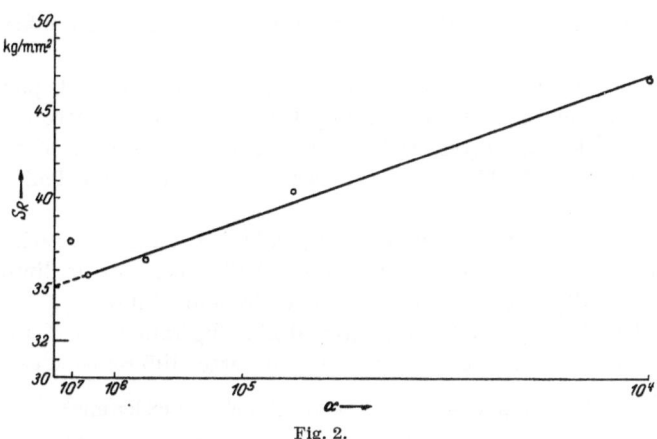

Fig. 2.

Les points correspondant aux quatre vitesses les plus élevées paraissent sensiblement alignés mais une remontée se produit pour la vitesse la plus faible.

La méthode des moindres carrés conduit à la décomposition de variance du tableau 4.

La régression est largement significative; il en est de même de $s_2^2/s_3^2$, d'où il résulte que la régression ne peut être considérée comme linéaire. Ceci tient surtout au résultat relatif à la vitesse la plus faible. À $1,585 \cdot 10^{-7}$ $kg/mm^2/cycles$, la moyenne des contraintes de rupture dépasse en effet de $1,65\ kg/mm^2$ celle à $0,631 \cdot 10^{-6}\ kg/mm^2/cycle$ alors qu'elle devrait lui être inférieure.

Sans faire d'hypothèses sur les formes des distributions statistiques des contraintes de rupture $S_R$, on trouve par un test non paramétrique [2] que la première série est significativement supérieure à la seconde.

Tableau 4. *Régression de $S_R$ par rapport à $\sqrt{\alpha}$*

| | Somme des carré | | Degrés de liberté | Carré moyen | | Rapport des variances | Seuil de signif. de $F$ |
|---|---|---|---|---|---|---|---|
| Régression | $b^2 \Sigma (x - \bar{x})^2$ | 110.929 | 1 | $s_1^2 =$ | 110.929 | $\dfrac{s_1^2}{s_3^2}=813,7$ | $F_{0,01} = 6,63$ |
| Variation non linéaire | $\Sigma n_i (\bar{y}_i - y_i)^2$ | 4.176,5 | 3 | $s_2^2 =$ | 1.392,16 | $\dfrac{s_2^2}{s_3^2}= 10,2$ | $F_{0,05} = 2,60$ |
| Variance intraclasse | $\displaystyle\sum_{i,j} (y_{ij} - \bar{y}_i)^2$ | 8.997,1 | 66 | $s_3^2 =$ | 136,32 | | |
| Total | $\displaystyle\sum_{i,j} (y_{ij} - \bar{y})^2$ | 124.102,6 | 70 | | | | |

Cette anomalie, signalée par M. Davin [3] est bien confirmée par nos essais.

On peut remarquer que les essais très lents, surtout par paliers successifs, ressemblent à du coaxing. Or, la différence entre $S_R$ moyen à $1{,}585 \cdot 10^{-7}$ kg/mm²/cycle et la limite d'endurance déterminée à charge constante est de 5,59 kg/mm², différence dont on peut calculer la précision.

La variance de la moyenne de $S_R$ calculée d'après la série des observations faites à cette vitesse est de 0,173; celle de la limite d'endurance est déjà connue. La variance de leur différence, égale à la somme des deux précédentes, vaut 0,217 (kg/mm²)² et l'écart-type: 0,465 kg/mm². Il est donc probable que cette différence n'est pas inférieure à:

$$5{,}59\ \text{kg/mm}^2 - 1{,}96 \times 0{,}465\ \text{kg/mm}^2 = 4{,}68\ \text{kg/mm}^2$$

c) **Interprétation limitée aux vitesses pratiques d'utilisation.** Dans des essais industriels, on n'utiliserait pas une vitesse aussi faible que $1{,}585 \cdot 10^{-7}$ kg/mm²/cycle. Les autres points du diagramme paraissant sensiblement alignés, nous avons calculé la régression de la contrainte de rupture par rapport à la racine carrée de la vitesse en faisant abstraction de la plus faible:

$$S_R = 35{,}10 + 1161 \sqrt{\alpha}$$

L'analyse de la variance (Tableau 5) montre que le quotient $s_2^2 / s_3^2$ dépasse légèrement le seuil de signification de $F$ à 0,05. Cependant, la comparaison des machines entre elles nous ayant révélé à plusieurs reprises, des différences significatives de sens et d'importances variables, il ne faut pas attacher un sens trop strict au résultat de ce test car la variance intraclasse est alors un peu trop faible. Nous croyons que l'équation de régression linéaire constitue un ajustement valable en première approximation.

Tableau 5

*Régression de $S_R$ par rapport à $\sqrt{\alpha}$ d'après les quatre vitesses les plus élevées*

| | Somme des carrés | | Degrés de liberté | Carré moyen | | Rapport des variances | Seuil de signif. de $F$ |
|---|---|---|---|---|---|---|---|
| Régression | $b^2 \Sigma (x - \bar{x})^2$ | 107.376,38 | 1 | $s_1^2 =$ | 107.376,38 | $s_1^2/s_3^2 = 921,13$ | $F_{0,01} = 7,08$ |
| Variation non linéaire | $\Sigma n_i(\bar{y_i}-y_i)^2$ | 771,12 | 2 | $s_2^2 =$ | 385,56 | $s_2^2/s_3^2 = 3,30$ | $F_{0,05} = 3,15$ |
| Variance intraclasse | $\underset{i,j}{\Sigma} (y_{ij} - \bar{y_i})^2$ | 6.294,77 | 54 | $s_3^2 =$ | 116,57 | | |
| Total | $\underset{i,j}{\Sigma} (y_{ij} - \bar{y})^2$ | | 57 | | | | |

On peut calculer la précision de l'ordonnée à l'origine $E'$ de la droite. On lui trouve un écart-type de 0,224 kg/mm² et par suite l'intervalle de confiance à 0,95 suivant:

$$34,66 < E' < 35,54$$

On peut aussi calculer l'écart-type du coefficient de régression $C$ de $S_R$ par rapport à $\sqrt{\alpha}$. L'application de la formule classique [1] donne:

$$s_C = 39,9$$

D'où l'intervalle de confiance:

$$1083 < C < 1239$$

Enfin, la variance d'erreur (ou résiduelle) a pour estimation:

$$s' = 1,122$$

## 4. Comparaison des résultats de ces divers essais

**a) Considérations générales.** On peut prendre comme caractéristiques fondamentales du comportement d'un matériau à la fatigue, celles qui résultent d'essais à charge constante effectués dans la zone d'endurance et au-dessus.

On peut ensuite, à partir de ces données et selon la théorie que l'on adopte, établir ce que devraient être les résultats d'essais différents tels que ceux en charge progressive.

Les paramètres caractéristiques du diagramme $S$-$N$-$P$ interviennent donc dans les résultats des essais en charge progressive et peuvent être mis en relation avec eux.

---

[1] $s_b = \dfrac{s}{\sqrt{\Sigma (x-\bar{x})^2}}$

2*

Nous partirons de ceux de la courbe de Wöhler et de la zone d'endurance: $E'$, $\mu$, $k$ et $\sigma$. Nous les comparerons aux paramètres caractéristiques de l'essai Prot:

> L'ordonnée à l'origine $E'$
> La pente $C$
> L'écart-type de l'erreur résiduelle $\sigma'$.

**b) Comparaison de $E'$ et de $E$.** Ayant fait abstraction de l'anomalie constatée à la vitesse la plus réduite, nous avons obtenu pour l'ordonnée à l'origine $E'$ une estimation $e'$ d'écart-type: $0{,}224\ \mathrm{kg/mm^2}$.

La variance de $e$ obtenue par la méthode à charge constante étant connue, on en déduit celle de la différence $(e' - e)$:

$$\sigma_{e'-e} = 0{,}308$$

La différence $(e'-e)$ égale à $3{,}17\ \mathrm{kg/mm^2}$ a donc l'intervalle de confiance à $0{,}95$ suivant:

$$2{,}57 < E' - E < 3{,}77$$

**c) Comparaison de $C$ et $K$.** La linéarité de la variation de $S_R$ en fonction de $\sqrt{\alpha}$ est basée sur les hypothèses suivantes:

1. La courbe de Wöhler est une hyperbole équilatère: $N(S-E) = K$.

2. La rupture a lieu lorsque: $\int_{O}^{N} (S - E)\, \mathrm{d}N = K$ intégrée pour les valeurs $S \geqq E$.

Sous ces conditions, l'équation de la droite de Prot est:

$$S_R = E + \sqrt{2\alpha K}$$

mais si l'on fait une hypothèse un peu plus générale sur la courbe de Wöhler, par exemple:

$$N = K(S - E)^{-\mu}$$

tout en conservant la deuxième hypothèse, on obtient l'équation:

$$S_R = E + [(\mu + 1)\,\alpha\, K]^{\frac{1}{\mu+1}}$$

dans laquelle la contrainte de rupture est linéaire en fonction de

$$\alpha^{\frac{1}{\mu+1}}$$

Il importe alors de noter que lorsque l'on maintient que le dommage est exprimé par la formule: $\int \dfrac{\mathrm{d}N}{N}$

le coefficient angulaire de la droite a pour expression:

$$C = [(\mu + 1) \cdot K]^{\frac{1}{\mu+1}}$$

Nous avons deux raisons de penser que $\mu$ est voisin de 1 pour cet acier:

1. L'estimation de $\mu$ d'après l'ajustement de la courbe de Wöhler a donné:

$$m = 1,075$$

2. La contrainte de rupture $S_R$ varie à peu près linéairement en fonction de $\sqrt{\alpha}$.

Avec $\mu = 1$, la formule précédente donne:

$$C = \sqrt{2K}$$

Comme nous avons, d'après les expériences, des estimations indépendantes de $C$ et de $K$ et leurs précisions, on peut tester la validité de cette formule.

En passant aux logarithmes, on devrait vérifier que dans la limite des erreurs probables:

$$2 \log C - \log K - \log 2 = 0$$

On calcule que:

$$\text{Var} (2 \log c) = 0,0009$$
$$\text{Var}\, k \qquad = 0,0615$$

d'où:

$$\text{Var} (2 \log c - k) = 0,0624$$
$$\text{Écart-type} = \sqrt{0,0624} = 0,250$$

or, avec les estimations de $C$ et de $\log K$, on a:

$$2 \log c - k - \log 2 = -0,5974$$

soit 2,29 fois l'écart-type.

*La valeur du coefficient angulaire de la droite de* PROT *est donc significativement différente de celle que lui attribue la théorie.*

D'après une théorie différente du dommage (voir le travail de M. BASTENAIRE) la relation entre $S_R$ et $\alpha^{\frac{1}{\mu+1}}$ serait encore approximativement linéaire mais le coefficient angulaire serait égal à:

$$(\mu K)^{\frac{1}{\mu+1}}$$

On est donc conduit à tester que $C = \sqrt{K}$ c'est-à-dire à voir si $(2 \log c - k)$ dont nous avons calculé l'écart-type (0,250) diffère significativement ou non de zéro.

On trouve que: $2 \log c - k = -0,2964$, soit à peine plus d'un écart-type.

Cette théorie attribue donc au coefficient angulaire une valeur qui ne diffère pas significativement de la valeur observée.

Il faut remarquer toutefois que la droite de PROT ayant une ordonnée à l'origine différente de $E$, sa pente devrait être plus accentuée. L'accord avec la nouvelle théorie du dommage n'en serait que meilleur mais la valeur trouvée d'après la théorie classique ne serait peut-être plus significativement différente de la valeur observée.

**d) Comparaison des écarts-types.**   Dans l'hypothèse où les distributions statistiques de $S$ pour une valeur donnée de $N$ ont même dispersion quel que soit $N$, on peut trouver de cette dernière deux estimations différentes.

La première résulte de la méthode à charge constante arrêtée à trente millions de cycles.

La deuxième est la variance résiduelle de la méthode Prot car, pour les faibles vitesses, la distribution de $S_R$ devrait, en l'absence d'understressing, (c'est-à-dire si $E$ était égal à $E'$) être identique à celle que l'on obtient à charge constante.

Les deux estimations de l'écart-type figurent au tableau 6 avec leurs intervalles de confiance. On voit qu'elles peuvent être considérées comme égales.

*Tableau 6*

|  | Minimum | Estimation de $\sigma$ | Maximum |
|---|---|---|---|
| Méthode à charge constante | 0,42 kg/mm² | 1,21 kg/mm² | 2 kg/mm² |
| Méthode de charge progressive | 0,955  ,, | 1,122   ,, | 1,385  ,, |

## 5. Conclusions

L'interprétation des résultats relatifs aux trois parties de ce programme d'essais par les méthodes statistiques a permis d'arriver aux conclusions suivantes sur l'acier étudié :

a) On a pu prendre, pour la courbe de Wöhler, l'équation :

$$N (S - E) = \text{Constante}.$$

b) Dans les essais en charge progressive, il s'est produit aux faibles vitesses une remontée significative de la contrainte de rupture moyenne.

L'extrapolation de la partie à peu près rectiligne de la courbe représentative de la contrainte de rupture moyenne en fonction de la racine carrée de la vitesse de mise en charge a fourni une valeur significativement différente de la limite d'endurance déterminée par la méthode à charge constante.

Nous pensons pouvoir ultérieurement rechercher si cette différence peut être mise en relation avec le phénomène d'understressing.

c) La valeur du coefficient angulaire de la partie rectiligne de la courbe est en désaccord avec la théorie du dommage basée sur le rapport des cycles.

# 6. Notations

$S:$ Contrainte en kg/mm$^2$

$N:$ Nombre de cycles

$E:$ Limite d'endurance à 50% à $3 \cdot 10^7$ cycles (kg/mm$^2$)

$\mu:$ Exposant de $(S-E)$ dans l'expression $N\,(S-E)^\mu = K$

$K:$ Constante du second membre de $N\,(S-E)^\mu = K$

$e:$ Estimation statistique de $E$ (kg/mm$^2$)

$k:$ Estimation de $\log_{10} K$

$m:$ Estimation de $\mu$

$\sigma:$ Écart-type de la courbe sigmoïde donnant la proportion de rupture en fonction de $S$ pour $3 \cdot 10^7$ de cycles

$s:$ Estimation de cet écart-type (kg/mm$^2$)

$\alpha:$ Vitesse de mise en charge (kg/mm$^2$/cycle)

$S_R:$ Contrainte de rupture dans l'essai PROT (kg/mm$^2$)

$E':$ Ordonnée à l'origine de la courbe de régression de $S_R$ par rapport à $\sqrt{\alpha}$ (kg/mm$^2$)

$C:$ Coefficient angulaire de la droite de PROT

$e':$ Estimation statistique de $E'$

$c:$ Estimation statistique de $C$

$\sigma':$ Variance de $S_R$ pour une valeur donnée de $\alpha$

$s':$ Estimation de $\sigma'$

NOTA — Dans les tableaux d'analyse de variance, $x$, $y$ et $b$ désignent de façon générale: la variable indépendante, la variable dépendante et le coefficient de régression de $y$ par rapport à $x$.

## Bibliographie

[1] WEIBULL, W.: KTH Handl. (Trans. Roy. Inst. Tech.) (Stockholm) Nr. 27 (1949).

[2] MANN and WHITNEY: Ann. math. Statist., 18, 309 (1947).

[3] DAVIN, M.: Rev. gén. Mécan., 38, (1954) Juin.

[4] HALD, A.: Statistical Theory with Engineering Applications, New York 1952, 374.

## Discussion

F. A. McCLINTOCK: It would be interesting to see what confidence limits for the endurance limit by the PROT method would be obtained if the exponent for the loading rate were allowed to vary rather than being assumed constant at $\frac{1}{2}$. As shown in the paper by CORTEN, DIMOFF, and DOLAN, and its discussion (Proc. ASTM, 1954) surprisingly broad confidence limits may be found.

F. GATTO: Peut-être que la différence entre la valeur de la limite de fatigue obtenue avec la méthode d'analyse Probit (charge constante) et la méthode de M. PROT est due à la valeur de l'exposant de $\alpha$ que vous avez considérée égale à $\frac{1}{2}$. Il suffit d'introduire un petit changement pour avoir une forte variation de courbure à l'origine.

Je pense qu'il serait intéressant de comparer les valeurs du tab. 2 avec $E$ estimé par la méthode Probit et d'essayer la linéarité de vos quatre dernières valeurs avec celui-ci en changeant, naturellement, la valeur de l'exposant de $\alpha$.

Si cette dernière linéarité était admissible d'après les tests statistiques, vous n'auriez pas de différence entre la méthode PROT et la méthode de charge constante.

F. BASTENAIRE: Le calcul doit être effectué pour pouvoir conclure définitivement mais la disposition des points sur le diagramme ne suggère pas une amélioration sensible de la linéarité en changeant l'exposant de $\alpha$. On peut penser que son estimation conduirait à une valeur voisine de $\frac{1}{2}$ et que l'ordonnée à l'origine ne s'en trouverait guère affectée.

# Contribution à l'étude de la fatigue des matériaux avec essais à charge progressive

Par

**A. Ferro[1] et U. Rossetti[1]**

Avec 5 figures

La présente recherche a été effectuée sur une machine de type PROT [1], [2], installée au Centro di Studio sugli Stati di Coazione Elastica CNR, auprès de l'École Polytechnique de Turin [3].

Dans cette étude on s'est proposé d'étudier de manière détaillée les différences qui peuvent exister entre les résultats des essais conduits sous charge constante suivant la méthode classique et les essais sous charge progressive [1], [2].

On a effectué, en même temps, une analyse critique de la méthode proposée par PROT [2] pour déterminer la limite de fatigue et qui, comme on le sait, consiste à extrapoler, jusqu'à vitesse de charge nulle, la courbe des résultats expérimentaux sur un diagramme portant en abscisse les racines carrées de la vitesse de charge, et en ordonnées les contraintes à rupture.

La recherche a été précédée par un examen du comportement de la machine d'essai et par une analyse statistique de la dispersion des résultats, respectivement dans les méthodes sous charge progressive et sous charge constante.

## 1. Effectuation des essais et résultats

L'étude a été effectuée pour deux métaux:

1. Acier 35 CM4 au Cr-Mn composition: C 0,35%, Cr 1%, Mn 0,9%, traité avec résistance 105 kg/mm², limite de fatigue sur éprouvettes normales (diamètre 8 mm, longueur 100 mm) 48 kg/mm².

2. Duralumin extrudé et vieilli, résistance 42 kg/mm², limite de fatigue à $10^7$ cycles sur éprouvettes normales: 15 kg/mm².

Pour chaque matériau on a determiné, toujours par flexion rotative:

a) la courbe de fatigue normale de Wöhler effectuée avec éprouvette et machine PROT fonctionnante sous charge constante;

b) la nouvelle courbe de fatigue suivant la méthode sous charge progressive sur la même machine PROT. Pour l'acier les essais à charge pro-

---

[1] Absents. Présenté par M. L. LOCATI.

gressive sont effectués avec deux valeurs de précharge : 40 et 45 kg/mm² ;
pour le duralumin les essais sont effectués avec une seule précharge de
12 kg/mm².

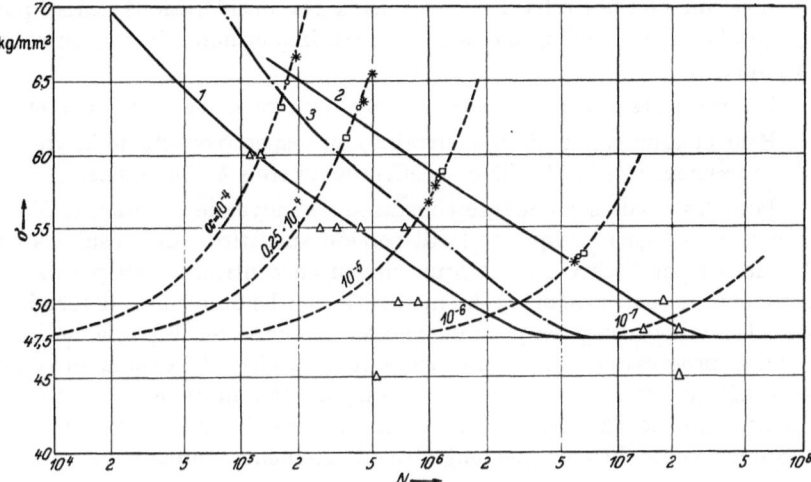

Fig. 1. Courbes de fatigue de l'acier.

*1* sous charge constante (Wöhler)
*2* sous charge progressive (PROT), avec les valeurs moyennes selon les deux précharges.
*3* sous charges progressive, calculée d'après les valeurs sous charge constante.

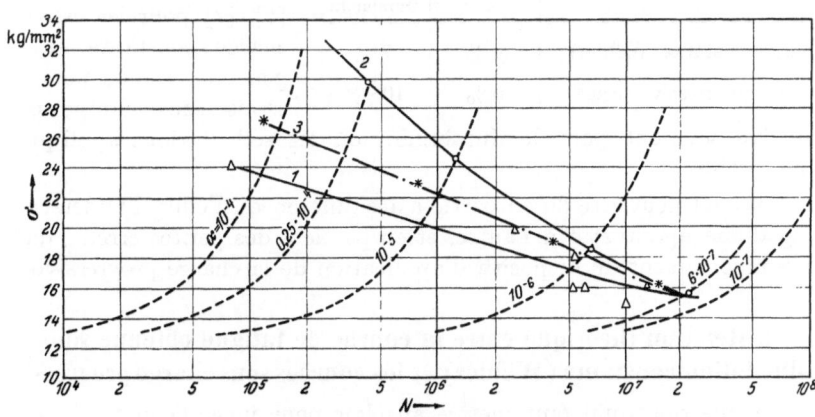

Fig. 2. Courbes de fatigue du duralumin.

*1* sous charge constante (Wöhler)
*2* sous charge progressive (PROT)
*3* sous charge progressive, calculée d'après les valeurs sous charge constante.

Les éprouvettes sont du type CAQUOT (voir fig. 1 du travail de MM.
BASTENAIRE, CAZAUD et WEISZ) avec diamètre de 2,58 mm dans sa section
minima. Les éprouvettes sont prélevées sur les mêmes barres, traitées et

usinées de manière identique de façon à assurer le maximum d'homo-
généité des groupes eux-mêmes.

Pour les valeurs de la sollicitation de rupture on a toujours assumé,
selon ce que l'on fait d'habitude en base à des considérations statistiques
[5], [6], la valeur rapportée à la section minima et non à la section réelle
de rupture.

Les résultats expérimentaux obtenus sont reportés dans fig. 1 et 2.

Pour chaque valeur de la contrainte ou respectivement de la vitesse
d'accroissement de la charge on a effectué de trois à cinq essais.

Pour les essais sous charge constante, la moyenne des durées $N$ est
la moyenne logarithmique et la dispersion statistique des résultats est
définie [5] par l'écart quadratique moyen en contrainte des points expérimentaux par rapport à la meilleure courbe moyenne, déterminée
selon la méthode proposée par Peterson [6]. Pour les essais par la méthode
à charge progressive, la moyenne des contraintes à rupture est la moyenne
arithmétique et la dispersion statistique des résultats est définie par
l'écart-type de la contrainte. Comme il est évident les écarts relatifs
aux deux types d'essais peuvent être directement comparés entre eux.

Dans nos essais les écarts trouvés en pourcent de la limite de fatigue
sont respectivement:

| Type d'essai | Écart quadratique moyen | |
|---|---|---|
| | Acier | Duralumin |
| charge constante (Wöhler) | 4 % | 7 % |
| charge progressive (Prot) | 5 % | 10 % |

La dispersion est donc
tout à fait normale [5],
[6], [7] pour les essais à
charge constante et un
peu plus grande pour les
essais sous charge pro-
gressive sourtout pour le duralumin, où les sollicitations appliquées
sont petites.

Cet effet peut être dû en partie à des différences d'effet d'understressing d'une éprouvette à l'autre, et en partie à des petites erreurs dans
le comportement du dispositif d'application de la charge progressive.

## 2. Relation théorique entre la courbe de fatigue obtenue sous sollicitation constante (Wöhler) et les courbes sous charge progressive

La question qu'il faut mettre au clair pour juger la méthode sous
charge progressive, c'est de voir si la limite de fatigue obtenue avec ce
type d'essais coïncide avec la limite déterminée de la façon normale, et
si les résistances obtenues pour différentes vitesses de charge, peuvent
être réduites à des valeur correspondantes sur la courbe de Wöhler sous
charge constante.

Prot [2] a donné la solution de ce problème dans le cas particulier que la courbe de fatigue normale puisse être représentée par une hyperbole du type:

$$(S - S_f) N = K \tag{1}$$

où $N$ est le nombre d'alternances, $S_f$ est la limite de fatigue et $K$ une constante de proportionnalité.

Dans cette hypothèse il a pu démontrer par des considérations géométriques que les points de la courbe représentés sur le même diagramme de fatigue, et pour la valeur de précharge égale à la limite de fatigue elle-même, sont encore alignés suivant une hyperbole du même type, mais un peu déplacée à droite de la courbe sous charge constante. Dans cette hypothèse PROT a aussi remarqué que les points expérimentaux des résistances à rupture reportés en fonction de la racine carrée de la vitesse d'accroissement de la charge sont alignés selon une ligne droite. La méthode de PROT d'extrapolation pour déterminer la limite de fatigue est basée sur ce résultat.

Les considérations faites dans l'ouvrage de PROT peuvent être reprises analytiquement et conduites de manière tout à fait générale pour n'importe quelle forme de la courbe de fatigue, si l'on admet l'hypothèse de MINER [10] du dommage cumulatif; cette hypothèse est en général celle que l'on adopte dans l'analyse des résultats d'essai avec charge variable. Si dans ces conditions on indique par l'unité le dommage cumulatif faisant briser l'éprouvette, la résistance à rupture à terme $S_t$, sera donnée par

$$\int_{S_o}^{S_t} \frac{\mathrm{d}N}{N(S)} = 1 \tag{2}$$

où $S_o$ est la précharge et $N$ est la durée notée pour chaque valeur de la sollicitation dans l'essai de Wöhler.

Pour le cas de charge progressive avec vitesse uniformément croissante $\alpha$, on a

$$S = \alpha\, n + S_o \tag{3}$$

et donc la résistance à rupture est immédiatement donnée par l'équation.

$$\int_{S_o}^{S_t} \frac{\mathrm{d}S}{\alpha\, N(S)} = 1 \tag{4}$$

C'est évident que l'intégrale peut être écrite de façon identique avec une autre limite inférieure, c'est-à-dire la précharge, arbitraire, pourvu qu'elle soit inférieure à la limite de fatigue; en effet, jusqu'à cette valeur $N = \infty$, soit le dommage par cycle, est nul.

Dans les limites de cette hypothèse il est démontré que, pour n'importe quelle vitesse d'accroissement, la valeur de la résistance à fatigue déterminée par la méthode à charge progressive ne dépend pas de la précharge.

Mais, l'hypothèse de la constance du comportement du matériau n'est valable qu'en première approximation: en fait, il y aura toujours d'effets d'understressing qui vont modifier un peu les résultats théoriques. Quand même si l'on néglige ce dernier effet on peut, dans l'hypothèse du dommage cumulatif, déterminer analytiquement la correspondance entre la courbe de Wöhler et la courbe à charge progressive.

Du point de vue analytique par exemple, si la courbe de fatigue à charge constante est une hyperbole d'ordre $(a + 1)$

$$(S - S_f)^a \cdot N = k \qquad (5)$$

de la courbe de fatigue à charge progressive resulte encore une hyperbole du même ordre mais un peu deplacée à droite, c'est-à-dire on a:

$$(S - S_f)^a \cdot N = (a + 1)\,k \qquad (6)$$

La courbe de la sollicitation à rupture, dans la représentation de Prot, en fonction de la racine carrée de la vitesse d'accroissement de la sollicitation par cycle, est une ligne droite pour une hyperbole de $2^e$ ordre; c'est le cas discuté par Prot, et elle est en général plus ou moins recourbée avec concavité vers le bas pour des exposants $a$ plus elevés. Cette courbe devient une droite si l'on la trace avec en abscisse la racine $(a + 1)$ de la vitesse au lieu de la racine carrée.

Pour le cas que la courbe de Wöhler en échelle semi-logarithmique est une ligne droite qui se prolonge jusqu'à atteindre la valeur de limite de fatigue, ce qui correspond d'habitude à la meilleure approximation que l'on peut faire des courbes expérimentales, surtout s'il s'agit d'aciers, on trouve encore que la courbe de fatigue à charge progressive est de forme très proche à celle sous charge constante et deplacée à droite. Dans la représentation de Prot en fonction de la racine carrée la ligne est aussi recourbée avec concavité vers le bas.

Mais en général l'integration de la (4), la courbe de Wöhler étant expérimentale, sera effectuée par voie numérique sans cependant tenir compte, dans ce second essai, des cycles exécutés audessous de la limite de fatigue.

## 3. Discussion des résultats expérimentaux

Les courbes de fatigue respectivement sous charge constante et sous charge progressive sur acier et duralumin sont reportées aux figures alléguées 1 et 2; dans ces figures sont aussi tracées les courbes théoriques sous charge progressive déduites par intégration numérique.

De l'examen des figures on remarque comme la transformation théorique de la courbe de fatigue sous charge progressive se trouve à la droite de la courbe de Wöhler et a presque la même allure. Pour l'acier les courbes experimentales sous charge croissante ne coïncident avec les courbes calculées que pour des vitesses d'accroissement très élevées; pour des vitesses d'accroissement moyennes et basses, elles sont remarquablement déplacées, et cette différence donne la mesure de l'effet d'understressing obtenu sur le matériau dans ce second type d'essai. Les différences relevées entre les valeurs calculées et les valeurs expérimentales sont reportées au tabl. 1.

*Tableau 1*

| α kg/mm²/cycle | Sollicitation de rupture kg/mm² | | | Effet d'understressing kg/mm² | | Effet moyen d'understressing | |
|---|---|---|---|---|---|---|---|
| | calculée | moyenne remarquée | | précharge 40 kg/mm² | précharge 45 kg/mm² | kg/mm² | % |
| | | précharge 40 kg/mm² | précharge 45 kg/mm² | | | | |
| 1/10.000 | 65 | 66,6 | 63 | + 1,6 | — 2 | — 0,2 | — 0,5 |
| 1/25.000 | 60 | 65,4 | 61 | + 5,4 | + 1 | + 3,2 | + 5,5 |
| 1/100.000 | 56 | 56,8 | 59,5 | + 0,8 | + 3,5 | + 2,2 | + 4 |
| 1/1.000.000 | 49,5 | 52,8 | 53,2 | + 3,3 | + 3,7 | + 3,5 | + 7 |

Par contre, pour le duralumin l'allure des effets d'understressing résulte très différente de celle remarquée sur l'acier: on a des effets d'understressing très forts pour les vitesses de charge très élevées, et understressing nul pour les vitesses d'accroissement basses.

Les résultats concernant le duralumin sont reportés au tabl. 2.

Tableau 2. *Duralumin*

| α kg/mm²/cycle | Résistance à rupture | | Effet d'understressing moyen | |
|---|---|---|---|---|
| | calculée | moyenne remarquée | kg/mm² | % |
| 1/10.000 | 27 | 37,7 | + 10,7 | + 40 |
| 1/25.000 | 25,5 | 29,5 | + 4,0 | + 16 |
| 1/100.000 | 23 | 24,5 | + 1,5 | + 6,5 |
| 1/1.000.000 | 19 | 18,25 | ~ 0 | ~ 0 |
| 1/6.000.000 | 16 | 15,7 | ~ 0 | ~ 0 |

Ces résultats ne peuvent être directement comparés avec ceux obtenus dans d'autres essais d'understressing effectués par d'autres auteurs [4], [11] sur le duralumin et sur l'acier. En effet, il est probable que les effets d'understressing dépendent beaucoup du programme par lequel on fait varier la sollicitation appliquée à l'éprouvette, ce qui fait que des différences très remarquables peuvent se vérifier de fois en fois.

A la fin du jugement de la méthode PROT pour effectuer l'essai de fatigue on peut de toutes façons conclure qu'il existe des effets d'understressing assez importants pouvant déplacer en mesure remarquable les différentes valeurs de la résistance à fatigue pour un nombre limité d'alternances.

Ces effets d'understressing en correspondance de la limite de fatigue seront en général encore sensibles, comme il est bien connu [11], seulement si la précharge est inférieure à la limite de fatigue même et seront évidemment nuls si celleci coïncide avec la limite.

Pour la comparaison des essais sous charge progressive avec les essais à charge constante il faut encore faire une remarque: les essais de fatigue sous charge progressive sont en fait des essais dans lesquels le nombre de cycles produisant la plupart de la fatigue elle-même dans l'éprouvette est relativement petit: c'est-à-dire qu'ils correspondent à des essais sous charge constante effectués dans le domaine de la résistance à nombre limité d'alternances comme il apparaît bien évident par exemple, dans le tabl. 3.

Tableau 3. *Acier. Précharge 45 kg/mm²*

| $\alpha$ kg/mm²/cycle | Sollicitation à rupture kg/mm² | N° de cycle total dans l'essai sous charge progressive | N° de cycles dans les essais sous charge constante |
|---|---|---|---|
| $10^{-4}$ | 63,1 | $1,80 \cdot 10^5$ | $0,65 \cdot 10^5$ |
| $10^{-5}$ | 58,7 | $1,370 \cdot 10^6$ | $1,80 \cdot 10^5$ |
| $10^{-6}$ | 52,8 | $7,800 \cdot 10^6$ | $7,40 \cdot 10^5$ |
| $10^{-7}$ | 47,5 | $30,00 \cdot 10^6$ | $4,00 \cdot 10^6$ |

Le nombre d'alternances nécessaires pour obtenir la rupture sous charge constante (Wöhler) est donc bien plus bas que dans un essai sous charge progressive et, avec une évaluation en première approximation, on peut le retenir égal à l'inverse de la vitesse d'accroissement de la sollicitation dans ce second type d'essai. La raison de la différence est due en bonne partie au fait que dans la méthode sous charge progressive, un nombre élevé de cycles ne donne aucune contribution à la fatigue de l'éprouvette. Ceci, bien entendu, abstraction faite de toute considération pratique sur la possibilité de déterminer la limite de fatigue avec un moindre nombre d'éprouvettes.

## 4. La réprésentation des résultats par la méthode Prot et la détermination de la limite de fatigue

Comme on a vu, aussi les résultats obtenus par la méthode sous charge progressive peuvent être reportés comme ceux des essais sous charge constante en échelle semi-logarithmique. Pour les points expérimentaux on peut alors tracer une courbe très semblable à la courbe de fatigue normale, de laquelle on peut déduire la limite de fatigue en extrapolant les résultats à une vitesse d'accroissement infinitésimal.

Dans ce cas l'extrapolation est cependant plus difficile à effectuer que pour les courbes de Wöhler, car l'inclinaison des courbes sous charge progressive décroît très lentement même pour les plus basses valeurs de la vitesse d'accroissement de la charge. Ce fait est physiquement bien compréhensible parce que dans les essais à charge progressive, comme on a déjà vu, le nombre de cycles produisant la plupart du dommage est relativement petit.

La méthode PROT pour extrapoler les résultats et déterminer la limite de fatigue, consiste à reporter les valeurs de la résistance obtenues en fonction de la racine carrée de la vitesse d'accroissement; la limite de fatigue est celle que l'on obtient en extrapolant la courbe expérimentale à vitesse d'accroissement de la charge nulle (fig. 3 et 4). On peut remarquer que la méthode PROT est assez voisine à la méthode déjà proposée par LEHR [8] et par AMBRUSTER [9], où, en admettant que les courbes de fatigue sous charge pussent être représentées par une hyperbole, on déterminait les valeurs de la limite en reportant les valeurs des sollicitations à rupture en fonction de l'invers des durées respectives. Cette méthode donnait, dans beaucoup de cas, des résultats satisfaisants, pourvu que les points expérimentaux fussent compris dans l'intervalle entre $10^5$ et $10^7$ alternances.

De façon tout à fait

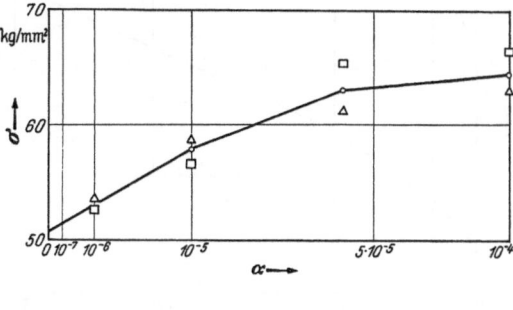

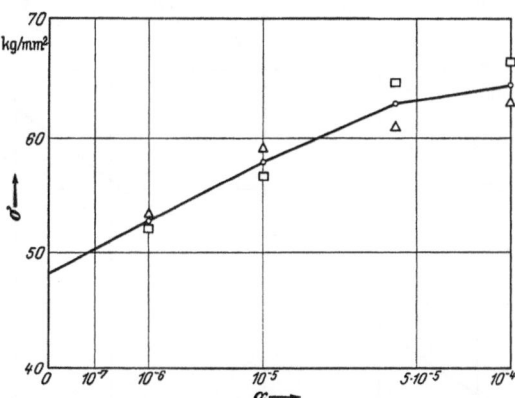

Fig. 3. Courbes de fatigue de l'acier. Essais sous charge progressive, valeurs moyennes pour les deux précharges. Courbes en fonction des racines carrées (partie supérieure) et des racines cubiques (partie inférieure) de la vitesse d'accroissement de la charge $\alpha$ en kg/mm²/cycle.

analogue, comme on a déjà dit, la ligne reliant les points expérimentaux aux différentes vitesses d'accroissement de la charge, dans la représentation de PROT est une ligne droite si la courbe de fatigue sous charge constante est une hyperbole de 2ᵉ ordre.

Comme les courbes de fatigue de Wöhler ne sont en général pas des hyperboles de 2ᵉ ordre, les courbes de PROT, faute d'effet d'understressing, seront en général recourbées avec concavité vers le bas comme on a déjà vu avant, en utilisant des approximations analytiques des courbes de Wöhler. L'extrapolation à vitesse de charge nulle serait donc possible seulement si l'on dispose d'un suffisant nombre de points à vitesse de charge très basse. Par exemple, pour l'acier que nous avons essayé, la ligne obtenue est très recourbée; pour le duralumin elle est également recourbée, et il faut remarquer qu'elle le serait davantage, si ce matériau ne présentait pas, comme on a déjà vu, d'importants effets d'understressing. De façon analogue, le fait que les courbes de nombreux matériaux — alliages légers et aciers — reportées par PROT, sont assez proches à des lignes droites sur un long trait, est probablement dû à des effets d'understressing aux vitesses élevées d'accroissement de la charge.

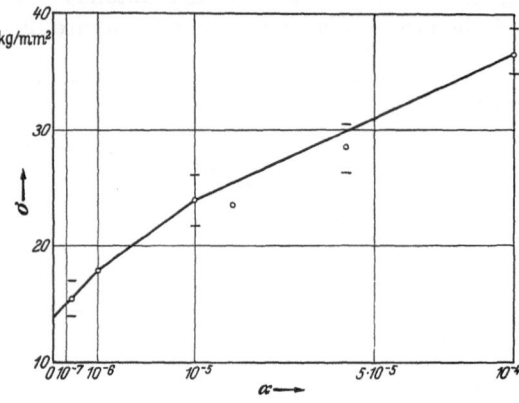

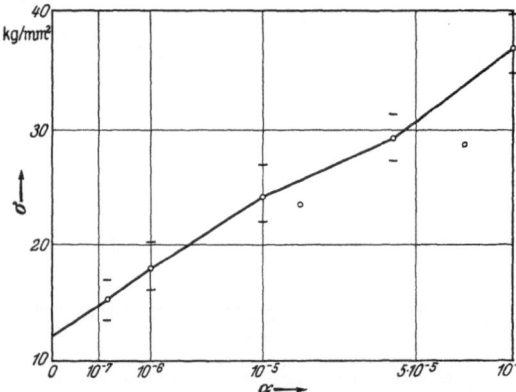

Fig. 4. Courbes de fatigue du duralumin, essayé sous charge progressive, en fonction des racines carrées (partie supérieure) et des racines cubiques (partie inférieure) de la vitesse d'accroissement de la charge α en kg/mm²/cycle.

Dans nos essais en ayant à disposition des points expérimentaux jusqu'à une vitesse de moins de $10^{-6}$ kg/mm²/cycle l'extrapolation à la limite de fatigue peut être considérée bonne comme il résulte des fig. 1 et 2, mais elle n'aurait pas été possible si l'on avait fait seulement des essais avec vitesse plus grande ($10^{-4}$ au $10^{-5}$ kg/mm²/cycle).

Pour l'acier la limite de fatigue PROT est un peu plus haute de la limite observée sur la courbe de Wöhler et pour le duralumin est pratiquement coïncidente. Les difficultés que l'on a mis en evidence dans l'extrapolation des résultats par la méthode PROT ne permettent pas de dire si pour l'acier les différences observées doivent être toutes attribuées à l'effet d'understressing.

Par contre, si l'on tient compte de la forme réelle plus fréquente de la courbe de Wöhler qui, comme on peut voir en fig. 5, est beaucoup plus proche à une hyperbole du troisième ordre qu'à une de 2ᵉ, on peut remarquer après les considérations analytiques déjà faites que les diagrammes de PROT doivent être plus proches à une ligne droite si on reporte en abscisse la racine cubique de la vitesse au lieu de la racine carrée. Cela est en effet ce que l'on trouve avec la représentation de nos résultats en fonction de la racine cubique (fig. 3 et 4 en bas): les lignes tracées sont beaucoup plus proches à des droites pour un long trait. Avec une représentation ainsi modifiée, en extrapolant les résultats à une vitesse d'ac-

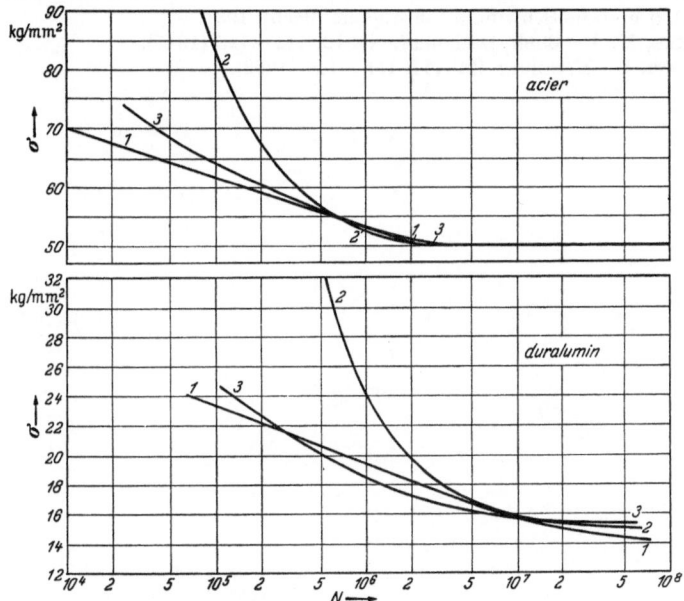

Fig. 5. Comparaison entre les courbes de fatigue
1 sous charge constante réelles
2 leurs approximations analytiques $(S - S_f) N = $ const.
3 leurs approximations analytiques $(S - S_f)^2 N = $ const.

croissement nulle, on obtient, pour l'acier, une limite de fatigue coïncidant avec celle de Wöhler et pour le duralumin une valeur plus basse.

Ce dernier type de représentation semble cependant peut-être préférable à celle originaire de PROT, aussi par le fait que les points correspondants aux vitesses basses sont maintenant bien plus écartés. En se rappelant alors, comme on a dit avant, que le nombre d'alternances à rupture dans l'essai sous charge constante coïncide avec l'inverse de la vitesse d'accroissement, on pourra par exemple donner, selon les conventions habituelles [4], la limite de fatigue à $10^7$ ou à $10^8$ cycles, au lieu de celle pour un nombre d'alternances infini qui, en fait, n'existe que pour la plupart des matériaux ferreux, tandis que pour beaucoup d'autres il représente une extrapolation qui n'est pas tout à fait sûre.

## Bibliographie

[1] PROT, M.: Comptes Rendus, **225**, 669 (1947).

[2] PROT, M.: Mes. et Cont. industr. (1948) Sept.

[3] ROSSETTI, U. P.: Atti e rassegna tecn. Soc. Ing. Archit. (Torino) **6**, 356 (1952).

[4] LOCATI, L.: La fatica dei materiali metallici, Hoepli 1950.

[5] EPREMIAN, E. et F. R. MEHL: NACA TN 2719, 1952.

[6] PETERSON, R. E.: Bull. ASTM Nr. 156, 50 (1949).

[7] RAVILLY, E.: Publ. sci. techn. Ministère de l'air (Paris) Nr.120, 52—70 (1938).

[8] LEHR: Dr. diss. Stuttgart 1925.

[9] ARMBRUSTER, E.: Einfluß der Oberflächenbeschaffenheit auf den Spannungs-verlauf und die Schwingungsfestigkeit, Berlin 1931.

[10] MINER, M. A.: Mach. Design **17**, Nr. 12, 111—115 (1945).

[11] LOCATI, L.: Metallurg. ital.,**44**, 135—144 (1952).

# Theories relating to fatigue of materials under combinations of stress

By

## W. N. Findley

With 1 figure

Analysis of available data suggests that the phenomenon of fatigue of materials results primarily from alternating shearing stress producing cracks along shear planes, and that the resistance to fatigue fracture is influenced by other factors. Some of these factors are: changes in structure of the material resulting from heat treatment, elastic distortion from applied stresses (or residual stresses), or plastic deformation; the mode of crack propagation (by shear or by separation); and the normal stress on planes of principal shear stress (called here the complementary normal stress).

A review of the literature on fatigue under combined stress, published in 1953 [1], shows that the test data obtained by various investigators support a variety of different theories. In fact, it was concluded by one investigator that no single rational theory, such as the principal shear stress theory, could explain fatigue under combined stress.

However, it was observed by the writer that certain modifying factors such as anisotropy, which were not fully considered in the literature, might be responsible for the divergent results. It was further observed that the data of several investigations agreed with a principal shear stress theory as well as with the theory proposed by the investigators. And in a recent study of fatigue under combined bending and torsion [1] an examination of the fractures disclosed that the fatigue fracture in every combination of stresses probably originated on planes of principal shear stress, while the propagation of the fracture changed from shear to tension at different stages in the fracture, depending on the magnitude of the alternating shearing stress and on the normal stress on planes of principal shearing stress.

## 1. Mode of fracturing

The study of fractures suggests the following sequence in formation of fatigue cracks. Under repeated stressing, slip occurs in crystal grains favorably oriented in or near planes of principal shear stress and which have relations with neighboring grains (such as a free surface on one side) which permit slip under the applied stress.

Repeated stressing causes repeated or reverse slip in some grains resulting first in a disruption of the ordered atomic array along planes of slip, and finally in the formation of a crack. The removal of restraint resulting from the initial crack permits slip to occur more readily in adjacent crystals so that the crack tends to spread roughly in the plane of shear.

As the crack becomes larger, the shearing displacement between the faces of the crack increases with a consequent mechanical interference between the irregularities left in the wake of the crack. The resulting abrasion causes fine particles of the material to be torn loose and exude from the crack as dust.

As long as (a) the alternating principal shear stress and (b) the ratio of the alternating principal shear stress to the alternating plus mean principal stress are larger than certain values the crack propagates in shear. But if either becomes less than this value, the propagation changes soon to tensile separation.

## 2. Effect of static stresses

These observations, together with studies of the effect of static stresses on fatigue [1], [2], led the writer to suggest that fatigue results from alternating shearing stress as the prime factor, with superimposed static stresses, complementary normal stress and anisotropy as modifying factors which alter the fatigue strength of the material.

Studies of the influence of static stresses [1], [2], showed that the fatigue strength of some materials particularly in torsion was not influenced much by static stresses, whereas for other materials and other states of stress a substantial influence was found. This suggested that the effect might be caused by (a) changes in structure of the material resulting from either elastic or plastic deformation under action of the static plus alternating stress and (b) the influence of the complementary normal stress. The latter stress would be altered by superimposing static stresses for most states of stress but not for torsion.

To examine these possibilities, fatigue tests in tension and in torsion were made on a material having a substantial decrease in tensile fatigue strength with static tension, 75 S-T aluminum [3]. Three series of tests were performed both in tension and torsion: (a) Tests at zero mean stress, (b) tests at zero mean stress after loading the specimen into the yielding range then reverse loading it as far as the minimum stress to be used in fatigue at zero mean stress, (c) tests at a high mean stress following the same pre-loading cycle as in (b). In tension the fatigue strength was reduced 30 per cent by the pre-loading alone and 60 per cent by the pre-loading and mean stress combined. In torsion the fatigue strength was reduced by 4 and 11 per cent respectively by the pre-loading and pre-loading plus mean stress.

From these results it may be concluded that: (A) the mean stress alone in the case of torsion, where the complementary normal stress is zero, caused a small effect (a decrease of about 9 per cent) resulting from the static elastic distortion; (B) the structural change resulting from yielding produced a small decrease (4 per cent) in the fatigue strength in torsion; and (C) when a tensile complementary normal stress was added, as in bending, the decrease in fatigue strength was substantially greater.

## 3. Programming fatigue tests

The method of programming these tests was to establish the approximate shape of the $S$-$N$ diagram in the desired region by 3 to 5 tests while trying to establish one test point at the desired number of cycles. Then three or more tests were run at the same stress. This stress was the one estimated to yield a mean $\log N$ at the desired number of cycles. From the resulting mean $\log N$ and approximate slope of the $S$-$N$ diagram the fatigue strength at the desired number of cycles was obtained by a slight extrapolation.

## 4. Effect of extreme compression

To further study the influence of the complementary normal stress, tests in axial loading were made of SAE 4340 steel at different static mean stresses, including extremely high values in compression [3]. A gradual increase in fatigue strength was noted as the mean stress (and hence the complementary normal stress) decreased from a high tension, to zero, to a high compression. Available data indicate that this change is probably due largely to the complementary normal stress.

The extreme compression tests were performed in an attempt to determine whether cycles of stress in which the entire cycle was a compression stress of 20,000 psi or greater would produce fatigue cracks. Cracks were produced and propagated transverse to the section but progressed only to a certain depth. Thus, the presence of high compressive normal stresses on planes of principal shear stress did not inhibit fracture. They may, however, have prevented cracks from progressing beneath a layer of surface weakness resulting from the unsupported free surface.

## 5. Effect of static torsion on alternating bending

Data are available from three investigators showing the effect of static torsion on alternating bending. Tests by GOUGH [4] on nickel-chromium-molybdenum steel show a decrease in fatigue strength of 7 to 8 per cent for static stresses which did not produce yielding, whether the static stresses were bending or torsion. If the complementary normal stresses are computed from these data it is observed that the reduction in the endurance limit corresponding to the complementary normal stress is in closely the same proportion whether the normal stress is produced by static bending or static torsion.

The data of LEA and BUDGEN [5] and ONO [6] show that the addition of static torsion to reversed bending in soft steels caused no change or a slight increase in endurance limit (depending on hardness) for nominal twisting stresses up to about 50 per cent above the yield stress followed by a marked reduction at higher stresses. The softer the steel the greater the increase in endurance limit resulting from static torsion. Examination of these data shows that the principal shear stress resulting from the combined loading was above the yield point for all values of static torsion employed, and at the highest static stresses employed by LEA and BUDGEN the combined loading would have produced large strains.

It may also be observed that the planes of the greatest principal shear stress resulting from the combination of bending and torsion loads, and hence the planes on which the greatest slip would occur during yielding, are different from the planes of principal shear stress resulting from the alternating bending.

The following explanations are offered for the above observations on soft steels: The static torsion produces an increase in the complementary normal stress on planes of alternating principal shear stress. This probably produces a tendency toward a lower resistance to fatigue. However, in the tests on soft steels yielding was produced on planes intersecting the planes of alternating principal shear stress as explained above. This yielding may have a work hardening effect for small strains whose strengthening effect on fatigue of the material may slightly exceed the weakening effect of the tensile value of complementary normal stress. At the large twisting strains the material may have been damaged by micro cracks, resulting in reduced fatigue resistance — especially under the influence of the higher normal stresses.

A question arises as to why do not static bending stresses also produce an increase in bending endurance limit in soft steels. The reason may be that yielding on planes which intersect planes of alternating principal shear planes produce increased resistance to fatigue on the latter planes, whereas yielding on the same planes does not increase the resistance to fatigue, or at least not to the same degree.

## 6. Effect of static bending on alternating torsion

GOUGH's data on nickel-chromium-molybdenum steel tested in torsion fatigue with superimposed static torsion or static bending show a decrease in endurance limit of about 8 per cent for static torsion stresses producing combined stresses above and also just below the yield point in torsion [4]. Static bending on the other hand produced a decrease in endurance limit of as much as 23 per cent for combined stresses up to about 2/3 the yield point. For the static torsion no complementary normal stresses were introduced. The effect observed may be attributed to the change in structure of the material resulting from the static stresses. For static bending, however, the complementary normal stress was increased from zero to $+69,000$ psi. Thus, most of the observed effect may be attributed to the tensile complementary normal stress.

## 7. Modified theories of fatigue under combined stress

Fatigue tests in bending $b$ and torsion $t$ obtained for many different materials by different investigators show a wide range of ratios of $b/t$ from less than 1 to more than 2. Since all of the rational theories of failure under combined stress require either a fixed value of $b/t$ or one which varies with one plus Poisson's ratio, the observed variation in $b/t$ needs explanation. Available data can be grouped by type of material to show a trend from small to large $b/t$ with progression from cast irons, to steel and aluminum alloys, to copper alloys, to laminated plastics [7]. This suggests that there may be different mechanisms of failure operating for different type materials. Or, perhaps more likely, the basic mechanism remains the same for all materials but the effect of certain influencing factors changes with material. It has also been observed that the same steel at different heat-treatments has different values of $b/t$.

It was suggested [1] that anisotropy of the material might be at least one factor in causing the variation in $b/t$. Following this suggestion, a method of correction of the rational theories of failure to bring them into agreement with data in bending and torsion was proposed. It was found that application of this correction reduced six of the eight rational theories considered to the same form as (1) below. In the form of the principal shear stress theory, the modified expression is

$$\tau_1 = \tfrac{1}{2}\sqrt{\sigma^2 + (b/t)^2 \tau^2} \tag{1}$$

All six of the equations (when rationalized if necessary) may be written as
$$\sigma^2/b^2 + \tau^2/t^2 = 1 \qquad (2)$$
(2) is identical with the empirical ellipse quadrant of GOUGH which agreed so well with data on combined bending and torsion fatigue of ductile metals.

The principal strain theory when modified in the same manner [7] may be reduced to
$$(b/t - 1)\,\sigma^2/b^2 + (2 - b/t)\,\sigma/b + \tau^2/t^2 = 1 \qquad (3)$$
which is identical to the ellipse arc proposed by GOUGH for brittle irons.

The principal stress theory modified in the same way [7] reduces to the parabola
$$\sigma/b + \tau^2/t^2 = 1 \qquad (4)$$
which describes data on iron and iron alloys even better than (3).

## 8. Influence of anisotropy

To further explore the influence of anisotropy, fatigue tests were made in bending and torsion on specimens having their axes parallel,

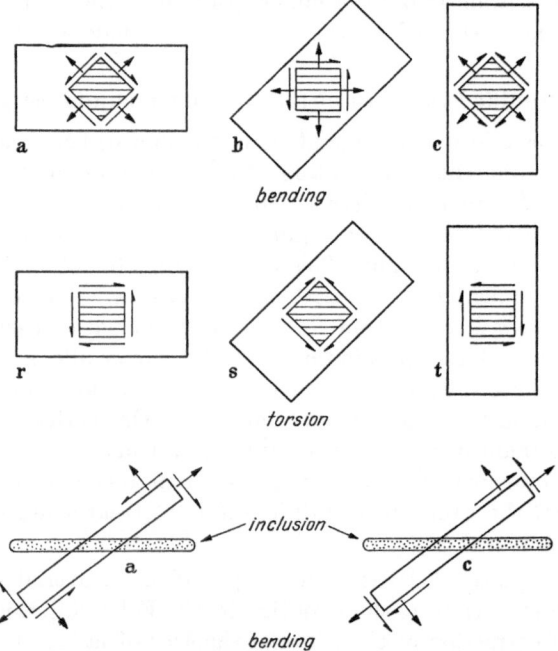

Fig. 1. Orientation of principal shear and complementary normal stresses relative to the texture of the material in tests for aniso-tropy in the fatigue properties. (The direction of the texture is horizontal.)

normal and at 45 degrees to the direction of rolling of the parent bar stock [8]. These tests were made on three alloys previously tested in combined bending and torsion fatigue. The results showed a small anisotropy in torsion, with maximum strength at 45 degrees for 2 of the 3 materials and minimum at 90 degrees, and a larger anisotropy in bending, with maximum strength parallel to the direction of rolling (direction of texture) and minimum at 90 degrees.

If alternating shear stress is the prime factor causing fatigue with complementary normal stress and anisotropy as modifying factors, then the following should be true because of similar orientation of stress and texture; see fig. 1: (a) the fatigue strength in torsion parallel (r, fig. 1) and 90 degrees (t, fig. 1) to the rolling direction should be equal (nearly true for two of the materials tested); (b) the shearing fatigue strength in bending of diagonal specimens b should be less than the fatigue strength in torsion parallel r and at 90 degrees t (as observed); (c) the shearing fatigue strength in bending parallel a and at 90 degrees c should be less than that of diagonal specimens in torsion s (as observed); and (d) the fact that the bending fatigue strength is greater parallel a than at 90 degrees c may be explained as follows. In specimens of both orientations, a and c, the planes of principal shear are at 45 degress. In parallel specimens a the complementary normal stress tends to open cracks between metal and elongated inclusions (for example) while shear stresses tend to close such cracks; see fig. 1. But in 90 degree specimens c, both normal and shear stresses tend to open such cracks. Thus, lower fatigue strength would be expected.

## 9. Explanations for variations in $b/t$

If the principal shear stress theory is accepted (or any of five other theories for that matter) the ratio $b/t$ must be constant; since it is not, explanations are needed. The above discussion suggests two sources of the variations: anisotropy and the complementary normal stress, the influence of both varying with material. In fig. 1 the difference between conditions in tests s and c are solely the tensile normal stress in c. It was found that the reduction in fatigue strength resulting from this normal stress was 34, 24, and 31 per cent respectively for the 76S-T61, 25S-T6 aluminum and SAE 4340 steel tested [8]. This is in accord with the results obtained by GOUGH, as described above, in which a reduction of 23 per cent in endurance limit resulted from superimposing a static bending stress on alternating torsion.

On the other hand, comparison of r and s or t and s (see fig. 1) shows that the only known difference lies in the orientation of shear stressing relative to texture. Thus, the ratio of the corresponding fatigue strengths represents the effect of anisotropy. Tests of the three materials mentioned [8] showed the effect of anisotropy alone to be small.

An examination of a, b and c of fig. 1 shows that the shear stress has progressed from an orientation of "down-grain" relative to the texture, to across-grain, to up-grain, as the fatigue strength has decreased. All this has been in the presence of a tensile complementary normal stress. On the other hand, during part of the cycle of stress of specimens represented by a the sense of all stresses was reversed. This yields the less favorable "up-grain" shear stressing of c. However, the complementary normal stress in this condition is compression, so that failure under this more severe shear stress condition is suppressed in favor of the less severe shear stress condition present with tensile normal stress.

The above explanation seems satisfactory. However, it was observed that the orientation of shear stress relative to texture in diagram s of fig. 1 was evidently less severe than that in r. Hence, it would seem that the condition represented by c should be less severe than b instead of the reverse. It appears that the presence of the complementary normal stress inverts the effect of the texture. It is not clear why. Thus, further study of this problem seems warranted.

## Bibliography

[1] FINDLEY, W. N.: NACA TN 2924, 1953.
[2] FINDLEY, W. N., F. C. MERGEN and A. H. ROSENBERG: Proc. ASTM 53, 768 (1953).
[3] FINDLEY, W. N.: Proc. ASTM 54, 836 (1954).
[4] GOUGH, H. J.: Proc. Instn mech. Engrs 160, 417 (1949).
[5] LEA, F. C., and H. P. BUDGEN: Engineering 122, 242 (1926).
[6] ONO, A.: Mem. Col. Engr Kyushi Imp. Univ., 2, No. 2, 117 (1921).
[7] FINDLEY, W. N., and P. N. MATHUR: Modified Theories of Fatigue Failure under Combined Stress, presented at the Soc. exp. Stress. Anal. meeting, Los Angeles 1955.
[8] FINDLEY, W. N., and P. N. MATHUR: Anistropy of Fatigue Strength of a Steel and two Aluminum Alloys in Bending and Torsion, to be presented at the ASTM meeting, Atlantic City 1955.

## Discussion

D. G. SOPWITH questioned the value of author's phenomenological approach and preferred considerations based on microscopic slip, as developed by TAYLOR and himself.

The influence of residual stresses on fatigue limit was discussed by P. P. BENHAM and E. GASSNER who pointed out that residual stresses at notches may start cracks at an early stage of the test. The cracks may then stop when stresses have become released.

W. N. FINDLEY: It will be interesting to study a report on the theories of TAYLOR and SOPWITH when it becomes available. I agree with the remarks of BENHAM and GASSNER. It is my opinion, however, that residual stresses were not the primary explanation for the fractures observed in fatigue under extreme compression.

# Effect of simultaneous cyclic variation of stress and temperature on a high temperature material

By

**A. Fransson**

With 9 figures

## 1. Introduction

For the purpose of showing experimentally, by laboratory tests, if a certain high temperature material is suitable for turbine blades in gas turbine engines, it has so far been customary to adopt creep tests and also, occasionally, fatigue tests at high temperatures. Thus, TOOLIN and MOCHEL [1], for example, have carried out extensive bending fatigue tests on a great number of high temperature alloys at 1,200 and 1,500°F (650 and 815°C).

Although the static (time dependent) creep test as well as the dynamic (cycle dependent) fatigue test are of great value, when judging the material, they do not give a complete picture of the behaviour of the material in, for instance, jet engines, where stresses and temperature often undergo rapid changes. The stresses in the turbine blades consist essentially of tensile stresses in the longitudinal direction of the blade, caused by the centrifugal force. The gas forces introduce a larger or smaller bending stress in the blade, the magnitude of the stress depending on the shape and design of the blade. To this are added mechanical stresses as a result of blade vibrations (vibration stresses), which at certain critical turbine speeds can reach relatively high values and sometimes cause fatigue failures in the blades.

At the same time as the turbine blades are subjected to such complex stresses, they are also exposed to the influence of high temperature, which can produce certain mechanical stresses due to temperature gradients in the geometrically irregularly shaped blade. Finally one must not disregard the chemical influence (high temperature corrosion) of the hot exhaust gas on the material of the turbine blades.

The relatively short operating periods, involving many starts, make the turbine operating conditions more complicated in jet engines (especially in fighter aircraft) than in stationary gas turbines. Furthermore, rapid changes of the turbine speed upwards or downwards have often to be made. At starting or when the turbine speed is changed rapidly, the tensile stress and the temperature of the turbine blade change quickly at the same time. This will also imply that several critical speeds are passed, giving vibrations, whether the rate of revolution is increasing or decreasing.

This gives a good reason to study how the turbine blade material behaves during simultaneous relatively rapid cyclic variation of tensile stress and temperature with or without influence of vibrations and possibly also corrosive gases. Cyclic variation of the stress (dynamic stress superimposed on static creep stress) at constant temperature has earlier been studied for instance by LAZAN [2]. Similar tests have also been carried out by GUARNIERI and YERKOVICH [3].

The object of this paper is partly to give a short description of a machine which allows simultaneous cyclic variation of tensile stress and temperature in a specimen, and partly to give a brief account of test results obtained so far.

## 2. Testing method

In the testing machine, designed and built at the Materials Laboratory Malmslätt, a specimen is simultaneously subjected to cyclic temperature variations and intermittent tensile stresses with or without

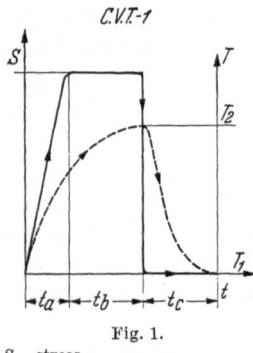

Fig. 1.

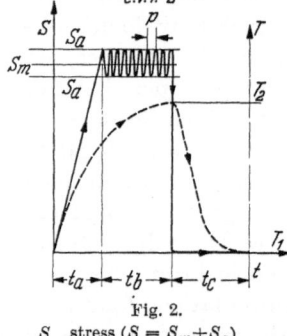

Fig. 2.

$S$   stress
$T$   temperature ($T_1$ resp. $T_2$)
$t$   time, 1 cycle $c = t_a + t_b + t_c$
$t_a$  time during which $S$ is increased from zero to the maximum value
$t_b$  time during which full load is imposed
$t_c$  time during which $S = 0$ and $T$ is decreased from $T_2$ to $T_1$
$t_a + t_b$ time during which $T$ is increased from $T_1$ to $T_2$.

$S$   stress ($S = S_m \pm S_a$)
$S_m$  mean stress or static pre-load imposed
$S_a$  alternating or cyclic stress superimposed on $S_m$
$f$   frequency (Hz) of the cyclic or vibratory stress
$t_b$  time during which $S_m$ and $S_a$ are imposed.

superimposed vibrations. The specimen which is tubular with very thin walls (about 0.5 millimeter) is heated by electrical high frequency induction which conveniently allows a rapid increasing and decreasing of the temperature.

The static tensile load is achieved by means of an electromagnet whose armature is connected to the specimen via a lower pull rod in the machine. Strain gauges, applied to the lower pull rod, enable occasional checking of the stress in the specimen. The same electromagnet makes it also possible to obtain vibrations by feeding the magnet with alternating current, superimposed on the direct current which gives the static load. The specimen together with the upper and lower pull rod and the armature forms a resonance system. The frequency of this system is 110 Hz.

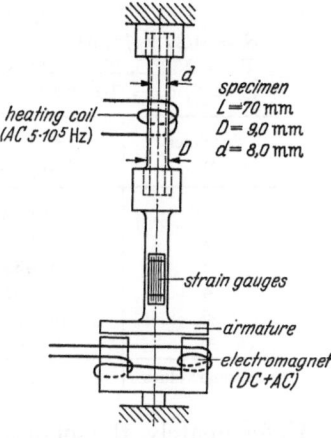

Fig. 3.
Schematic diagram of test equipment.

Each test is continued until fracture occurs and the machine is automatically stopped. The number of stress cycles is indicated on a counter. The principle of the so called Cyclic Variation Test, C. V. T., is presented in fig. 1 (C. V. T.-1) and fig. 2 (C. V. T.-2). The testing set up is shown in fig. 3.

## 3. Material and test results

The investigation was carried out on a Nimonic material with the following approximate composition: C 0.05, Cr 18, Ni 75, Ti 2.5, Al 1.0, Fe 0.25 per cent. Two different heats, "519" and "517", have been tested. The material was heat treated as follows: Solution heat treated at 1,080° C for 8 hours and aged at 750° C for 16 hours.

All the test specimens were machined in the solution treated condition, and after finishing they were aged before testing.

The investigation has included creep tests as well as tests under simultaneous cyclic variation of stress and temperature. The creep test was performed at 750° C and 27 kg/mm² and gave for material "519" the following results:

> Time to rupture 750 hours
> · Time to reach the third creep stage 560 hours
> Creep rate in the second stage 0.0006 per cent per hour

These figures represent the average of several determinations.

The cyclic variation of stress and temperature has been carried out according to fig. 1. The results of these tests are given in table 1. The material "519" used in the these two investigations (creep and C. V. T.-1) was taken from the same rolled and heat treated bar and can therefore be considered entirely comparable.

### Table 1. C. V. T.—1

$S = 0/27$ kg/mm$^2$
$T_1 = 550°$C, $T_2 = 750°$C
$t_a = 6$, $t_b = 10$ and $t_c = 10$ seconds

| Specimen No. | Number of cycles $(t_a + t_b + t_c)$ to rupture | Total time to rupture, hours | Time at full load, $\Sigma (t_b)$ hours |
|---|---|---|---|
| 1 | 29,653 | 216 | 82 |
| 2 | 31,347 | 228 | 88 |
| 3 | 30,438 | 222 | 86 |
| 4 | 32,751 | 239 | 92 |
| 5 | 30,288 | 221 | 85 |
| 6 | 35,405 | 256 | 98 |
| Average values | 31,647 | 230 | 89 |

Unfortunately, the quantity of material "519" was not sufficient for further investigations which were therefore continued on a similar material, originating from another heat, called "517". The only deviation, however, between the two materials was a slight difference in the Ti- and Al-content.

The creep characteristics are very much the same for both materials. Thus, the following mean values were obtained during creep testing at 750° C and 27 kg/mm$^2$:

    Time to rupture 730 hours
    Time to reach the third creep stage 380 hours
    Creep rate in the second stage 0.0015 per cent per hour

The material "517" has been tested under cyclic variation of stress and temperature according to fig. 2, i. e., with superimposed vibrations. The following stresses $(S_m \pm S_a)$ have been choosen: $25\pm2$, $27\pm2$ and $29\pm2$ kg/mm$^2$. The results are given in table 2.

The same table also shows a comparison between the three different testing methods (Creep, C. V. T.-1, and C. V. T.-2).

### Table 2. C. V. T.—2

$T_1 = 550°$C, $T_2 = 750°$C
$t_a = 6$, $t_b = 10$ and $t_c = 10$ seconds

| Spec. No. | $S_m$ kg/mm$^2$ | $S_a$ kg/mm$^2$ (frequency 110 Hz) | Number of cycles $(t_a + t_b + t_c)$ to rupture | Total time to rupture, hours | $\Sigma (t_b)$ hours |
|---|---|---|---|---|---|
| 78 | 25 | $\pm 2$ | 110,568 | 830 | 320 |
| 76 | 27 | $\pm 2$ | 36,941 | 272 | 105 |
| 73 | 29 | $\pm 2$ | 14,725 | 108 | 42 |

|  | Creep | C.V.T.-1 | C.V.T.-2 |
|---|---|---|---|
| Temperature, °C . . . . . . . | 750 | 550/750 | 550/750 |
| Stress (load), kg/mm² . . . . | 27 | 0/27 | $0/25 \pm 2$ |
| Time to rupture, hours . . . . | 740 | 230 | 830 |

The simultaneous cyclic variation of stress and temperature (C.V.T.-1) has produced a considerable decrease of the rupture life in relation to the time to rupture obtained during creep testing. The rupture life has decreased with about 60 per cent, in spite of the lower average temperature during this test. It is unlikely that this is due to any "metallurgical effect" in the material; the effect observed may probably be considered as some sort of fatigue phenomena.

If, on the other hand, superimposed vibrations are present, as in the C.V.T.-2, the result will be quite different. In this case no decreasing effect has been observed on the rupture life which even slightly exceeds that obtained during creep testing. In order to find an explanation to this rather unexpected test result much more work must be carried out. It looks however possible that the vibrations in this particular case have some favourable influence on the fine dispersion of the precipitated phase in the matrix. HIGNETT [4] has stated that alloys of this type owe their high strength to the precipitation of an intermetallic compound $\gamma'$ based on the cubic $Ni_3Al$ phase but with aluminium more or less replaced by titanium and also some chromium ($Ni_3M$). This substitution, which increases the misfit between the lattices of the phase and the matrix, raises the creep strength of the alloy. NORDHEIM and GRANT [5] found that this substitution also decreases the creep rate, the elongation at rupture and the tendency to transcrystalline fracture, and further also decreases the rate of growth and coalescence of the precipitated phase.

TAYLOR and FLOYD [6] have studied the constitution of nickel-rich alloys of the Ni-Cr-Al system. They found that the $\gamma'$-phase is formed during solidification of low-chromium alloys containing 20—30 atomic per cent aluminium via a peritectic reaction. In such alloys, annealed at 850° C, the $\gamma'$-phase was sometimes found precipitated in regular rows along crystallographic planes of the matrix. TAYLOR and FLOYD stated that the precipitate in a finely dispersed form appears to lie on the octahedral (111) slip planes of the matrix.

For metallographic examination a longitudinal section near the fracture of the specimen No. 78 (C.V.T.-2) was etched anodically in the following reagent: Aqueous solution of 10 per cent glycerine and 5 per cent hydrofluoric acid. As shown in fig. 4, a frequently occurring precipitated phase, probably $\gamma'$, is found in the matrix, while no tendency of coalescence can be observed. For comparison a sample from the not tested bar material of the same alloy was prepared and etched as previously described. This material was heat treated in the same way as that earlier

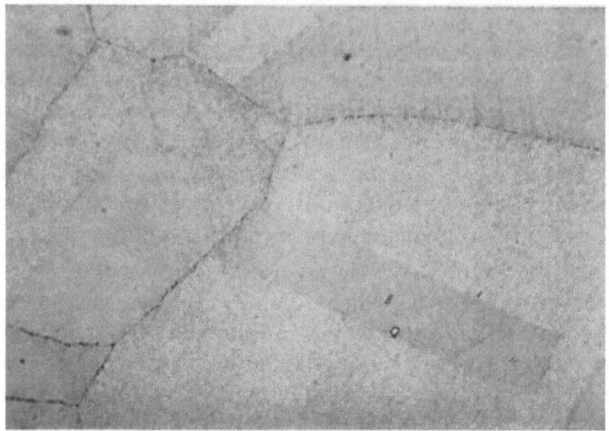

Fig. 4. Sample from C. V. T.-2, 830 hours. Hardness 453 HVP. Precipitate in the matrix, probably consisting of $\gamma'$ -phase. × 400.

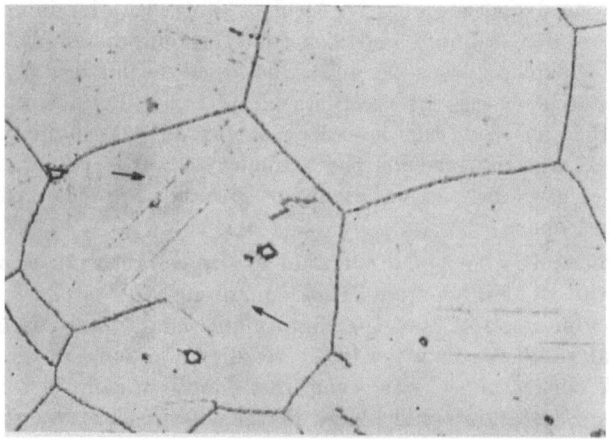

Fig. 5. Untested bar, solution heat treated at 1080°C and aged at 750°C 16 hours. Hardness 350 HVP. Clear "envelopes", probably consisting of $\gamma'$-phase. × 400.

tested (solution heat treatment at 1,080° C for 8 hours, then aging at 750° C for 16 hours). The matrix is in this case practically free from visible precipitated phases, but small clear "envelopes" can be seen, which, according to FLOYD [7], may indicate the presence of $\gamma'$-phase, (fig. 5).

It is also of interest to compare the hardness of the different specimens. In table 3 are collected the average of the hardness values, determined at room temperature on metallographically prepared surfaces near the fracture. The average grain size is also given.

*Table 3*

| Material from | Untested bar | Creep test | C.V.T. -1 | C.V.T. -2 |
|---|---|---|---|---|
| Hardness, $H_v$ . . . . . . . . | 350 | 364 | 427 | 453 |
| Grain size, ASTM E 19—46 . . | 0—1 | 0—2 | 2—3 | 5—6 |
| Sample No. . . . . . . . . . | (4328) | (4326) | (4168) | (4322) |

The exceptionally high hardness value of the C. V. T.-2 sample indicates that no overaging or coalescence of the precipitated phase has occurred.

The larger part of the fracture of creep testing specimens usually

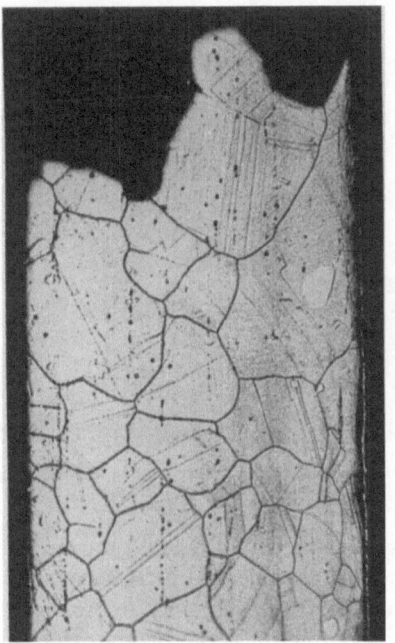
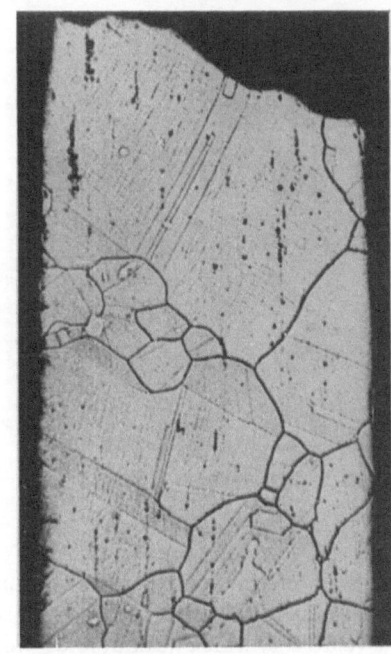

Fig. 6. Intercrystalline part of fracture in a C.V.T. specimen. Oxidized fracture. No necking. × 80.

Fig 7. Transcrystalline part of fracture in a C.V.T. specimen. Slight necking. × 80.

will be intercrystalline (at 27 kg/mm² and 750° C), while cyclic variation testing gives approximately 60 per cent transcrystalline and 40 per cent intercrystalline fracture. The intercrystalline part of the fracture is

formed first and has the character of brittle fracture without necking,
fig. 6. This part of the fractured surface is oxidized. The transcrystalline
part of the fracture is formed instantaneously, and is therefore free from
oxide. It shows a slight amount of necking, fig. 7. Neither of the two
cyclic variation tests (C. V. T.-1 and C. V. T.-2) result in a true fatigue
fracture. This could possibly be expected at C. V. T.-2, but the stress
amplitude $S_a$ is probably too small in relation to the steady stress $S_m$
to give a typical fatigue fracture.

As all the specimens have been exposed to the air under atmo-

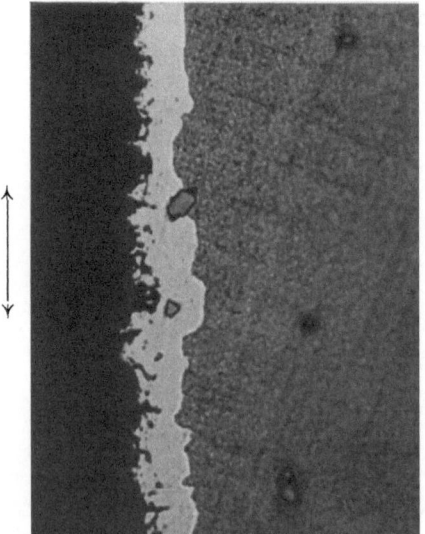

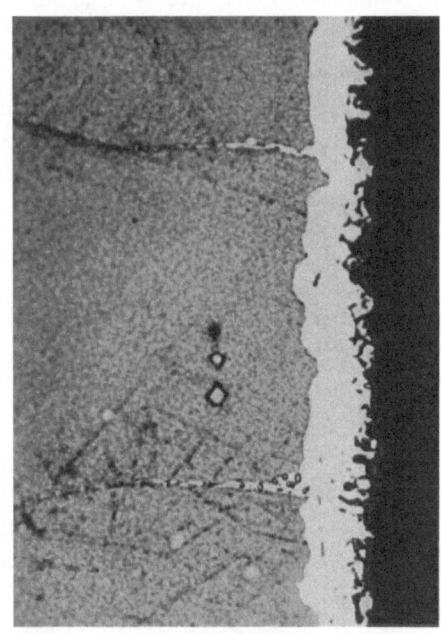

Fig. 8. Nickel layer due to oxidation of the specimen in air at 750°C. × 750.

Fig. 9. Diffusion of Ni into grain boundaries, perpendicular to the stress direction. × 750.

spheric pressure during testing, a certain amount of oxidation on the
surface of the specimen has occurred. This has resulted in an extremely
thin and brittle outer layer of chromium oxide, $Cr_2O_3$, and, underneath,
a relatively thick (about 0.01 millimeter) ductile layer of almost pure
nickel. This is shown in fig. 8 and 9. Figure 8 shows also how some
cyanonitrides, precipitated in the matrix, have been surrounded by the
nickel layer. The nickel layer seems to have a marked tendency to diffuse
into the grain boundaries, particularly if these are perpendicular to the
main direction of stress, see fig. 9.

That the surface layer mainly consists of nickel has been confirmed

by X-ray diffraction measurements with $CrK_\alpha$-radiation, which gave
the following result.

|  | Lattice parameter, Å |
|---|---|
| The matrix of the alloy . . . . . . . . | 3.574 |
| The surface layer[1]) . . . . . . . . . . | 3.532 |
| Pure cubic Ni . . . . . . . . . . . . | 3.517 |

## 4. Conclusions

a) Simultaneous relatively rapid cyclic variation of tensile stress
and temperature gives a considerably shorter rupture time than does
static creep testing, other conditions being equal. It is likely that the
phenomenon occurring here is near related to fatigue, although the
amplitude of stress is too high and the frequency too low to give a
typical fatigue fracture [see c) below].

b) If vibrations of the order of 110 Hz are superimposed on the
cyclic tensile stress, the interesting unexpected effect is obtained that
no decrease of the rupture life occurs. Instead, a slight increase in time
to rupture can be observed in relation to that obtained during the static
creep test. It is supposed that this may be due to the fact that the relatively
high frequency vibrations facilitate the proper dispersion of the $\gamma'$-phase
in the matrix. The result of hardness measurements is supporting this
view.

c) The fractured surface of the specimens subjected to cyclic variation
of stress and temperature will always show the same type of fracture
whether vibrations are superimposed or not. Thus, the fractured surface
consists to approximately 40 percent of the intercrystalline type without
necking. This part of the fractured surface is oxidized which indicates
that the failure has started in an intercrystalline crack. The other part
of the fracture is transcrystalline with a slight amount of necking and
has occurred instantaneously. In general, the type of fracture seems
to correspond more to creep fracture than to fatigue fracture.

d) The surface of the specimens has during testing been affected
by the oxygen in the air, forming an extremely thin brittle layer of
chromium oxide in the outer area. As a consequence of this, another
layer of almost pure ductile nickel, about 0.01 millimeter thick has
occurred in this surface area. The almost pure nickel shows a marked
tendency towards diffusing into grain boundaries, perpendicular to the
principal direction of the tensile stress. This effect has also been observed
in creep specimens.

The work described in this paper was carried out in the Materials Laboratory at Malmslätt and the author is indebted to the Royal Swedish

---

[1] The presence of hexagonal $Cr_2O_3$ has also been established.

Air Board for permission to present and publish the paper. Grateful acknowledgment is due to Mr. B. BURMAN, Mr. T. GÖRANSON, Mr. E. JANSSON and Mr. G. LÖFSTEDT for their valuable contributions, and to several other members of the staff of the Materials Laboratory, who have assisted in the work.

### Bibliography

[1] TOOLIN, R. R. and N. L. MOCHEL: Proc. ASTM **47**, 677—694 (1947).
[2] LAZAN, B. J.: Proc. ASTM **49**, 757—787 (1949).
[3] GUARNIERI, G. J. and L. A. YERKOVICH: Proc. ASTM **52**, 934—950 (1952).
[4] HIGNETT, H. W. G.: High Temperature Alloys in British Jet Engines. Presented at the meeting of the Detroit Chapter of Amer. Soc. Metals, Nov. 1951.
[5] NORDHEIM, R. and N. J. GRANT: Aging Characteristics of Nickel-Chromium Alloys Hardened with Titanium and Aluminium, Mass. Inst. Tech., 1952.
[6] TAYLOR, A. and R. W. FLOYD: J. Inst. Metals **82**, 451—464 (1952—53).
[7] FLOYD, R. W.: J. Inst. Metals **80**, 551—553 (1951—52).

### Discussion

G. V. UZHIK asked for the scatter in the tests CVT-2.

A. FRANSSON: Only a small number of test pieces has been tested so far.

C. E. PHILLIPS remarked that, at the MERL, the creep strengthening effect of vibrations had been observed for Nimonic as well as for other materials.

R. E. PETERSON: Author's test apparatus, which approximates service conditions represents an important addition in the testing field. In general we have attempted to evaluate the requirements of high temperature elements, for example gas turbine blades, by means of creep rupture tests and high temperature tests. More recently we have found it necessary to add a third test, namely a "thermal cycling" test. In this we used a test piece about the size of a coin like a Swedish krona but somewhat thicker. No mechanical loading is applied. The periphery is inductively heated rapidly to 1,500° F, cooled to 800° F, reheated cyclicly with a period 3—4 seconds until cracking of the rim occurs: sometimes in 50 to 100 cycles. This test very often rates materials in a different order from other tests mentioned. Our tests have been used largely as a basis of selecting materials. It would be interesting to know how materials would be rated in a test of the kind used by the Author. We may consider making some tests of this kind.

R. B. HEYWOOD: The Author has shown that in the second series of tests in which loading was at $25 \pm 2$ kg/mm², an appreciably longer life was obtained than in the first series in which loading was at 27 kg/mm². From a fatigue point of view this result might appear surprising, but if behaviour were to be attributed to a predominant creep effect, then one would expect that specimens tested at the higher mean stress would fail first, as in fact was obtained. Perhaps the Author would kindly give his opinion as to whether this might explain the results.

A. FRANSSON: I am very grateful for PETERSON's kind contribution to the discussion and for his opinion about our testing method. The question how to rate different materials in our test can not be answered before we have got the opportunity of testing other materials than Nimonic.

In reply to HEYWOOD's question I wish to refer to the fact that the load $0/27 \pm 2$ kg/mm² has given about 15 percent longer life than $0/27$ kg/mm² (table 2). It is likely that the explanation — as already has been mentioned — is to be found in certain structure changes due to the superimposed vibrations.

# Physical and statistical aspects of cumulative damage

By

**A. M. Freudenthal**

The problem of prediction of the fatigue life under repeated stress-cycles of varying amplitude, generally referred to as the problem of "cumulative damage", can be approached either from the point of view of a definite underlying physical process of progressive damage, or by assuming that the large number of variables known to affect the fatigue life in rather complex ways can only be dealt with summarily by simple probability considerations or, finally, by deriving an improved probability model from the statistical interpretation of fatigue data. Using the 3 alternative approaches it is therefore possible to arrive at a physical, a probabilistic and a statistical formulation of the problem and of its solution. Comparison of the alternative approaches, in the light of similarities and differences in their results, provides an interesting insight into the problem of cumulative damage.

## 1. The physical aspect

The physical formulation is based on the concept of progressive damage accumulating at a certain rate in each and every stress-cycle. Assuming a constant amplitude $S$ of the repeated stress, the increment $\triangle D$ of damage per stress cycle is necessarily a function of the number $N$ of prior stress repetitions. Hence,

$$\triangle D = \mathrm{d}D/\mathrm{d}N = f(N)_S \tag{1}$$

where the parameters of $f(N)_S$ are functions of $S$. If $N = V_S$ denotes the expected fatigue life, total damage is defined by

$$D_{VS} = \int_{N_{OS}}^{V_S} (\mathrm{d}D/\mathrm{d}N)\,\mathrm{d}N = \int_{N_{OS}}^{V_S} f(N)_S\,\mathrm{d}N = 1.0 \tag{2}$$

The damage thus increases from $D=0$ during the "incubation period" of fatigue [1], when $1<N<N_{OS}$, to $D=1.0$ at fracture. The existence of a minimum life $N_{OS}>0$ would suggest that the first $N_{OS}$ stress cycles do not actually cause fatigue damage, but only prepare its initiation by changes in the crystal structure. It has been observed that, with increasing stress-amplitudes, $N_{OS}$ tends towards small values that do not significantly differ from zero.

On the basis of recent studies of the changes produced in the crystal structure by repeated stressing [2], [3], [4] it appears fairly well established that:

a) the principal feature of these changes, characteristic of fatigue stressing alone, is the gradual intensification and widening into "striations" of slip-bands formed during an initial, relatively short stage of cyclic stressing;

b) irrecoverable fatigue damage within the striations in the form of cracks of optically unresolvable magnitude, probably formed as a result of sharply localized high temperatures (heat-flashes) due to the sharply localized reversed slip, and associated with relatively steep temperature and thermal stress gradients [5] occurs very early, probably within the first 10 percent of expected fatigue life;

c) fatigue cracks of resolvable magnitude appear only after more than one-half of the expected life has been expended;

d) the distance between the developed striations shows a fairly close relation to the distance between slipbands formed during the initial period of fatigue stressing.

The form of $f(N)$ should mainly reproduce the fact that the damage rate appears to be very small within a range considerably exceeding half the expected fatigue life, but increases rather rapidly as $N$ approaches $V_S$. Defining the "cycle ratio" $x$ by

$$x = (N - N_{OS})/(V_S - N_{OS}) \tag{3}$$

the simplest function fulfilling this condition is

$$dD/dN = \frac{\alpha}{V_S - N_{OS}} x^{\alpha-1} \text{ and } D = x^\alpha \tag{4}$$

with $\alpha = \alpha(S) > 1$. For $\alpha = 1$ equation (4) degenerates into the straight line relation $D = x$, with the constant damage rate $1/(V_S - N_{OS})$ for $N > N_{OS}$.

It has generally been assumed that the damage rate at one stress-amplitude is independent of that at any other stress-amplitude. The total fatigue damage from $N_i$ cycles at $i$ stress-amplitudes $S_i$ would, under this assumption, accumulate according to the relation

$$D = \sum_i x_i (N_i, S_i)^{\alpha_i(S_i)} \tag{5}$$

fracture being associated with $D = 1.0$.

When the stress-amplitudes vary in a well defined sequence, the sum in (5), because of the nonlinearity of the damage rate, necessarily reflects the effect of this sequence and can, therefore, not give a stable value of $D$. For random loading, however, defined by a histogram of relative frequencies of the stress-amplitudes $p_i(S_i)$, or by a continuous distribution function $p(S) = \frac{d}{dS} l(S)$, where $l(S)$ denotes the frequency of stress levels $>S$, for which, therefore, no characteristic sequence can be defined, the sum in (5) should tend towards a stable value. Hence an expected equivalent or "reduced" constant stress-amplitude $S_R$ which, after a total number of stress cycles $V_{SR} = \Sigma N_i$ would produce the same total damage as the random stress spectrum, can be computed from the sum

$$D = \Sigma_i x_i \, (p_i V_{SR}, \, S_i)^{\alpha_i(S_i)} = 1 \qquad (6)$$

or from the integral

$$D = \int x \, (p \cdot V_{SR}, \, S)^{\alpha(S)} \, dS = 1 \qquad (6a)$$

introducing $V_S = V_{SR}$ into the general $S$-$V_S$-relation (ref. [6])

$$V_S - N_{OS} = [k \, (S - S_0)]^{-\varrho} \qquad (7)$$

where $S_0$ denotes the expected "endurance limit". For $\alpha = 1$ the procedure is considerably simplified, leading to the conventional "linear damage law"

$$\Sigma_i x_i = 1 \qquad (8)$$

The expected fatigue life for random loading, assuming $N_{OS} \to 0$, would therefore be

$$V_{SR} = 1 / \Sigma_i (p_i / V_{Si}) \qquad (8a)$$

The equivalent stress is obtained, as before, by using (7).

It is well known that (8) is quite unreliable for the prediction of fatigue life under random loading; this is generally assumed to be due to its linearity. Several attempts have been made to use (6) or equivalent equations based on alternative non-linear damage laws, such as (ref. [7])

$$dD/dN = \frac{\gamma}{V_S - N_{OS}} e^{\gamma x} / (e^{\gamma} - 1) \text{ and } D = \frac{e^{\gamma x} - 1}{e^{\gamma} - 1} \qquad (9)$$

with $\gamma > 0$, retaining the assumption of the independence of the damage rates under different stress-amplitudes. It appears likely, however, on the basis of results of recent random fatigue tests [8] that the error introduced by the linearization of the damage functions (4) is less significant than the assumption of the independence of damage rates.

Assuming that the density of striations is proportional to the density of slip-lines produced in the initial stage, the number $n$ of which per unit length is (ref. [9]) $n = k \, (S - S_0)$, and assuming, furthermore, that the number of fatigue cracks initiated is roughly proportional to the density of striations and inversely proportional to the number $(N - N_0)$ of stress-cycles leading to fracture, it appears that the density of slip-bands at a stress-amplitude $S_i$ will be significantly increased by intermittent stress-amplitudes $S_{i+k} > S_i$, but will hardly be affected by $S_{i-k} < S_i$. Hence it might be considered that the expected fatigue life $V_{Si}$ at constant stress-amplitude $S_i$ is reduced by all stress-amplitudes $S > S_i$, the more so the larger the excess of $S$ over $S_i$, but remain practically unaffected by amplitudes $S < S_i$. The effect of such stress interaction could most simply be introduced in the form of a factor $\omega_i$ which indicates the reduction of $V_{S_i}$ by stress-amplitudes $S > S_i$; this factor is some function of the "overstress" intervals $(S_{i+k} - S_i)$ and of the relative frequencies of the stress-amplitudes $S < S_i$. The larger the sum

$$\sum_k p_k (S_{i+k} - S_i)$$

the more pronounced the reduction of $V_{S_i}$ and the larger therefore the value of $\omega_i$. It might be assumed that one of the effects of intermittent high stress-amplitudes is to eliminate the incubation period $N_{0S_i}$ at the constant stress-amplitude $S_i$; the non-linear damage law with expected lives adjusted for stress interaction can therefore be written in the form:

$$V_{SR} = 1/\sum_i (\omega_i p_i / V_{S_i})^{\alpha_i} \tag{10}$$

Random fatigue test results suggest that the expected fatigue lives at low stress-amplitudes are significantly reduced by relatively infrequent high stress-amplitudes. Hence, while "interaction factors" $\omega_i = 1$ might be expected at stress-amplitudes close to the yield-stress, these factors might be one order of magnitude larger ($\omega_i \sim 10$) close to the (true or designated) endurance limit $S_0$. It is obvious that stress interaction effects of such magnitude reduce to practical insignificance the possible effects of non-linearity of the damage-rate.

## 2. The probability aspect

A purely formal approach to the problem, unrelated to any physical mechanism, might be based on the assumption of a constant mean probability of failure $p$ in each cycle, related to the actual, variable probabilities of failure $p_m$ in the $m$-th out of an expected total of $N = V_S$ stress-cycles of amplitude $S$ by the relation $\sum_m p_m = p V_S$. This assumption disregards the progressive character of fatigue damage and considers the repeated stress-cycles as independent attempts to produce fatigue fracture. It is obvious that an interpretation of fatigue on this basis is rather far removed from a representation of the real phenomenon. The interesting point in this approach, however, is the fact that the result obtained is identical with certain limiting cases of the results of the physical and the statistical approaches to the problem.

Because of the relatively large number of stress-cycles required to produce fatigue fracture, $p_m$ and $p$ are necessarily very small; this creates the conditions for the application of Poisson's law governing the probability of "rare events". Hence, assuming that $N_{0S}$ can be neglected in relation to $V_S$

$$p(n) = \frac{1}{n!}(N/V_S)^n \exp(-N/V_S) \qquad (11)$$

With $n = 1$ this expression indicates the probability of occurence of failure (once) at $N$ stress-cycles; with $n = 0$ it establishes the probability function of survival at $N$ stress-cycles. Therefore

$$p(1) = (N/V_S)\exp(-N/V_S) = x\,e^{-x} \qquad (12)$$

represents the distribution of lives $N$ of fatigue specimens at a constant stress-amplitude $S$ as a function of the "cycle ratio" $x$ (with $N_{OS} = 0$), while

$$p(0) = \exp(-N/V_S) = e^{-x} = l(N)_S \qquad (13)$$

is the survivorship function at this stress-amplitude. The assumption $N_{OS} = 0$ is convenient, but not necessary; (12) and (13) are valid for any definition of $x$.

Obviously, the probability of survival under $i$ stress-amplitudes $S_i$, each applied $N_i$ times is

$$l(\varSigma N_i) = \Pi_i [\exp(-N_i/V_{Si})] = \exp[-\varSigma_i (N_i/V_{Si})] \qquad (14)$$

The equivalent or reduced expected constant stress-amplitude $S_R$ that can be repeated $N = \varSigma N_i$ times is obtained by first computing $V_{SR}$ from

$$l(\varSigma N_i) = l(N)_{SR} \text{ or } \exp(-N/V_{SR}) = \exp(-\varSigma N_i/V_{Si}) \qquad (15)$$

which, for $N = V_{SR}$, is transformed into $\varSigma x_i = 1$. Hence, with $N_i = p_i V_{SR}$

$$1/V_{SR} = \varSigma_i (p_i/V_{Si}) \qquad (16)$$

Introducing $V_{SR}$ into (7) the reduced stress is obtained. The identity of (16) and (8a) illustrates the fact that the assumptions of a constant damage rate and of a constant mean probability of failure in every stress cycle are equivalent, both leading to the linear damage law. The exponential survivorship function which is rather widely used in the "lifing" of parts of aircraft [10] as the basis for the estimate of replacement rates of such parts, can thus also be considered as implying a constant damage rate in such parts.

If it is assumed that the mean probability of failure in a cycle of constant stress-amplitudes $S_i$ may be increased by intermittent cycles of amplitudes $S > S_i$ by a factor $\omega_i$, from $1/V_{S_i}$ to $(\omega_i/V_{Si})$, eq. (10) with $\alpha_i = 1$ is obtained from (16).

## 3. The statistical aspect

The statistical approach is based on the interpretation of actual observations of the distribution of fatigue lives $N$ under constant stress amplitudes. Analysis of fatigue data has shown that the observed survivorship functions at constant stress-amplitudes $S_i$ can be fairly well represented by the so-called third asymptotic probability function of extreme (smallest) values

$$l\,(N_i)_S = \exp\left[-\left(\frac{N_i - N_{OSi}}{V_{Si} - N_{OSi}}\right)^{\alpha_{Si}}\right] = e^{-x_i^{\alpha_{Si}}} \qquad (17)$$

where $N_i > N_{OS}$, and $N_{OS} \neq 0$ at small stress-amplitudes, decreasing with increasing stress-amplitudes towards $N_{OS} = 0$. For $N_{OS} = 0$ the parameter $1/\alpha_{Si}$ is proportional to the standard deviation of the logarithms of $N$; $[1/\alpha_S = \pi/\sqrt{6} \cdot (s_{\log N})]$; for $N_{OS} > 0$ the characteristic number $V_S$ (which for $N_{OS} = 0$ is the mode of the distribution) and the parameter $1/\alpha_S$ are no longer independent, and the relation between the standard deviation $s_{\log N}$ and $1/\alpha_S$ is less simple, involving ($V_S - N_{OS}$). The survivorship function (17) is transformed into the exponential function (13) for $\alpha_{Si} = 1$; with $\alpha_{Si} = 2$ it represents the probability function associated with a specific distribution function known as the Rayleigh distribution, which has recently been used in studies of fluctuating pressures on flight structures arising from jet exhausts ("jet-buffeting").

As in the case of the exponential distribution, the probability of surviving a stress spectrum of $i$ stress-amplitudes $S_i$ each applied $N_i$ times can be expressed by:

$$l\,(\Sigma N_i) = \Pi_i\, l\,(N_i)_{Si} = \Pi_i\left(e^{-x_i^{\alpha_{Si}}}\right) = \exp\left[-\Sigma x_i^{\alpha_{Si}}\right] \qquad (18)$$

The effective or reduced constant stress-amplitude $S_R$ which might be expected to produce failure after $N = \Sigma\, N_i$ stress cycles is associated with a survivorship function

$$l\,(N)_{SR} = \exp\left[-\frac{N - N_{OSR}}{V_{SR} - N_{OSR}}\right]^{\alpha_{SR}} \qquad (19)$$

Assuming that $N_i = p_i N$, and therefore for the expected life $N_i = p_i\, V_{SR}$, the effective stress $S_R$ is obtained from the condition $l\,(N)_{SR} = l\,(\Sigma\, N_i)$ and (7). Hence

$$\Sigma_i x_i^{\alpha_{Si}} = \Sigma_i\left|\frac{p_i V_{SR} - N_{OSi}}{V_{Si} - N_{OSi}}\right|^{\alpha_{Si}} = \left[\frac{N - N_{OSR}}{V_{SR} - N_{OSR}}\right]^{\alpha_{SR}} \qquad (20)$$

For $N = V_{SR}$ the right side of (20) is equal to one, producing the relation $\Sigma_i x_i^{\alpha_{Si}} = 1$; with $N_{OSi} \to 0$ the relation is simplified to

$$\left(\frac{p_i\, V_{SR}}{V_{Si}}\right)^{\alpha_{Si}} = 1 \qquad (20\,\text{a})$$

$V_{SR}$ represents the characteristic value of the resultant distribution $l\,(N)_{SR}$ at the quantile $l\,(V_{SR})_{SR} = 1/e$; for $N_{OSR} = 0$ it represents the mode of the distribution. This value can therefore be determined by trial and error from (20a), since it is independent of the parameters $\alpha_{SR}$ and $N_{OSR}$. The probability function $l\,(N)_{SR}$ itself, however, could only be established if $\alpha_{SR}$ and $N_{OSR}$ were known functions of $\alpha_{Si}$ and $N_{OSi}$. Assuming that a general effect of damage-interaction at different stress-levels is the elimination of $N_{OS}$ for the low stress levels at which the minimum life is significant, the functions $l\,(N)_{Si}$ are simplified by $N_{OSi} = 0$. Introducing, moreover, for the sake of expediency the (physically probably unjustified) assumption $N_{OSR} = 0$, an approximation for $\alpha_{SR}$ is obtained when considering that, — since for $N_{OS} = 0$, $1/\alpha_S$ is proportional to a standard deviation and therefore $(1/\alpha_S)^2$ proportional to a variance, — a reasonable superposition procedure for $\alpha_S$ would be, in analogy to the superposition of variances,

$$(1/\alpha_{SR})^2 = \sum_i (1/\alpha_{Si})^2 \tag{21}$$

Thus an approximation of the function $l\,(N)_{SR}$ is obtained, valid for $N_{OSR} = 0$. It appears likely, however, that even if all $N_{OSi} = 0$, the minimum life at the "reduced" stress-amplitude $N_{OSR} > 0$, the actual value of $N_{OSR}$ depending on the shape of the distribution function $p\,(S)$ of the applied stress-amplitudes.

Eq. (20a) is identical with (6) obtained by a basically different approach. This identity suggests the identification of the parameters of dispersion $\alpha_{Si}$ with the exponents $\alpha_i$ defining the non-linearity of the physical damage rate at constant stress-amplitudes $S_i$. Considering that statistical analysis of fatigue test results indicates that $\alpha_S$ varies roughly between 2 and 6, with high stress levels usually associated with the higher values of $\alpha_S$, these results suggest that the non-linearity of the damage rate increases with increasing stress levels.

In order to consider stress interaction effects the probability of survival according to (17) could again be adjusted by a factor $\omega_i$ within the bracket, indicating the reduction of $(V_{Si} - N_{OSi})$ resulting from this interaction. (20a) would then be replaced by

$$\sum_i (\omega_i x_i)^{\alpha_{Si}} = 1 \tag{21a}$$

which is identical with (10).

Since with $\alpha_{Si} = 1$ equation (17) degenerates into the exponential distribution and (20) into the linear damage law, it is interesting to note that observed values of $\alpha_{Si} = 1$ are very infrequent. They characterize results of fatigue tests that have been performed under conditions of inadequate experimental control. Under such conditions therefore fatigue appears to be predominantly a probability effect, to be dealt with by Poisson's law rather than by considering a physical mechanism. The increasing significance of the actual fatigue mechanism is associated with values $\alpha_S > 1$.

## 4. Cumulative damage equation in terms of stress-amplitudes

The cumulative damage equation (10) or (21), formulated in terms of the number $N_i$ of cycles at various stress-amplitudes $S_i$, can be transformed into an equivalent equation in terms of stress-amplitudes by using the general relation between $S$ and $N$, which is determined by the condition that the probability function $l\,(N)_S$ of the number of stress cycles at constant stress-amplitude must be compatible with the probability function $l\,(S)_N$ of stress-amplitudes at constant number of stress cycles. Assuming that $l\,(S)_N$ can be represented by a function of the same type as $l\,(N)_S$, specified by (17), with $S$, $S_V$, $S_{ON}$ and $\beta_N$ replacing $N$, $V_S$, $N_{OS}$ and $\alpha_S$ respectively, the compatibility condition takes the form:

$$\exp\left[-\left(\frac{N-N_{OS}}{V_S-N_{OS}}\right)^{\alpha_S}\right]=\exp\left[-\left(\frac{S-S_{ON}}{S_V-S_{ON}}\right)^{\beta_N}\right] \tag{22}$$

along any line $l=$ const. The characteristic $S$-$N$-curve for $l=1/e$ can be determined, provided the coordinates are known of an arbitrary reference point along this curve. Introducing these coordinates into (22) the $S$-$N$-relation along $l=1/e$ is obtained (ref. [6]).

$$(V_S-N_{OS})=\text{const}\,(S-S_{ON})^{-\varrho} \tag{23}$$

where $\varrho\,(N,S)=\beta_N/\alpha_S$; the value of the constant is determined by the coordinates of the reference point. Neglecting, in first approximation, the dependence of $\alpha_S$, $\beta_N$ and $S_{ON}$ on $S$ and $N$ respectively, and considering them as true constants $\alpha_S=\alpha$, $\beta_N=\beta$ and $S_{ON}=S_0$, (23) becomes identical with (7), with $\varrho=\beta/\alpha$. Hence, for any stress level $S_i$ the characteristic number of cycles

$$(V_{Si}-N_{OSi})=\text{const}\,(S_i-S_0)^{-\varrho} \tag{24}$$

Combining this equation with (21) for $N_{OSi}=0$, the cumulative damage equation in terms of the stress-amplitudes is obtained:

$$\underset{i}{\Sigma}\left[\omega_i\,p_i\left(\frac{S_i-S_0}{S_R-S_0}\right)^{\varrho}\right]^{\alpha}=\underset{i}{\Sigma}\left[(\omega_i\,p_i)^{\alpha}\left(\frac{S_i-S_0}{S_R-S_0}\right)^{\beta}\right]=1 \tag{25}$$

Hence the reduced stress-amplitude

$$(S_R-S_0)=\left[\underset{i}{\Sigma}\,(\omega_i\,p_i)^{\alpha}\,(S_i-S_0)^{\beta}\right]^{1/\beta}=\sqrt[\beta]{\underset{i}{\Sigma}\left[\omega_i\,p_i\,(S_i-S_0)^{\varrho}\right]^{\alpha}} \tag{26}$$

can be directly determined from the distributions of $\omega_i$, $p_i$ and $S_i$ provided two of the parameters $\alpha$, $\beta$ and $\varrho$ are known from experiment. $\alpha$ can be obtained from the statistical interpretation of repeated fatigue tests at constant stress-amplitudes $S_i$, while $\varrho$ represents the (negative) slope of the observed trend of the $S$-$N$-relation for $l=1/e$ when plotted in double-logarithmic scale.

The spread of the distribution of $N$ at constant $S$, which is proportional to $1/\alpha_S$ is, in general, much wider than the spread of the distribution of $S$ at constant $N$, which is proportional to $1/\beta_N$, hence $\beta_N > \alpha_S$ and $\varrho > 1$. Since values of $\alpha_S$ derived from fatigue tests on small specimens of technical metals vary roughly between $2 < \alpha_S < 6$, depending on material and stress-amplitude, while the trend of observed $\log N$-$\log S$ diagrams suggest values of $3 < \varrho < 10$, the parameter $\beta > 6$, which indicates a narrow range of variation of $S$ at constant $N$.

Considering (25) in the light of the above values of the exponents, it is obvious that, since each term of the sum must be smaller than one, the individual terms must be governed by the inequality

$$(S_i - S_0)/(S_R - S_0) << (1/\omega_i\, p_i)^{1/\varrho} \tag{27}$$

Because of the large value of $\varrho$ the contribution to the cumulative damage of stress-amplitudes $S_R > S_i > S_0$ will be small, even if, in the vicinity of $S_0$, the factors $\omega_i$ may be relatively large. For the same reason a small number of cycles of stress-amplitudes $S_i > S_R$ may produce substantial fatigue damage. It would therefore appear, on the basis of (25), that high stress-amplitudes shorten the fatigue life out of all proportion to their number of application or their cycle-ratio.

### Bibliography

[1] FREUDENTHAL, A. M. and E. J. GUMBEL: J. Amer. statist. Ass. 49, 575 (1954).
[2] WOOD, W. A., F. P. BULLEN and A. K. Head: Proc. Roy. Soc. (A) 216, 332 (1953).
[3] FORSYTH, P. J. E.: J. Inst. Metals 82, 449 (1953—54).
[4] WADSWORTH, N. J. and N. THOMPSON: Phil. Mag. 45, 223 (1954).
[5] FREUDENTHAL, A. M. and J. H. WEINER: To be published in J. appl. Phys. 27 (1956).
[6] FREUDENTHAL, A. M.: Fatigue, Handb. Physik, vol. 7, Berlin 1955.
[7] SHANLEY, F. R.: RAND Corp. Rep. (U. S. A.) P-350 (1952).
[8] FREUDENTHAL, A. M.: Proc. ASTM 53, 896 (1953).
[9] BROWN, A. F.: J. Inst. Metals 80, 115 (1952).
[10] TYE, W. and H. B. CUNDALL: J. Roy. aeronaut. Soc. 57, 391 (1953).

### Discussion

E. GASSNER hob hervor, daß die Beanspruchungen unter der Ermüdungsgrenze bei der Teilschadentheorie unberücksichtigt bleiben. Diese niedrige Beanspruchungen haben jedoch einen entscheidenden Einfluß auf die Lebensdauer.

J. SCHIJVE: I would like to have some comments on the physical meaning of $N_{0S}$ as it seems that there is no damage created between $N = 0$ and $N = N_{0S}$

A. M. FREUDENTHAL: If damage $D$ is plotted against number of cycles $N$ the real behaviour of metals would be according to the dotted curve of left figure, next page, whereas WEIBULL's approach assumes a curve of the type $W$.

F. R. SHANLEY: At different stress levels one would expect damage lines according to the right figure below.

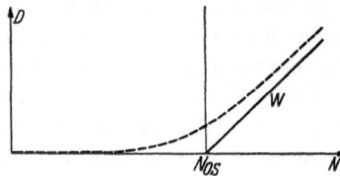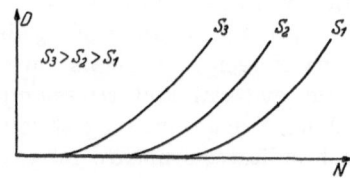

L. LOCATI: The first stage of damage doesn't correspond to zero value but rather to a negative one, because the fatigue resistance is increased by "understressing".

A. M. FREUDENTHAL: GASSNER's remark correctly refers to the shortcomings of a damage theory without interaction factors $\omega_i$. The "endurance limit" does not remain unaffected by intermittent higher stress amplitudes and is therefore no longer the same constant as under conventional tests. We are at present performing random fatigue tests to study this phenomenon. The indications are that if one stress level of the spectrum is below the conventional endurance limit, and therefore assumedly irrelevant on the basis of a simple cycle ratio theory, its elimination does actually not remain without influence on the life under random loading.

LOCATI's remarks can only refer to strain aging materials where coaxing may be important.

# Ermüdungsfestigkeit
## bei statistisch veränderlichen Spannungsamplituden[1]

Von

### E. Gassner

Die für die Bemessung wiederholt beanspruchter Konstruktionsteile verwendeten Festigkeitswerte (Zeitfestigkeit, Dauerfestigkeit) entstammen vorwiegend Versuchen, bei denen die Belastung (oder Spannung) zwischen zwei während des Versuchs gleichbleibenden Grenzwerten $P_u$, $P_o$ (bzw. $\sigma_u$, $\sigma_o$) wechselt (Wöhlerkurve $= S\text{-}N\text{-}$Kurve). Eine sinnvolle Anwendung derartiger Festigkeitswerte ist jedoch nur für solche Konstruktionsteile möglich, deren Betriebsbeanspruchungen ähnlich ablaufen wie in den sogenannten Wöhler-Versuchen.

Demgegenüber stellen die Betriebsbeanspruchungen der meisten Konstruktionsteile, insbesondere des Straßen-, Schienen- und Luftfahrzeugbaues, eine mehr oder weniger regellose Folge von seltenen hohen und häufigen niedrigen Werten dar. Dabei zeigt die statistische Auswertung von Langzeitbeanspruchungsmessungen, daß in sehr vielen Fällen die Häufigkeitsverteilungen der Beanspruchungen sehr gut durch Normal- oder logarithmische Normalverteilungen angenähert werden können [1], [2].

Die neuere Konstruktionspraxis sieht sich nun der Aufgabe gegenüber, an Hand experimentell ermittelter Wöhlerkurven und gemessener Beanspruchungs-Häufigkeitsverteilungen eine Bemessungsmethode zu finden, die Ermüdungsbrüche gerade noch vor Ablauf einer geforderten Lebensdauer ausschließt. Anhaltspunkte für die von einer Konstruktion bis Bruch ertragbaren Lebensdauerwerte sollte die von PALMGREN und von MINER aufgestellte und heute allgemein bekannte Schadensakkumulationstheorie liefern.

Die wesentlichste Voraussetzung für die Gültigkeit dieser Theorie, nämlich das Vorhandensein einer linearen Schädigung ist schon sehr bald auf Grund umfangreicher Versuche gefallen; an dieser Tatsache hat auch die Anwendung statistischer Hilfsmittel, wie sie in den USA sehr weit verbreitet ist, nichts geändert.

---

[1]) Gedruckt nach dem Vordrucksmanuskript 'des Verfassers. Eine erweiterte Fassung des Vortrags erscheint demnächst in der Zeitschrift „Konstruktion", Springer-Verlag, Berlin.

Ob durch Einführung gültiger Schädigungs- und Verfestigungs-funktionen in absehbarer Zeit Methoden für eine zuverlässige Abschätzung von Lebensdauerwerten gefunden werden können, erscheint fraglich.

Eine für die besonderen Belange des Flugzeugbaues entwickelte Methode der experimentellen Lebensdauerbestimmung besteht seit etwa 1938 und hat sich inzwischen vielfach bewährt [3].

Das wesentliche Merkmal dieser Versuchsmethode (,,Betriebsfestig-keits-Versuch") besteht darin, daß alle im Betrieb des betrachteten Kon-struktionsteils zu erwartenden Beanspruchungen nach Größe und Häu-figkeit, betriebsähnlich vermischt, in hierfür geeigneten Prüfmaschinen reproduziert werden.

Am Beispiel eines idealisierten Konstruktionsteils — Rundstab mit Querbohrungen — wird für zwei aus der Praxis des Fahrzeugbaues übernommene und dafür typische Beanspruchungs-Häufigkeitsvertei-lungen (Normal- und logarithmische Normalverteilungen) das Ergebnis solcher Betriebsfestigkeits-Versuche und ihre Darstellung in Lebens-dauerfunktionen erörtert [3]. Die Exponenten dieser Lebensdauerfunk-tionen werden durch die Form der Häufigkeitsverteilung stark beein-flußt, während der Werkstoff, die statische Festigkeit und vorhandene Spannungskonzentration sich nur auf den Spannungsmaßstab der Funktion auszuwirken scheinen.

Der Einfluß sehr kleiner, weit unterhalb der Dauerfestigkeit liegender Spannungsamplituden, die nach den Ansätzen der Schadensakkumula-tionstheorie unberücksichtigt bleiben, konnte bei den untersuchten Häufigkeitsverteilungen, insbesondere im Bereich hoher Lebensdauer-werte, als stark schädigend nachgewiesen werden.

### Literaturverzeichnis

[1] GASSNER, E: Luftwissen 6, 61—64, (1939).

[2] GASSNER, E: Auswirkung betriebsähnlicher Belastungsfolgen auf die Festig-keit von Flugzeugbauteilen. Dr. diss T. H., Darmstadt 1941.

Auszugsweise Wiedergabe im Jb. Deutsch. Luftf.-Forschg., I 972—983, 1941, Vollständige Fassung im Bericht FB 1461 Deutsche Versuchsanstalt für Luftfahrt, 30. 8. 41.

[3] GASSNER, E: Konstruktion 6, 97—104, (1954).

### Diskussion

B. LUNDBERG: Testing with varying load amplitudes, or program testing, is of great importance for particular applications, but it has also many limitations which should not be forgotten. If program testing is made in the normal way by repeating a number of program cycles or program blocks, it is necessary to make each block so small that the blocks can be repeated at least say 20 to 50 times before failure occurs in order to reduce the error due to failure within a block. It follows that such program testing can be represented by the parallel lines in the figures, each representing one program block. In the often common cases where such a block simulates the history of random loads on a structure, for instance the gust loads acting on an aeroplane wing, during a certain part of the service life, it is evident that it also represents the probability of the occurrence of loads of various magnitudes. It thus follows that a repetition of loading blocks in program testing, by which the smallest possible number of the highest load applied in each block is one, necessitates the exclusion of all the still higher loads which on the average must be assumed to occur during the total service life. This is indicated by the dotted lines in the figure, which show that a considerable part of the load spectrum has to be excluded in program testing and that this part is larger the larger the number of applied blocks are before failure.

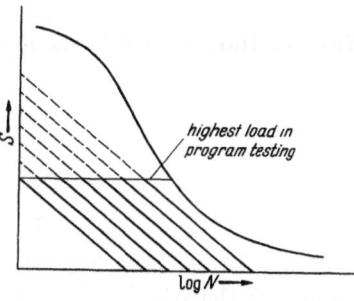

This exclusion of the upper part of the load spectrum might be of great significance as those high loads often might cause the largest deviations with regard to the simple cumulative damage law. This difficulty might be overcome to some extent by using a random loading machine, but apart from the complication of such a machine it is of little use for detail studies of the influence of the high loads, in particular the influence of the sequence of high and low loads.

I strongly believe that the fact that the simple cumulative damage law is not always valid is not a reason for abandoning $S$-$N$ testing or even limiting the scope of such testing. No doubt there is a great need for extended research with varying amplitude loading, but it must be remembered that $S$-$N$ testing should form the main basis in fatigue research as it gives the pure fatigue qualities of a material or a specimen, whereas program testing gives the combined results of the qualities of the material and the external loading. Program testing is therefore of a more applied nature. Its importance lies firstly in connection with research in cumulative damage and secondly in "check testing", i.e. testing of samples of designed and manufactured structural parts. For the very important topic of establishing design information for sound design of structural parts in order to prevent fatigue within a given service life, I believe that $S$-$N$ testing should remain the main basis of information.

E. GASSNER: Der von Herrn LUNDBERG erwähnte Mangel im Ablauf der üblichen Programm-Belastungs-Versuche wurde frühzeitig erkannt; eine 1941 in der Deutschen Versuchsanstalt für Luftfahrt durchgeführte Versuchsreihe bezog den „oberen Teil des Lastspektrums" ein. Wegen des geringen Gewichtes, das diesen seltenen Belastungen im Rahmen des Gesamtkollektivs zukommt, war ihr Einfluß auf die ertragbaren Spannungen gering.

Der Vortragende stimmt mit Herrn LUNDBERG darin überein, daß der Wöhler-Versuch seine dominierende Bedeutung für die Grundlagenforschung behalten muß. Die kritische Situation, der sich der Flugzeugbau und der Fahrzeugbau zur Zeit gegenübersehen, zwingt die angewandte Forschung zu einer stärkeren Heranziehung des Programm-Belastungs-Versuches; die ihm in seiner jetzigen Form möglicherweise noch anhaftenden Mängel stehen in keinem Verhältnis zu dem Gewinn an Sicherheit und grundsätzlichen Erkenntnissen. Es sind Fälle bekannt, in denen die Überprüfung konstruktiver Maßnahmen durch Wöhler-Versuche zu falschen Folgerungen führt und auch erklärlicherweise führen muß.

# New statistical methods applied to the analysis of fatigue data

By

**F. Gatto**

With 6 figures

## 1. Introduction

The analysis of fatigue data is liable to serious uncertainty owing to the fact that the random dispersion of results, as already well known, attains a relatively great magnitude, as compared with values of test data and even with the variations due to systematic modifications of test conditions.

Therefore, in order to obtain a rating criterion for the data evaluation it is necessary to perform the tests on large series of specimens, and organize them on statistical considerations.

In the last few years, there have been many researches on the application of the statistical approach to the planning and interpretation of fatigue tests and several methods have been devised [8].

In this work, after a brief description of two new methods, which we recommend for the analysis of fatigue data, we report some applications.

## 2. Methods for interpolation of the average curve

The methods devised to individuate the central tendency of the test points of fatigue diagrams, may be grouped into two main classes:

a) methods of average life

b) methods of functional interpolation

The first group is mainly based on the carrying out of tests on predetermined stress levels and on the determination of the average life of the test specimens in each group (by the arithmetical, logarithmical and reciprocal logarithmic average etc.). The trend of the average points to collect in the immediate proximity of the average curve contributes to decrease the dispersion and makes the laying out of the interpolating curve easier.

The main undesirable point of this method, consists in the reduction of the number of available points for the graphic interpolation, thus reducing the advantage obtained by the decrease of dispersion range.

The mathematical interpolation methods are based on the systematic use of arbitrary functional formulas, chosen with a criterion of formal simplicity and with the aim of introducing an easier approximation to the presumed position of points; the determination of the parameters of the formulas is obtained, as well known, by means of the position of experimental points.

By considering that the number of experimental points greatly exceeds that of the parameters, it becomes necessary [3], in order to deal with a solvable system, to adopt the "criterion of least squares" or similar devices, or any of the following methods proposed by the "statistical adaptation" theory [7]:

a) method of the sums                          (RING)
b) method of the differences                   (GINI)
c) method of the areas                         (CANTELLI)
d) method of the moments                       (PEARSON)
e) method of the maximum likelihood            (GAUSS-FISHER)
f) the graphic method                          (CASTELLANO)

To increase the statistical power of the functional method, it is preferable to carry out the tests for a number of levels equal to the number of parameters present in the general equation, and to conduct the calculation for the curve to pass through the average points at each level [4], [5].

Two methods, recently proposed by the author [8], are the following ones which are very simple both from the theoretical and the operative point of view:

a) method of the local averages,

b) method of the data rearrangement.

In the first method the $(N - n + 1)$ couples of average values:

$$\bar{x}_i = \frac{\sum\limits_{m=-n}^{n} x_{i+m}}{2n+1} \; ; \quad \bar{y}_i = \frac{\sum\limits_{m=-n}^{n} y_{i+m}}{2n+1} \tag{1}$$

are substituted for the $N$ couples $(x_i; y_i)$ of experimental values.

This is correct for linear relationship or, for non-linear, provided $(2x_i - x_{i+n} - x_{i-n})$ is small.

In such a way, it becomes possible to reduce the statistical variance to about $\frac{1}{2n+1}$ of the original value.

The data rearrangement method, is based on a "global" property, i.e. the monotonous and decreasing character of fatigue diagrams.

This method has been first proposed by C. GINI [1] for the general application to monotonous increasing functions, but its extension to the decreasing ones follows immediately.

Let us consider the problem of the deduction of the relationship between two variables where this relationship is certainly known to be an increasing function: if one orders values of the first variable in increasing succession, the correspondent ones of the second variable should be equally increasing.

If we dispose of a sufficient number of data, in order to reduce the entity of errors affecting the variables, the two groups may be separately ordered in two rising successions, and a new correspondence can be established between terms equally placed in the two rearranged series.

In the application of this method to fatigue tests, in which the function is a monotonous decreasing one, the same procedure may be applied with a simple alteration of the method [8]: i.e. after having disposed the values of the first variable (e.g. the number of test cycles) in a rising order, the values of the second one (the test load) should be ordered in a decreasing manner and the correspondence is to be established between the shorter rod life and the higher applied load and so on.

The basic assumption of the method consists essentially in postulating that among all the $N!$ possible rearrangements of the data, the actual physical bond between variables, is best approximated by the correspondence obtained between monotonously rearranged series.

The theoretical basis for the rearrangement method (the same may be said about every other above mentioned method), consists in the exploitation of a "global" property [6] of the bond, i.e. the monotonous character of the functional relationship; the analytical relationship deduced by means of the rearranged values, will therefore have a character of "global" relationship, in the sense of loc. cit.

### 3. Properties of the rearranged points

We will now consider a few properties of the rearranged points, in order to allow for a better critical evaluation of the formal advantages presented by the method described.

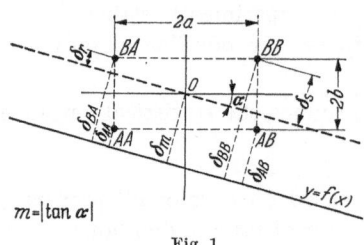

Fig. 1.

Let us take two couples of experimental data $AA \equiv (x_1;\ y_1)$ and $BB \equiv (x_2;\ y_2)$, with $x_1 < x_2$ and $y_1 < y_2$ (fig. 1).

When the interpolating function is a non-rising one, we consider for simplicity only the case of a linear relationship, the average square distance between points (which may as well express the square standard deviation of the points) will be given by the following expression:

$$\delta_s = (b + ma) / \sqrt{(1+m^2)}$$

$$\sum \delta^2 = \delta^2_{AA} + \delta^2_{BB} = 2(\delta^2_m + \delta^2_s) =$$

$$= \frac{2}{\sqrt{(1+m^2)}} \cdot \left[ \sqrt{(1+m^2)} \cdot \delta^2_m + b^2 + m^2a^2 + 2mab \right]$$

while the square distance of the rearranged points will be expressed by:

$$\delta_r = (b - ma) / \sqrt{(1+m^2)}$$

$$\sum \delta^2 = \delta^2_{BA} + \delta^2_{AB} = 2(\delta^2_m + \delta^2_r) =$$

$$= \frac{2}{\sqrt{(1+m^2)}} \cdot \left[ \sqrt{(1+m^2)} \cdot \delta^2_m + b^2 + m^2a^2 - 2mab \right]$$

Hence follows that rearrangement, by reducing the square distance of points from all monotonous non increasing functions, greatly improves their central trend.

The above demonstration is valid for any number of points, as the total rearrangement may always be expressed in terms of a succession of dual rearrangements.

As the number of points increases, the decrease of the square deviation is ever more emphasized, as a consequence of the more regular succession achieved.

Anyway, we ought to point out that such a property can not, by itself, be a guarantee that the interpolating function of the rearranged points will be identical, or even very near, to the true one. Much more the rearrangement is very likely to induce some arbitrary local deformation, the more so as the data are limited in number. Such deviations are inevitable in connection with "global" functions, and can not be avoided whatever method is adopted (minimum square method, local means ... etc.) [6].

However, in its practical applications it is quite immaterial which method, out of a given cathegory, is chosen, if the differences between functions are kept within the interval of statistical insignificance. In order to justify the adoption of the rearrangement method, it will be sufficient to prove the practical coincidence of the final results, as compared with those obtained by employing other methods of more immediate physical interpretation (as pointed out in par. 5).

A remarkable property of the method, consists in the fact that the points will tend to crowd, as the rearrangement is carried out, in the proximity of the curve connecting the local centroid of the experimental points.

This may easily be demonstrated though only by the way of intuition, considering that the coordinates of the centroid of $N$ points, depend only on the analogous coordinates of the points (thus its abscissa is derived from the abscissas of the points and not from their ordinates), and the value is independent of the succession in which such coordinates are ordered:

$$X_B = \overline{x} = \frac{\sum\limits_{i=1}^{N} x_i}{N}$$

$$Y_B = \overline{y} = \frac{\sum\limits_{i=1}^{N} y_i}{N}$$

Consequently, the rearrangement operation does not modify the position of the centroid of the points.

Thus, if the whole set of experimental points is divided into $n$ groups, and the rearrangement is carried out within each group, the points will all lay on a discontinuous line (dotted curve in fig. 2) and the centroids of the segments will coincide with those of their respective groups, however the grouping is made.

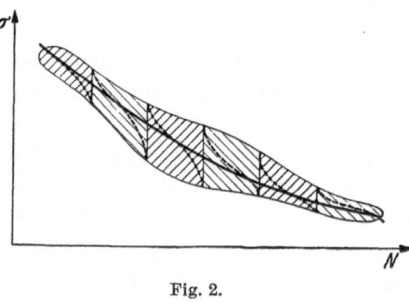

Fig. 2.

All discontinuous lines referred to all possible kinds of grouping gather to a single curve as the groups are enlarged. The final curve will therefore lay very near to the local centroid of the points.

Now, if we keep in mind that the passage from the points $AA$ and $BB$, to the points $AB$ and $BA$, may be visualized as an inversion of the abscissas:

$$AA \rightarrow AB$$
$$BB \rightarrow BA$$

or of the ordinates:

$$AA \rightarrow BA$$
$$BB \rightarrow AB$$

it becomes immediately evident that the rearrangement operation is symmetrical towards the reference directions, and that the rearranged points will crowd in an intermediate position between the two interpolating lines which are obtained by the method of least squares applied to the abscissas or to the ordinates.

This is a very precious property indeed as it makes the curve independent of the reference system.

## 4. Methods to estimate the dispersion range

Several methods have been devised for the calculation of the statistical dispersion of results from fatigue tests; an obvious distinction can be made depending on whether the departures are measured in a horizontal (number of cycles) or in a vertical (stress) direction.

Within the limits of the present work, we will examine only two methods, both within the last group. These have earlier been described in [8].

Once the mean course of the experimental points is known (after the drawing of the average curve as above described), it becomes possible to express the randomness of the points as their vertical distance from the curve.

As already pointed out in [8] the investigation of the variation of the range as a function of the number of cycles, may be of great interest, due to the formal simplicity that could be attained if the range could be considered as independent of the life of the specimens.

For this purpose, if we plot the absolute values of the deviation or, better, the square of the deviation from the average curve versus the number of cycles by means of the method of local averages, we easily obtain the mean absolute deviations (or, respectively the least square deviation).

A direct method for the determination of statistical dispersion without the previous determination of the average curve, may consist in the application of successive differences:

$$\triangle y_{i + 1/2} = y_i - y_{i - 1}$$

Very likely such differences are independent of the systematic tendency of the points.

The variance of such differences is twice as great as that of the points, and therefore it becomes quite possible to deduce the dispersion of the points, from that of the successive differences.

## 5. Applications

The usefulness and efficiency of the above mentioned methods, has been demonstrated for a large series of fatigue data at the ISML laboratories in Novara.

Fatigue tests had been carried out on 9 different alloys of the Ergal type (Al-Zn-Cu-Mg alloys), with a varying zinc content (6%, 7%, 8% about), and with varying amount of Fe + Si. The total number of tests was 313.

Taking into account all the points, the average fatigue curves for all 9 alloys have been drawn. Subsequently, the vertical distance of the points from the curve, have been directly measured and analysed in order to investigate the differences in the behaviour of the alloys. The conclusions arrived at will shortly be published separately.

In such a way systematic influences have been minimized and sta-

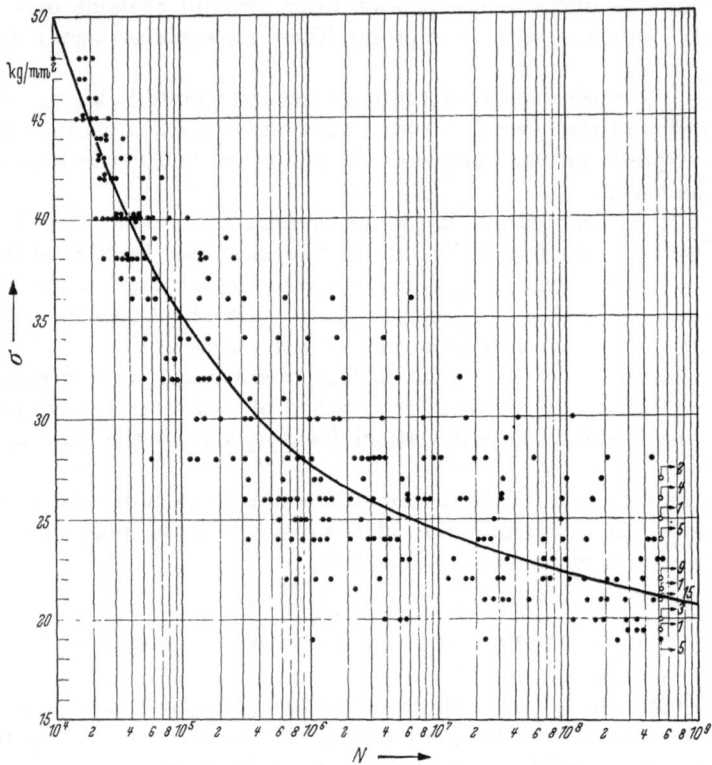

Fig. 3. Experimental results for 9 different Ergal type alloys.

tistical comparison has been possible, enabling conclusions as to the relative statistical significance of the differences.

The first part of the problem consisted in devising the most reliable graphical lay-out of the mean line of the points.

The occurence of appreciable random departures, in addition to the systematic ones due to the different chemical composition of the alloys, contributed to broaden considerably the spread of the points. It is quite selfevident (fig. 3) that every direct endeavour to draw the average curve, should have involved a rough approximation.

But, by calculating the local mean for 5 points, it became possible to reduce by half the width of the statistical range. Actually, as shown in fig. 4, the object was attained but the closeness of the points could not yet be taken as satisfactory in spite of the very considerable amount of work spent in calculating the $2 \times 309$ mean values by means of (1).

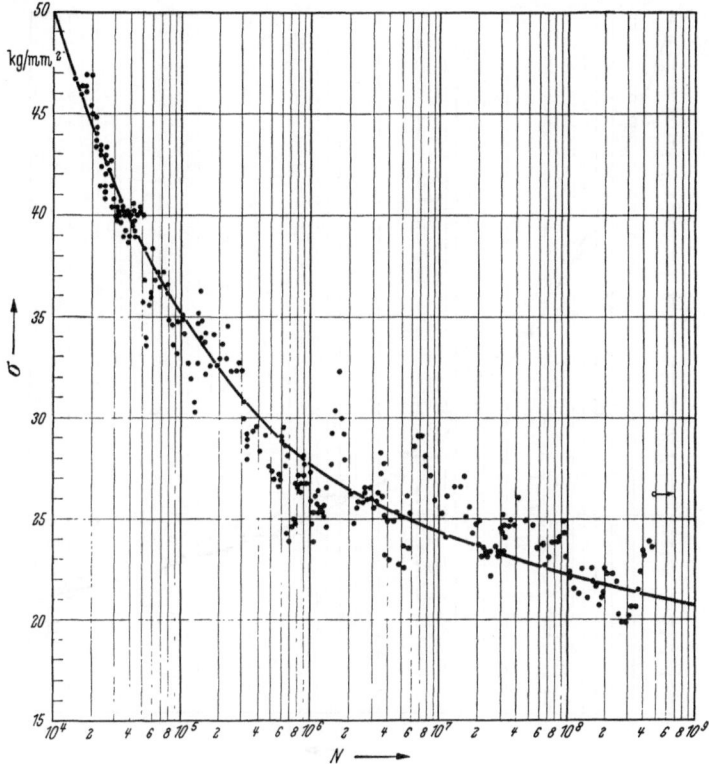

Fig. 4. Method of local averages.

With the rearrangement method, however, a sufficiently condensed pattern was obtained in a remarkably short time and without mathematical calculations. Then it was quite easy to draw the interpolating curve (fig. 5). This curve was then superposed on the two previous diagrams, to make a direct comparison possible.

As may be seen, the agreement is quite satisfactory, thus providing an experimental evidence to our previous deductions and demonstrating the applicability of the method to the fatigue tests analysis.

The analysis of the random dispersion was carried out both with

the method of successive differences and with that of the vertical departures from the average curve. As may be seen in fig. 6a), the range
of the dispersions is quite independent of the life of specimens, thus
giving an additional evidence of the opportunity of modifying the
Peterson "projections method" [2], by the adoption of the parallel

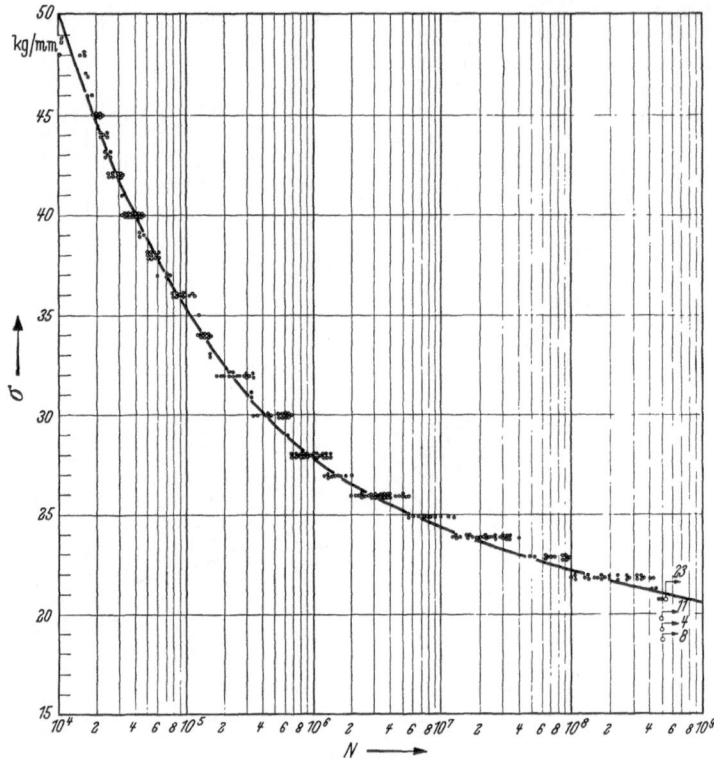

Fig. 5. Rearrangement method.

projection of the points ([8] par. 6), which, besides, brings about a
greater operative simplicity.

In the graphical representation of the figures of successive differences we have reduced the ordinate scale by $1/\sqrt{2}$ in fig. 6a) in order
to achieve an approximate comparability between fig. 6a) and 6b). As
already mentioned, the variance of successive differences, amounts
effectively to twice the simple departures of points.

For all the points, a partial correction of the systematic effect, has
been automatically achieved, as they do not represent the distances

of experimental points from the average curve, but from the average curve for each alloy.

The scatter diagram of vertical distances (fig. 6b) seems to show a slight bending which should indicate a systematic difference between

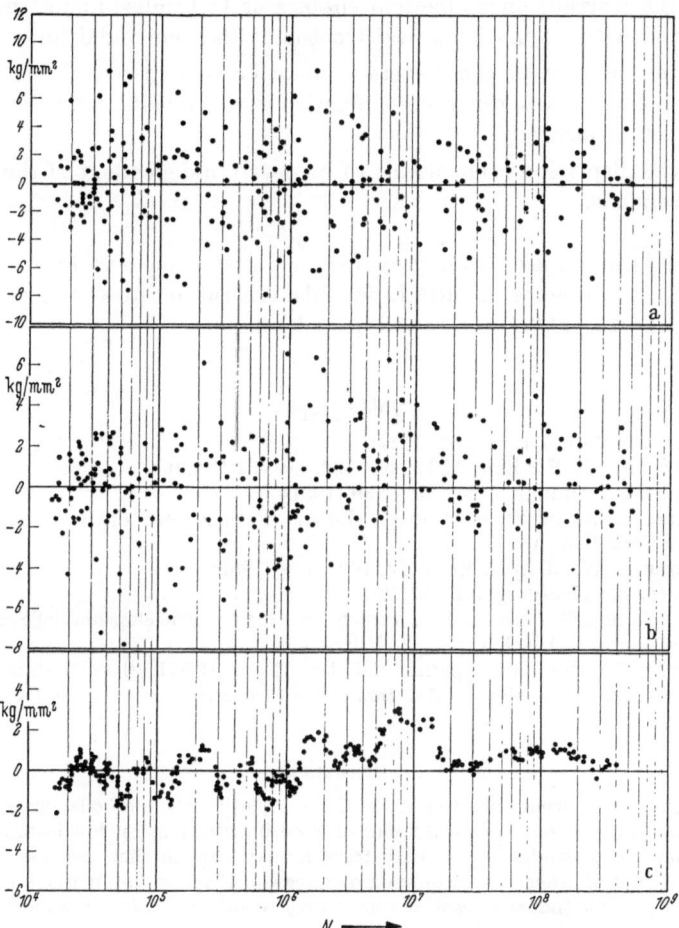

Fig. 6. Random dispersion determined by, a successive differences, b vertical deviations, c local mean of vertical deviations.

the average curve obtained with the "rearrangement method" and the centroidal line of the points. It seems, anyhow, that it is only an apparent effect, as it is shown by the relative local mean (for 10 values) (fig. 6c).

This is a more rigorous proof that the rearrangement method allows to obtain the centroidal line.

## 6. Conclusions

The following conclusions have been reached:

a) the method of local averages, is less efficient and more hard than the rearrangement method;

b) the rearrangement method enables us to localize almost immediately and without mathematical treatment the centroidal line;

c) the analysis of the dispersion may be carried out either by the method of successive differences, or, with better results, with the parallel projection method;

d) the dispersion range seems to be nearly independent of the life of the specimens.

The Author wishes to express his deep gratefulness to Prof. C. Panseri D. E. Director of ISML for his critical interest and the kind permission to publish the experimental results.

### Bibliography

[1] Gini, C.: Metron 4, 1—162 (1924).
[2] Peterson, R. E.: Bull. ASTM No. 156, 50—52 (1949).
[3] Gatto, F.: Alluminio, 20, 533—539 (1951).
[4] Weibull, W. in W. M. Murray (Edit.): Fatigue and Fracture of Metals, New York 1952, 182—196.
[5] Weibull, W.: J. appl. Mech. 19, 109—113 (1952).
[6] Gatto, F.: Metallurg. ital. 44, 391—398 (1952).
[7] Gini, C. and G. Pompilj in L. Berzolari (Edit.): Enciclopedia delle matematiche elementari, vol. 3, part. 3, Milano 1953.
[8] Gatto, F.: Rep. Istit. sperim. Met. leg. (Novara) 541110/4907. Presented at the Congr. intern. Matér. l'Aviation et les Projectiles-fusées, Paris 1955.

### Discussion

J. Schijve: I would like to ask Dr. Gatto whether the methods mentioned by him, may be used for a small number of experimental results. For instance if an S-N curve is determined by twenty tests, it may happen that one test result is completly out of order, say by an unknown reason. If the second method is applied it will be possible that this result becomes a reasonable test result. I wonder if that would be correct.

F. Gatto: The method does offer little advantage if the number of tests is small, i. e. less than 30.

B. Lundberg: Gatto's method appears to be a supposingly rational method of determining the mean S-N curve. This is naturally of some importance, but the engineer must also have knowledge of the scatter, for instance expressed in standard deviation or by S-N curves for different probability levels, i. e., the P-S-N family of curves. In particular, P-S-N curves for rather low P values are of interest for the designer and if tests with large sample sizes are made, the results should of course be utilized for determining also such P-S-N curves.

F. GATTO: For the computation of scatter one has to go back to the original observations, cf. fig. 6.

F. A. McCLINTOCK: In interpreting fatigue data, one needs not only an estimate of the central tendency, but also some knowledge of the variance of that estimate, or how far that estimate may be from the true value. For instance, when the individual alloys are analyzed, can one determine whether or not apparent differences between alloys are really significant?

Also, one needs to know in many cases an estimate of the variability of the population about its central tendency. Can this be obtained from only the fitted curve, such as fig. 5, or must original data be used?

F. GATTO: To estimate the random variability of points it is possible to employ the differences among the experimental values of either coordinates (abscissas or ordinates) and the value of the rearranged coordinate; for example in the case of fatigue tests it is preferable to calculate the difference, for each value of the experimental number of the cycles, of the experimental and the rearranged value of the stress. But the theoretical aspect of this problem is still not completely solved. I think that it is preferable to calculate the vertical variances with the method described in par. 4.

To determine whether or not two alloys give significant difference, one can determine the rearranged curve of all points. Then measuring the vertical distances of points and considering these differences as a new statistical variable you can determine the significance of mean values, or of the coefficients of more general interpolation curves.

# Über Verformungserscheinungen in Stählen bei der Wechselbeanspruchung

Von

## M. Hempel

Mit 9 Abbildungen

## 1. Einleitung

Die theoretische Behandlung der Vorgänge in einem wechselbeanspruchten Werkstoff erfolgt meist unter Berücksichtigung atomarer Vorgänge. Doch fehlen noch genauere Vorstellungen über die Bedingungen, durch die der Vorgang des Dauerbruchs oder das Auftreten der ersten Anrisse eingeleitet wird, da sowohl strukturelle Änderungen als auch Verformungserscheinungen in einem Werkstoff während der Wechselbeanspruchung eintreten. Vielfach werden daher physikalisch-metallkundliche Untersuchungsverfahren zur Bestimmung dieser Veränderungen und zur Deutung der im Werkstoff ablaufenden Vorgänge herangezogen. Insbesondere zeigen röntgenographische und metallographische Beobachtungen, daß die Ursache dieser Eigenschaftsänderungen in Veränderungen des Kristall- und Gefügezustandes einzelner Kristallite zu suchen ist. Über einige Ergebnisse der im Max-Planck-Institut für Eisenforschung, Düsseldorf, zur Klärung dieser Zusammenhänge ausgeführten Untersuchungen wird im folgenden zusammenfassend berichtet.

## 2. Kristallzustand

Die Untersuchungen der Verformungserscheinungen bei der Wechselbeanspruchung wurden zunächst mit Hilfe der Röntgen-Interferenzverfahren an grob- und feinkörnigem Stahl ausgeführt. Die Versuche an grobkörnigem Stahl mit ungestörtem Kristallgitter bieten den Vorteil, daß die Verformung für jeden einzelnen Kristalliten des Werkstoffes mit Hilfe des zugehörigen Röntgen-Interferenzfleckes verfolgt werden kann. Das Verfahren ist aber an Werkstoffen im kaltverformten Zustand nicht mehr anwendbar, weil diese durch die Kaltverformung so feinkristallin sind, daß sie geschlossene Interferenzringe liefern. Durch die Ausbildung von Gitterstörungen infolge von Kristallitverformungen werden die $K_\alpha$-Dublettlinien in den Röntgenaufnahmen so verbreitert, daß sie unscharf erscheinen.

Die Röntgenuntersuchungen brachten die Erkenntnis, daß der Wechselfestigkeitswert eine deutliche Grenze im Verhalten der Kristallite eines Werkstoffes darstellt und daher als eine Verformungsgrenze angesehen werden muß. Bei Belastungen *unterhalb* der Wechselfestigkeit werden im allgemeinen keine Veränderungen des Kristallitzustandes beobachtet. *Überschreitet* die Belastung jedoch die Wechselfestigkeit, so erkennt man im Röntgenbild schon nach wenigen tausend Lastspielen an zahlreichen Interferenzpunkten kleine Verbreiterungen und Verzerrungen. Daraus geht hervor, daß in den zugehörigen Kristalliten bildsame Verformungen eingetreten sind, die zu Störungen im Kristallgitter geführt haben. Diese Kristallitverformungen treten vorwiegend an den Stellen des späteren Dauerbruchs auf, während der Kristallzustand an den Stellen ohne Dauerbruchansätze bis zum Gewalt-

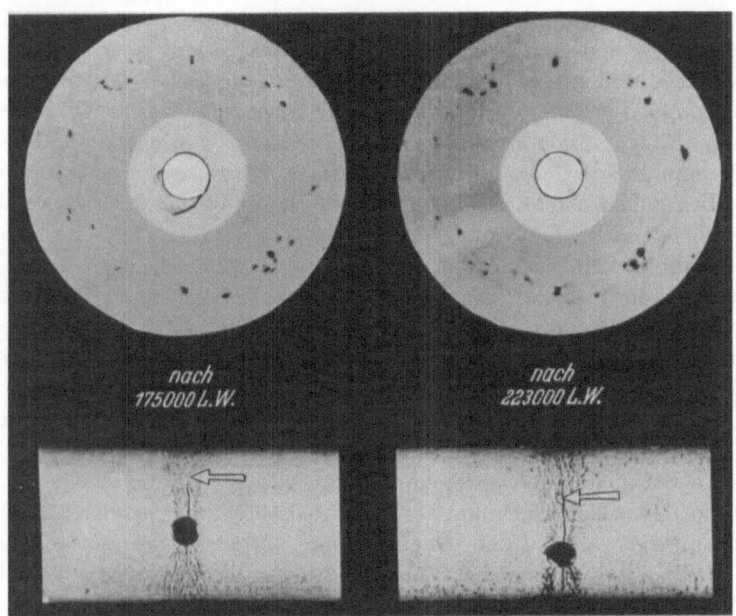

Abb. 1. Änderung des Kristallitzustandes beim Dauerbruch-Anriß. Umlaufbiegeversuche: $n = 4000$ r/min. Stahl mit 0,02 % C. Stabdurchm. = 7,52, Bohrung = 1,0 mm.

bruch praktisch unverändert bleibt. Eine Probe wurde mit $\pm$ 24 kg/mm² bis $N = 0,5$ Mill. Lastspielen oberhalb der Wechselfestigkeit belastet, die Kristallitverformungen wurden an verschiedenen Stellen des Probenumfanges röntgenographisch verfolgt. Verwaschungen der Interferenzpunkte sind nur an solchen Stellen zu erkennen, wo der Dauerbruch eingetreten war, während an der Stelle des Gewaltbruches fast keine Veränderungen eingetreten sind.

Abb. 1 läßt den Grad der Gitterstörungen nach dem Auftreten eines Anrisses erkennen. Bevor der Anriß die Aufnahmestelle — durch Pfeil gekennzeichnet — erreicht, zeigen die Interferenzpunkte praktisch keine Veränderungen in ihrer Schärfe gegenüber dem Ausgangszustand. Durchschreitet der Anriß die Aufnahmestelle, so sind Verwaschungen und periphere Verbreiterungen der Interferenzpunkte sowie schwach angedeutete Debye-Scherrer-Ringe deutlich zu erkennen.

Aus diesen Beobachtungen folgt, daß der Anriß bereits eingetreten sein muß, wenn die Gitterstörungen noch verhältnismäßig klein oder noch nicht erkennbar sind und daß sich diese Gitterstörungen nur auf wenige örtliche Bereiche beschränken.

Weitere Versuchsreihen beschäftigten sich mit der Klärung der Frage, in welcher Beziehung die bei der Wechselbeanspruchung auftretenden, im Röntgenbild erkennbaren Kristallitverformungen zur Verfestigung des Werkstoffes einerseits und zur Zerrüttung oder Schädigung andererseits stehen. Im letzteren Fall wurden die Schwingungsversuche sowohl an Stäben, die durch Überlastung geschädigt waren, als auch an solchen Stäben vorgenommen, bei denen versucht wurde, die Schädigung durch eine Sonderbehandlung wie Wärmebehandlung und Entfernen der Oberflächenschicht zu beseitigen. Aus diesen Versuchen ergaben sich folgende Erkenntnisse: Die nach dem French-Verfahren bestimmte Schadenslinie fällt weder mit dem Beginn noch mit dem Ende der Kristallitverformung im Dauerschwingversuch zusammen; auch stellt sie keine Grenze dar, bei der eine unstetige Änderung im Ablauf der Kristallitverformung eintritt. Durch Glühen im $\gamma$-Gebiet oder durch Entfernen einer dünnen Oberflächenschicht von 0,03 bis 0,25 mm Dicke gelingt es, die Kristallitverformung zu beseitigen, doch wird hierdurch die Schädigung in keiner Weise beeinflußt. Erst nach sorgfältigem Entfernen einer dickeren Oberflächenschicht von $\geq$ 0,5 mm Dicke ist sowohl die Kristallitverformung als auch die Schädigung beseitigt. Daraus folgt, daß die während der Überbelastung aufgetretenen Schädigungen oder Risse eine Tiefe erreicht haben, die den Bereich der mit Gitterstörungen behafteten Kristallite um ein Vielfaches übertrifft.

In Verbindung mit Versuchen über die Beziehungen zwischen *Kristallitverformung und Verfestigung* wurde auch der *Einfluß des Vorschwingens* bestimmt. Das Vorschwingen erfolgte mit Beanspruchungen verschiedener Höhe und Dauer unterhalb der Wechselfestigkeit; danach wurden alle Stäbe oberhalb der Wechselfestigkeit mit $\pm$ 24 kg/mm² und 0,2 Mill. Lastspielen beansprucht. Abb. 2 zeigt den Einfluß verschiedener *Vorschwingzeiten* bei einer gleichbleibenden Vorschwinglast von $\pm$ 16 kg/mm². Zum Vergleich zeigt die erste Bildreihe die Kristallitverformungen bei unmittelbarer Überbelastung. Es ist ohne weiteres ersichtlich, daß mit wachsender Vorschwingzeit die Kristallitverformungen in der Überlaststufe geringer werden.

Während das Ausmaß der Kristallitverformung bei unmittelbarer Überlastung so groß ist, daß im Röntgenbild schon leichte Debye-Scherrer-Ringe auftreten, ist es nach der höchsten angewandten Vorschwingbeanspruchung noch so klein, daß die beiden Röntgenbilder vor und nach der Überbelastung kaum Unterschiede aufweisen. Bei kleinerer Vorschwingbeanspruchung ist die Verminderung der Kristallitverfor-

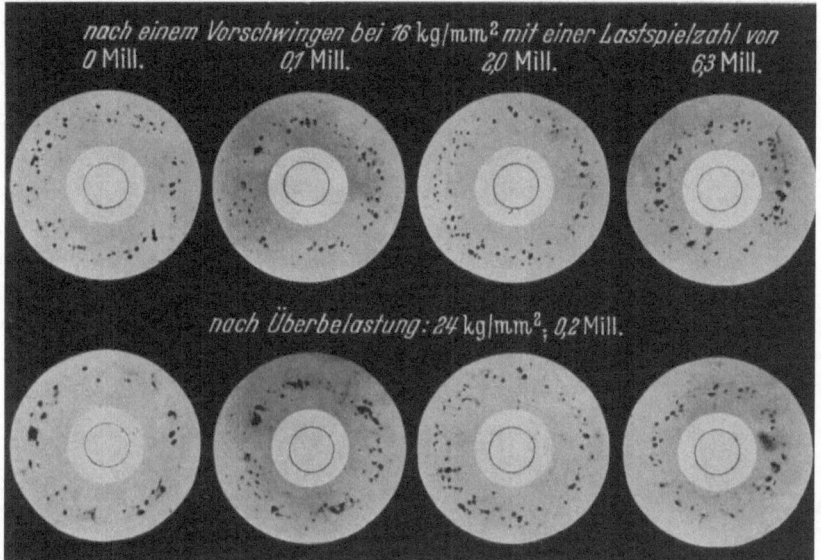

Abb. 2. Einfluß der Vorschwingzeit auf die Kristallitverformung durch Überbelastung.

mung in der Überbelastungsstufe zwar gering, doch ist der Einfluß des Vorschwingens sowohl nach 0,1 Mill. Lastspielen bei $\pm$ 16 kg/mm² als auch nach 6,3 Mill. Lastspielen bei $\pm$ 5 kg/mm² deutlich festzustellen. Daß selbst so kurze Vorschwingzeiten oder so niedrige Belastungen unterhalb der Wechselfestigkeit sich noch deutlich auf das Verhalten des Werkstoffes bei der nachfolgenden Überbelastung auswirken, sollte bei der Deutung der Vorgänge während einer Wechselbeanspruchung besonders beachtet werden.

Der an grobkristallinen Stahlproben mit ungestörtem Kristallgitter beobachtete Einfluß des *Vorschwingens* wird auch an feinkristallinen Proben *mit gestörtem Gitter* festgestellt. Durch die Kaltverformung werden die scharfen $K_\alpha$-Dublettlinien des Ausgangszustandes verbreitert. Bei unmittelbarer Beanspruchung oberhalb der Wechselfestigkeit nimmt die Schärfe der Interferenzringe erheblich zu. Nach einem Vorschwingen nahe unterhalb der Wechselfestigkeit, das selbst keine Änderung der Ringschärfe bewirkt, bringt die gleiche Überbeanspruchung trotz län-

gerer Beanspruchungsdauer nur eine sehr geringe Verbesserung der
Ringschärfe. Offenbar ist durch das Vorschwingen eine Erhöhung des
Fließwiderstandes und damit eine Verfestigung der einzelnen Kristallite
für die nachfolgende Überbeanspruchung bewirkt worden.

Aus diesen Versuchen ergibt sich ferner, daß durch die Wechselbeanspruchung auch eine Rückbildung der Gitterstörungen eintreten
kann, wenn nämlich das Kristallgitter im Ausgangszustand erhebliche
Störungen aufweist. Danach gehört anscheinend zu einer bestimmten
Wechselbeanspruchung im Gleichgewicht auch ein bestimmter Grad
von Gitterstörungen, dem der Kristallzustand während der Wechselbeanspruchung von beiden Seiten her, d. h. vom ungestörten wie vom
gestörten Kristallzustand aus, zustrebt.

### 3. Gleitlinien- und Rißbildung

Weitere wertvolle Aufschlüsse und Erkenntnisse über die Verformungserscheinungen bei der Wechselbeanspruchung brachten die metallographischen Beobachtungen. Dazu wurden glatte und gebohrte Flach-
proben aus St 37 mit mechanisch oder elektrolytisch polierter Oberfläche

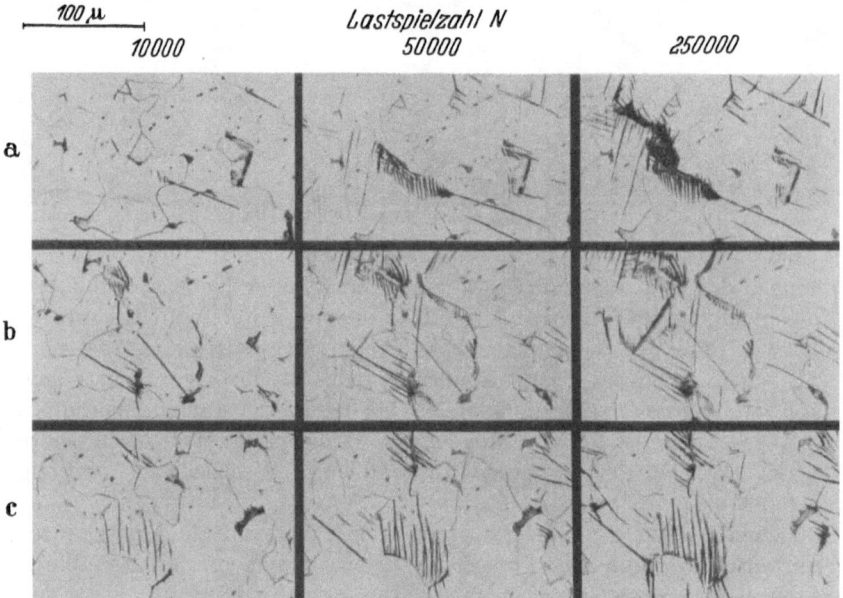

Abb. 3. Ausbildung von Gleitbändern bei hoher Wechselbelastung.
Stahl mit 0,09 % C. Biegewechselbelastung: $\sigma_a = \pm 24$ kg/mm².

im Biegewechselversuch beansprucht ($\sigma_m = 0$, $n = 1.500$ r/min) und die
an der Probenoberfläche eintretenden Gefügeänderungen in Abhängigkeit von den Beanspruchungsbedingungen metallographisch verfolgt.

Abb. 3 läßt die Ausbildung von Gleitlinien und ihre Verbreiterung zu Gleitbändern mit wachsender Beanspruchungszeit an drei Oberflächenstellen einer *oberhalb* der Wechselfestigkeit beanspruchten Probe erkennen. Art und Ausmaß der Gleitlinien und -bänder sind an allen drei Stellen praktisch gleich; auch ist ersichtlich, daß die Bildung dieser Gleitspuren nicht in allen Kristalliten erfolgt, sondern daß selbst nach 250.000 Lastspielen noch viele Kristallite frei von Gleitlinien sind.

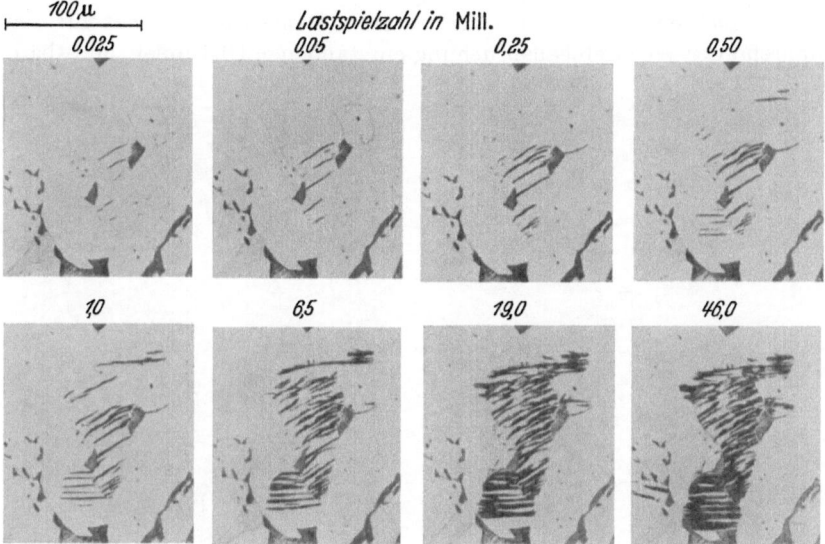

Abb. 4. Ausbildung von Gleitbändern bei niedriger Wechselbelastung.
Biegewechselbelastung: $\sigma_a = \pm 17,5 \ \text{kg/mm}^2$.

Die Ausbildung von Gleitlinien und -bändern an der Oberfläche einer *nahe unterhalb* der Wechselfestigkeit bis zu 46 Mill. Lastspielen beanspruchten, nicht gebrochenen Probe enthält Abb. 4. Im Vergleich zu der oberhalb der Wechselfestigkeit beanspruchten Probe ist hier nach der gleichen Belastungsdauer von 250.000 Lastspielen die Anzahl der Gleitbänder wesentlich geringer; doch nehmen Zahl und Ausmaß der Gleitlinien und -bänder im Laufe der Wechselbeanspruchung, selbst bis zu 46 Mill. Lastspielen, ständig zu.

Der Zeitpunkt des Auftretens der ersten Gleitspuren und die Geschwindigkeit ihrer Ausbreitung ist in besonderem Maße von der Belastungshöhe abhängig. Bei einer Belastung etwa 20% unterhalb der Wechselfestigkeit ist über viele Mill. Lastspiele keine Gleitlinienbildung festzustellen. Bei einer Belastung etwa 10% unterhalb der Wechselfestigkeit und einer Gesamtbeanspruchungsdauer bis 50 Mill. Last-

spiele treten die ersten Gleitlinien nach etwa 25.000 bis 50.000 Lastspielen
auf. Wird die Belastung über die Wechselfestigkeit hinaus gesteigert, so
können die ersten Gleitspuren bereits nach etwa 1.000 bis 2.500 Lastspielen, d. h. etwa nach 0,5% der Gesamtbruchlastspielzahl festgestellt
werden. Die gleiche Art der Gleitlinienbildung wird auch an *gekerbten
Proben* festgestellt. Durch die Spannungsspitzen an den Kerbstellen
wird das Auftreten der Gleitspuren allerdings zu niedrigeren Beanspruchungen hin verschoben.

In welch enger Weise der Verlauf eines Dauerbruchanrisses mit den
während der Wechselbeanspruchung entstandenen Gleitlinien und -bän-

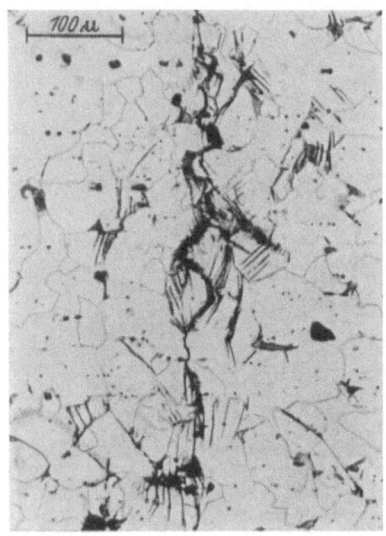 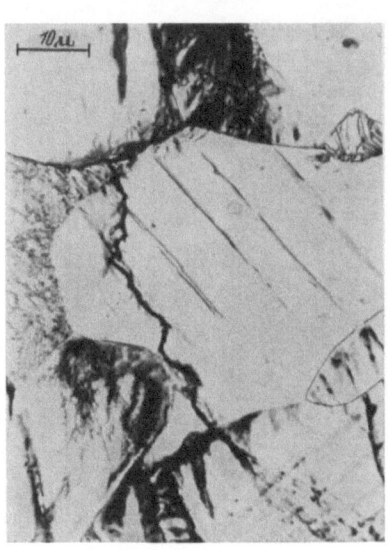

a                                    b

Abb. 5. Dauerbruchanriß in einem Bereich von Gleitbändern.
Beanspruchung: $\sigma_a = \pm 19$ kg/mm²; $N = 1,56$ Mill.

dern verbunden ist, läßt Abb. 5a erkennen. Ein Anriß schreitet im allgemeinen in der Ebene des höchstbeanspruchten Querschnittes nicht als
glatte Linie fort, sondern breitet sich zumeist in unregelmäßiger Zick-
zackform aus. Die Richtung des Fortschreitens wird vor allem durch
Störstellen der verschiedensten Art sowie durch die Orientierung der
Kristallite zur Beanspruchungsrichtung und durch die Gleitspuren
beeinflußt. Der unterschiedliche Anteil von verformten und unverformten
Kristalliten ändert die Spannungsverteilung weitgehend, wobei vor
allem hohe Zugspannungen Werkstofftrennungen innerhalb der Kristallite einleiten. Parallel mit einer Änderung der Spannungsverteilung
geht auch eine Erschöpfung des Formänderungsvermögens, wodurch

ebenfalls eine Werkstofftrennung begünstigt wird. Abb. 5b zeigt in stärkerer Vergrößerung, daß ein Mikroriß in einem Kristalliten nicht immer längs eines Gleitbandes verläuft. Er folgt diesem nur teilweise und stellt sich in den zwischen den Gleitbändern liegenden unverformten Ferritteilen immer wieder senkrecht zur Beanspruchungsrichtung ein.

Zur Prüfung der Frage, wie die Rißbildung mit den Gleitbändern zusammenhängt, wurde die Randzone einer wechselbeanspruchten Probe im Querschliff auf Anrisse untersucht. In einem Gleitlinienbündel zeigten sich zahlreiche Anrisse, deren Längen zwischen 2 und 150 $\mu$ lagen.

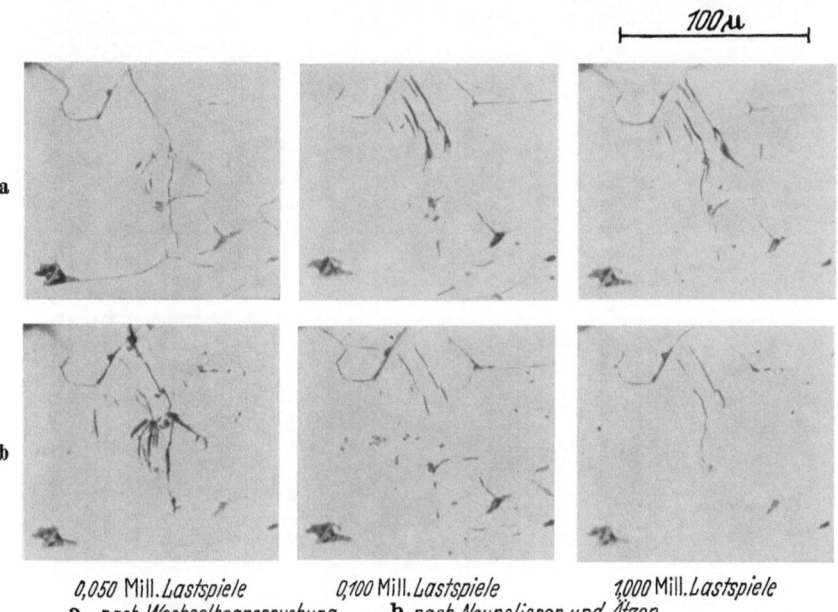

0,050 Mill. *Lastspiele*      0,100 Mill. *Lastspiele*      1,000 Mill. *Lastspiele*
a *nach Wechselbeanspruchung*   b *nach Neupolieren und Ätzen*

Abb. 6. Gleitbänder nach Wechselbelastung mit Zwischenpolieren und erneutem Ätzen.
Flachprobe mit 2 mm Bohrung.
Biegewechselbelastung: $\sigma_a = \pm\ 14$ kg/mm².

Zum Nachweis der unter Wechselbeanspruchung eintretenden Rißbildung wurde die Oberfläche der Probe nach verschiedenen Beanspruchungszeiten abpoliert und neu geätzt. Solange die Gleitbänder keine Mikrorisse enthalten, verschwinden die Gleitbänder nach kurzzeitigem Polieren. Beim Vorhandensein von Mikrorissen bleiben diese nach dem Abpolieren und Ätzen deutlich sichtbar. Bei der in Abb. 6 untersuchten Probe wurde das Zwischenpolieren mit erneutem Ätzen nach drei verschiedenen Beanspruchungszeiten durchgeführt. Es ist deutlich zu erkennen, daß bei dieser Behandlung nur ein Teil der Gleitbänder wieder zum Verschwinden gebracht werden kann. Darüber hinaus zeigen die

Teilbilder, daß sich bei Fortführung des Dauerversuchs das Fortschreiten der Gleitlinien vorwiegend auf diejenigen Kristallite beschränkt, die noch nicht mit feinen Mikrorissen durchsetzt sind.

Zur weiteren Auflösung und Kennzeichnung des Rißverlaufes in einem Gleitband reicht das lichtoptische Mikroskop nicht mehr aus, tiefere Einblicke in den Verformungsmechanismus werden erst unter

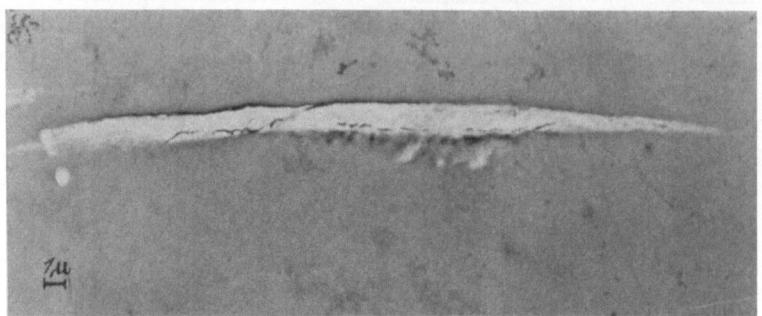

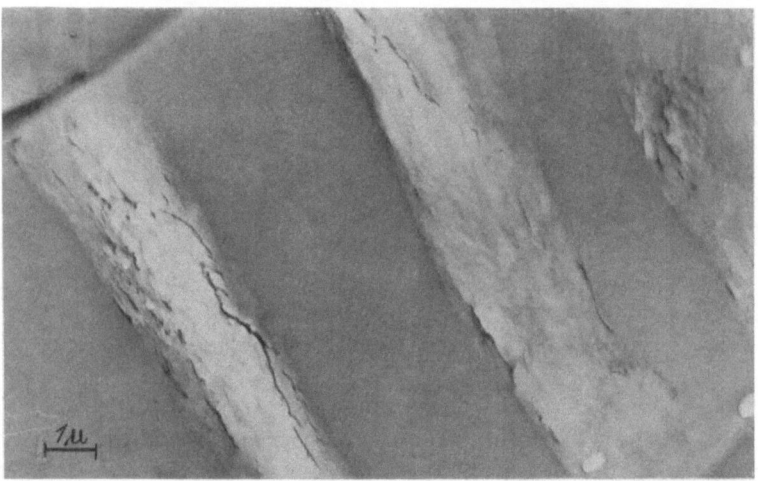

Abb. 7. Oberflächenrisse an Gleitbändern. Lackabdruck mit übermikroskopischen Aufnahmen.
Biegewechselbeanspruchung: $\sigma_a = \pm\ 19$ kg/mm² und $N = 1,56$ Mill. Lastspiele.

Heranziehung des Lackabdruckverfahrens in Verbindung mit übermikroskopischen Aufnahmen erhalten. Die in Abb. 7 wiedergegebene Probe wurde *oberhalb* der Wechselfestigkeit beansprucht; hier sind nun die aus dem Ferrit herausgewölbten Gleitbänder und deren narbige Oberflächen deutlich zu erkennen, die mit zahlreichen feinen Rissen

sowie tieferen Furchen oder Spalten durchsetzt sind. Ein weiteres Beispiel für das Auftreten von Oberflächenrissen in den Gleitbändern einer
Probe, die mit einer Belastung *nahe unterhalb* der Wechselfestigkeit bis
zu 19 Mill. Lastspielen beansprucht wurde, zeigt Abb. 8. Die lichtoptische und die Phasenkontrastaufnahme lassen wohl deutlich ausgebildete Gleitbänder, aber noch keine Anrisse erkennen, der Lackabdruck weist deutlich auf das Vorhandensein von submikroskopischen
Rissen hin. Die dieser Probe während des Dauerversuchs ständig zu-

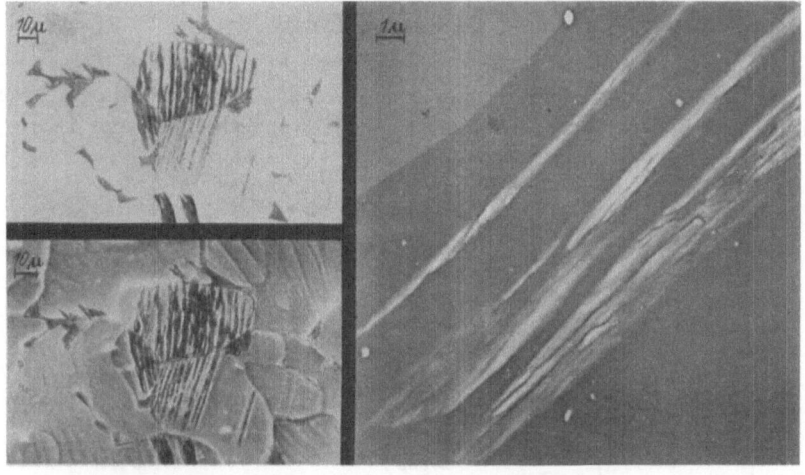

Abb. 8. Oberflächenrisse an Gleitbändern nach langzeitiger Wechselbeanspruchung.
Biegewechselbeanspruchung: $\sigma_a = \pm\ 17{,}5\ \mathrm{kg/mm^2}$ und $N = 19$ Mill. Lastspiele.

geführte Schwingungsenergie reicht jedoch nicht aus, um eine Vereinigung dieser submikroskopischen Risse in den einzelnen Gleitbändern zu
erzwingen und so einen Mikro- oder Makroriß und damit einen Dauerbruch hervorzurufen.

Aus den besprochenen Beobachtungen folgt, daß die Entstehung
eines Dauerbruchanrisses in ferritischen Werkstoffen mit ungestörtem
Kristallgitter die Bildung von Gleitlinien und -bändern zur Voraussetzung hat; im weiteren Verlauf der Wechselbeanspruchung bilden
sich in diesen Gleitbändern an zahlreichen Stellen feine rißähnliche Auf-
spaltungen aus. Diese submikroskopischen Risse vereinigen sich bei
entsprechender Höhe der zugeführten Schwingungsenergie zu Mikrorissen, die schließlich als Makroriß an der Probenoberfläche sichtbar
werden. Zu beachten ist hierbei, daß die Bildung von Gleitbändern und

submikroskopischen Rissen nicht in allen Kristalliten, sondern nur in kleinen örtlichen Bereichen erfolgt.

Eine Verallgemeinerung des Befundes über den Zusammenhang des Gleitmechanismus mit der Rißbildung ist jedoch nicht ohne weiteres möglich. Neben den im Bericht von F. WEVER mitgeteilten strukturellen Veränderungen der Werkstoffe nach langdauernder Beanspruchung in der Wärme und dem hier besprochenen Gleitmechanismus kann auch noch eine Zwillingsbildung als Verformungsmechanismus bei der Wechselbeanspruchung auftreten.

## 4. Zwillingsbildung

In diesem Zusammenhang sei daher noch kurz auf die Gefügeänderungen bei Dauerschwingversuchen im Bereich tiefer Prüftemperaturen eingegangen. Die Wechselfestigkeit verschiebt sich mit fallender Tempe-

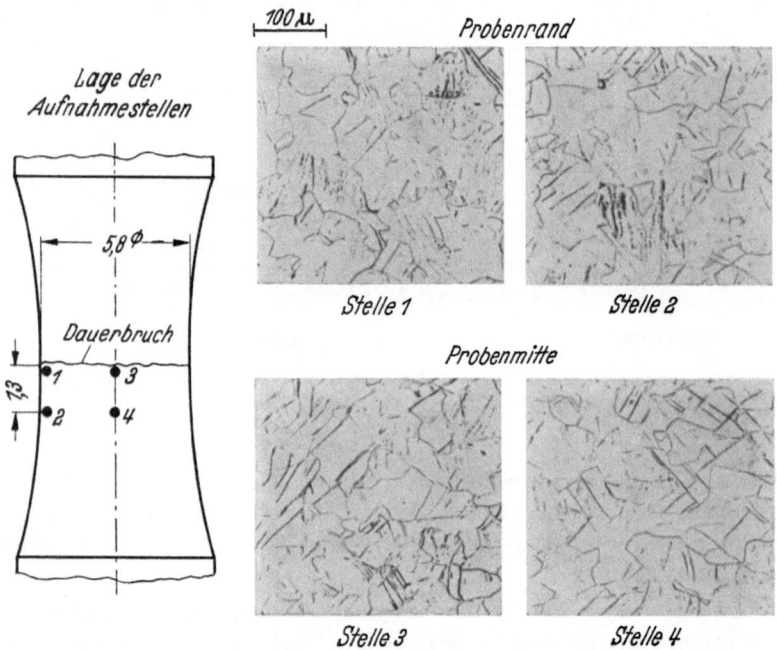

Abb. 9. Gefügeänderungen nach Kaltverformung bei + 20° und Wechselbelastung bei verschiedenen Temperaturen. Weicheisen: 18% stat. gereckt. Zug-Druck-Wechselbelastung: $\sigma_m = 0$, $\sigma_a = \pm 26,2$ kg/mm², $n = 2000$ r/min und $N = 2,08$ Mill. Lastspielen bei + 20° C vorbelastet und anschließend mit $\sigma_a = \pm 72,8$ kg/mm² und $N = 0,155$ Mill. Lastspielen bis zum Bruch bei − 180° C belastet.

ratur ebenso wie die Zugfestigkeit zu höheren Werten. So beträgt die Wechselfestigkeit kaltgereckter Weicheisenproben bei + 20° C rd. ± 25 kg/mm² und bei − 180° C rd. ± 61 kg/mm². Ebenso zeigen auch die

Gefügeaufnahmen einen deutlichen Unterschied. Bei einer Prüftemperatur von $+20°$ C treten in dem unteren Bereich der Zeitfestigkeit die von F. WEVER beschriebenen dunklen, punktförmigen Ausscheidungen im Gefüge hervor, dagegen ist in dem Gefüge der bei tiefer Temperatur $(-180°$ C) beanspruchten Proben eine deutliche Zwillingsbildung vorherrschend. Unter diesen Beanspruchungsbedingungen löst also die Zwillingsbildung den Gleitmechanismus als Verformungsmechanismus ab. Abb. 9 zeigt eine vorgereckte Probe, die bei Raumtemperatur so vorbelastet worden war, daß die Ausscheidung von Eisenkarbid in den Gleitlinien begonnen hatte, sie wurde dann bei tiefer Temperatur mit erhöhter Belastung bis zum Bruch weiter beansprucht. Dabei änderten sich die Ausscheidungen nicht mehr. Daneben trat die Zwillingsbildung deutlich hervor, die für eine bildsame Verformung unter Wechsellast bei tiefen Temperaturen kennzeichnend ist.

## 5. Schlußbemerkungen

Die mitgeteilten Beobachtungen lassen deutlich erkennen, wie komplex die Natur der Veränderungen ist, die während einer Schwingungsbelastung im Werkstoff auftreten. Eine befriedigende Einordnung dieser Versuchsergebnisse in die bestehenden Vorstellungen der Festkörperphysik mit Hilfe energetischer oder gittertheoretischer Überlegungen ist z. Zt. noch nicht ohne Widerspruch möglich. Aufgabe weiterer Untersuchungen wird es daher sein müssen, das vorliegende Beobachtungsmaterial zu ergänzen.

### Diskussion

D. R. HARRIES and G. C. SMITH, Department of Metallurgy, Pembroke Str., University of Cambridge (presented by L. HIMMEL):
The initiation and propagation of fatigue cracks in high-purity aluminium and certain aluminium alloys has recently been studied. Using metallographic techniques, many observations made by HEMPEL on mild steel and by THOMPSON on high-purity copper have been confirmed.
Experiments have been carried out upon the metallographic changes occurring during fatigue of pure aluminium and some aluminium alloys. The specimens were tested in plane bending at a frequency of 1,500 r/min. Before testing they were electro-polished, and etched with 50 % HF to remove the oxide film formed during electro-polishing. They were fatigued for small percentages of their total lives to fracture and then removed from the machine after which the deformation structure of slip lines etc. on the free surfaces was photographed. The specimens were then given a short time of electro-polishing followed by a light etch to reveal the grain boundaries. The average depth of metal polished away during the time taken to remove the majority of the slip markings was about $5\,\mu$. After this treatment the specimens were photographed, and then replaced in the machine and the fatigue test continued. After a further percentage of the fatigue life had elapsed, the specimens were again removed from the machine, photographed, electro-polished and etched and photographed again, the identical area of the surface

being examined each time. This process was repeated several times during the course of each test, until fracture occurred.

It has been found that certain of the slip markings produced during fatigue are very difficult to remove by further electro-polishing, even when only a few per cent of the life to fracture has elapsed. Furthermore these markings, within the grains and at the grain boundaries, develop clearly into cracks at a later stage of the test and join together to lead to major fatigue cracks in the specimens. The evidence which has been obtained indicates that the markings which are difficult to remove by electro-polishing, even after only a few per cent of the life to fracture, probably contain fine cracks. It has for example been found that these markings are still difficult to remove by electro-polishing, even if the fatigued specimen is annealed before the electro-polishing treatment. This indicates that fine cracks are probably responsible for the observed effects rather than regions of deformed metal, as the latter would be expected to be removed by an annealing heat treatment.

Furthermore a specimen which had been fatigued for about 15% of the life to fracture at room temperature was elongated 8% in tension. The markings at the grain boundaries and within the grains widened with this treatment, the former showing a more marked effect.

At room temperature cracks are formed both at grain boundaries and within the grains. Experiments over a range of temperatures have shown that at higher temperatures the amount of grain boundary cracking increases, whilst at lower temperatures the amount of cracking within the grains increases. On testing at $-180°$ C no grain boundary cracks are found. The earliest stage in the fatigue life at which cracks have been observed is 1%. The experiments show that the cracks grow slowly so long as their length is only of the same order of magnitude as the grain size of the material. This slow spreading and growth of the cracks continues throughout the major portion of the life. It is not until the last 20% or so of the life that the small cracks begin to link up to form major cracks of many grain diameters length, from which the final fatigue crack is formed.

The bulk of the work has been carried out using pure aluminium, but similar effects have been found with aluminium - 1% magnesium alloys.

In the case of pure aluminium some experiments have been carried out at low stresses where the total life to fracture is very large, being greater than $10^7$ cycles. At these stresses a slip line pattern is found similar to that observed at higher stresses, but not so marked in extent. However, if this pattern is removed by electro-polishing the markings which remain do not resemble cracks, but take the form of small pits distributed along the length of the slip bands and also at some grain boundaries. It has been found that if a specimen showing these pits is subsequently stressed at a higher stress where the life is much shorter, the pits extend along the slip lines with further fatiguing, and form cracks having an appearance identical with those formed when the specimen is stressed entirely at a high stress. T he pits thus appear to be a possible early stage in the formation of a crack. The pits can be observed in specimens where the deformation structure has been removed by mechanical polishing instead of electro-polishing and thus are not due to any etching effects occurring during the electro-polishing. They are also visible under the electron microscope on the as-deformed surface. In addition electron microscope examination has revealed the shape of the pits more clearly, and has shown them to be conical or cylindrically shaped cavities which are oriented so that their major axes are parallel to the operative slip plane. The pits lie within the width of the slip band, which in itself contains many individual slip planes, and they grow in width and depth until they link up to form a flat crack having its major plane parallel to the slip planes concerned.

Annealing experiments have shown that the pits are not removed by this treatment.

It has also been shown that protective coatings of rubber on the surfaces of the specimens have no effect on the appearance of the cracks at high stresses and the pits at low stresses. Thus the latter are not due to prolonged exposure of the specimens to the corrosive action of the atmosphere.

M. HEMPEL: Die von HARRIES und SMITH mitgeteilten metallographischen Beobachtungen über das Verhalten von Reinaluminium und einer Al-Mg-Legierung unter Biegewechselbeanspruchung bestätigen in bester Weise die an Stahl St 37 aufgetretenen Verformungserscheinungen. Faßt man die Ergebnisse der bisherigen Untersuchungen über das Auftreten von Gleitspuren unter Wechselbeanspruchung zusammen, so wird dieser Verformungsmechanismus sowohl unter verschiedenen Beanspruchungsarten wie Biege-, Verdreh- und Zugdruckwechselbeanspruchung, als auch an Werkstoffen unterschiedlichen Gitteraufbaues gefunden. Dabei ist das Auftreten der ersten Gleitspuren im wesentlichen von der Belastungshöhe abhängig und beträgt in einzelnen Fällen $\leq 1\%$ der Bruchlastspielzahl. Schon nach einigen wenigen Prozent der Gesamtlebensdauer können häufig die vorhandenen Gleitspuren nur zum Teil durch Abpolieren und Ätzen entfernt werden; in diesen beständigen Gleitbändern vermuten HARRIES und SMITH das Auftreten feiner Risse. Durch elektronenmikroskopische Aufnahmen von Gleitbändern an Stahl St 37 konnte das Vorhandensein submikroskopischer Risse in den Gleitbändern tatsächlich nachgewiesen werden. Diese Risse werden durch eine Glühbehandlung — ohne Anwendung eines äußeren Druckes — nicht beseitigt.

Über den Einfluß der Prüftemperatur auf die Rißausbildung an Aluminium berichten HARRIES und SMITH, daß bei Versuchen in der Wärme die Neigung zur Bildung von Korngrenzenrissen erhöht wird. In austenitischen Stahlproben, die bei Temperaturen von 550 bis 650° C unter Zugdruckwechselbelastung geprüft wurden, ergaben sich bei den bisherigen Untersuchungen vorwiegend Karbidausscheidungen in den Korngrenzen, und in einigen bei 500° C geprüften Proben eines Mo-Stahles mit 0,5% Mo verlief der Dauerbruchanriß intrakristallin. Bei Temperaturen von — 180° C wird in weichen Flußstahlproben der Gleitmechanismus durch eine Zwillingsbildung abgelöst. Hinsichtlich des Temperatureinflusses auf die Verformungserscheinungen ist bisher in dem Verhalten von Aluminium und Stahl keine Übereinstimmung festzustellen.

Besonders interessant sind die Hinweise auf die Bildung von konischen oder zylinderförmigen Narben oder Vertiefungen in den Gleitbändern, die dann auftreten, wenn langzeitig wechselbeanspruchte Proben anschließend poliert und geätzt werden. Eine derartige Verformungserscheinung konnte gleichfalls an Stahlproben, die bis zu 100 Mill. Lastspielen wechselbeansprucht worden waren, festgestellt werden.

# The effect of high loads on fatigue

By

## R. B. Heywood

With 7 figures

## 1. Introduction

At first sight, it might be thought that occasional high loads would have little influence on fatigue, so long as the damage as indicated by the cumulative damage rule was small. This supposition is supported by results of tests made at the Aluminium Laboratories [1] on plain aluminium alloy specimens, when a single initial stretch in axial tension slightly reduced the fatigue strength in rotating bending, the maximum reduction being 12%, see table 1.

Table 1. *Effect of pre-loading on the fatigue strength of B.S. L. 1. plain specimens tested in rotating bending (TEED [1]).*

| | Fatigue strength tsi for failure in $50 \times 10^6$ cycles | | | |
|---|---|---|---|---|
| Stretch produced by pre-load, % | 0 | 3 | 6 | 9 |
| When pre-loaded: | | | | |
| (A) Immediately after quenching and then allowed to age before test .. | ± 12.0 | ± 11.5 | ± 11.0 | ± 11.0 |
| (B) 1 hour after quenching and then allowed to age before test ...... | ± 12.0 | ± 11.8 | ± 11.3 | ± 10.5 |
| (C) After heat treatment and ageing ..................... | ± 12.0 | ± 12.0 | ± 11.5 | ± 10.5 |

For notched parts and structural members, the slightly damaging effect imparted to the material by a few high loads is dwarfed by other factors, which cause the high loads to exert a totally different influence on fatigue behaviour. In this paper a preliminary survey of these other factors is made, with special reference to the behaviour of representative aircraft parts.

## 2. Qualitative effect of high loads

A high load applied to a structure or structural element has two further effects — it produces residual stresses at notches, such as holes, fillets, etc., and it influences the load distribution due to redundancy in the structure.

The general pattern of residual stresses is well-known and is shown in fig. 1 a for a typical case. At the high load, the elastic stress distribution shown by curve I is modified by plastic flow to that shown by curve II, and upon removal of load, predominantly elastic recovery takes place to give residual stresses of the type shown by curve III. In the vicinity of the stress concentration, the residual stress is invariably of opposite sign to the imposed stress.

In a subsequent fatigue test at lower loads, the residual stresses shown by curve III in fig. 1 b combine with the fatigue mean stresses of curve IV to produce the resultant curve V. Clearly, if both the high and fatigue mean loads are applied in a given sense there is a reduction in stress at critical points. Thus at the critical point O in the notch, the mean stress is reduced from OA to OB. On the other hand, if the loads are of opposite sense, there is an increase in the local stress.

Alternating stresses are not affected by the preload, but are represented to some scale by the elastic curve I (assuming no cyclic plastic deformation occurs). For a tensile pre-load, the point of greatest alternating stress at O is matched by a reduced mean stress;

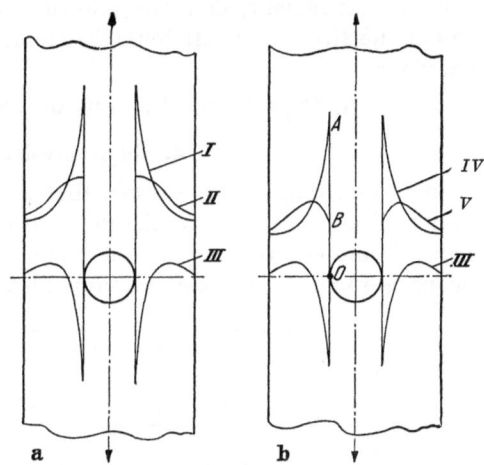

Fig. 1. Axial stress distributions in member with transverse hole.
a Application and removal of high load.
   I. Elastic stresses
   II. Plastic stresses
   III. Residual stresses
b Application of lower load.
   III. Residual stresses
   IV. Elastic stresses
   V. Resultant stresses

further away from the hole, a lower alternating stress is matched by the peak of the mean stress. Thus the fatigue life of the material at points within this region is approximately the same, and so an efficient utilisation of the material is achieved.

The behaviour due to redundancy in structures is similar in nature, except that, instead of dealing with variations in plastic strain within a part, we are now dealing with variations in plastic strain between individual structural members, and the resulting change in their length. This makes the load distribution become more uniform when the high and fatigue mean loads are applied in a given sense, but when loading is applied in opposite senses, the distribution would either be worse, or would be unaffected, depending on whether or not the effective lengths of members had been altered by the high loads.

The qualitative effects of high loads in producing residual stresses and in modifying load distributions are fundamental and unavoidable and indeed, both effects may be present simultaneously. From the fatigue viewpoint two issues remain to be solved, namely the quantitative values of these effects, and their degrees of persistence throughout the subsequent fatigue test. To throw light on these problems it was considered that practical fatigue tests were the best and most useful means of assessment, and the following results, obtained mostly from tests at the Royal Aircraft Establishment, give an indication of general behaviour.

### 3. Experimental results on effect of high loads

#### a. Single pre-load.

In 1946 FORREST [2] showed that a substantial increase in fatigue strength due to an axial tensile pre-load occurred in specimens containing a circumferential notch and tested in rotating bending. The specimens were made in the aluminium alloy B.S.6 L. 1, and for a pre-load

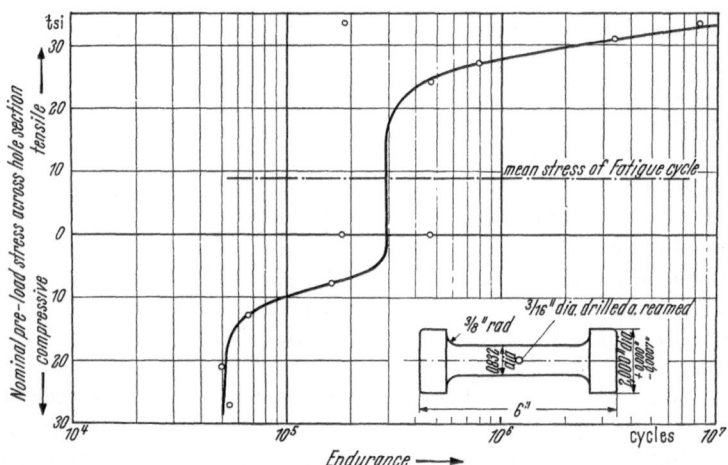

Fig. 2. Effect of pre-load on the endurance of round bars with a transverse hole.

equivalent to 25 tsi, the fatigue strength was doubled. These findings have since been confirmed by TEMPLIN [3] for similarly notched specimens made in the aluminium alloy 75S-T6.

The effect of magnitude of pre-load on the endurance of round bar transverse hole specimens is shown in fig. 2. The specimens, made in the aluminium alloy D.T.D. 683, were all tested in fatigue in axial tension at nominal stresses of $9 \pm 3.5$ tsi at the hole section. Insufficient specimens were available to establish results beyond question, but there is strong evidence that a tensile pre-load is beneficial, and that a compressive pre-load is harmful. It is interesting that specimens apparently identical in shape and material have given endurances covering the surprisingly wide range from 50,000 to 8,000,000 cycles. The exceptional result for the highest tensile load is in doubt, as flaws were present at the point of origin of the fatigue crack.

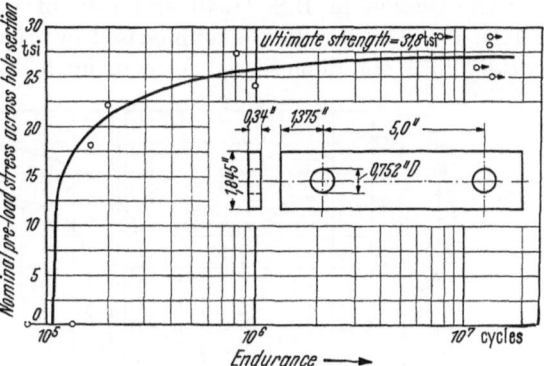

Fig. 3. Effect of pre-load on the endurance of lugs.

The harmful effect of a compressive pre-load has been confirmed by tests on D.T.D. 364 B flat plates with a $1/_4$ in. diameter transverse hole. Using the same fatigue stresses as before the geometric mean endurance was reduced from over 7.5 million to 325,000 cycles by a compressive pre-load of 20 t s i.

Fatigue tests on aluminium alloy lugs made in D.T.D 364 B and loaded through high tensile steel pins showed a spectacular increase in endurance

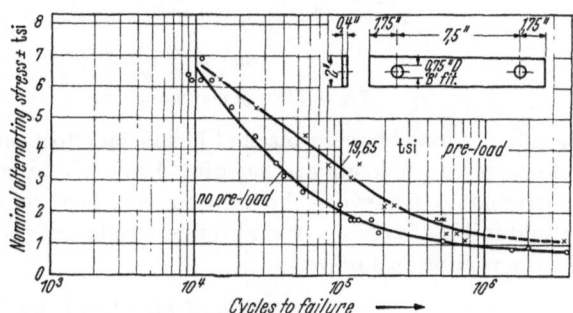

Fig. 4. Fatigue strength of lugs with and without pre-loading.
Nominal mean stress during fatigue test = 7.15 tsi
(Saunders-Roe tests).

due to tensile pre-loads above a certain amount, see fig. 3. A hundredfold increase in endurance was obtained for pre-loads equivalent to the 0.1% proof stress (26 tsi) of the material.

Aluminium alloy lugs in D.T.D. 683 tested by Saunders-Roe for the Ministry of Supply [4] enable endurances to be compared at various alternating stress levels due to a tensile pre-load of given amount. The pre-load was comparatively small, equivalent to 65% of 0.1% proof stress (20 tsi), yet for alternating stresses below $\pm 4.5$ tsi this caused an increase in life of two to three times, see fig. 4.

Tests on representative aircraft components have been made as follows: — (a) wing centre section spar boom of channel section made in the alloy D.T.D. 363A, with sheet webs riveted and bolted to boom, (b) three different designs of main spar wing root joints, two in D.T.D. 683 and one in D.T.D. 364B, with the load transmitted through bolts in shear to outer members, and (c) complete Meteor 4 tailplanes, with spars of angle section in B.S. 2L40 and skin of clad aluminium alloy to D.T.D. 390. The results are summarised in table 2, and are shown graphically in a non-dimensional form in fig. 5. The evidence shows that

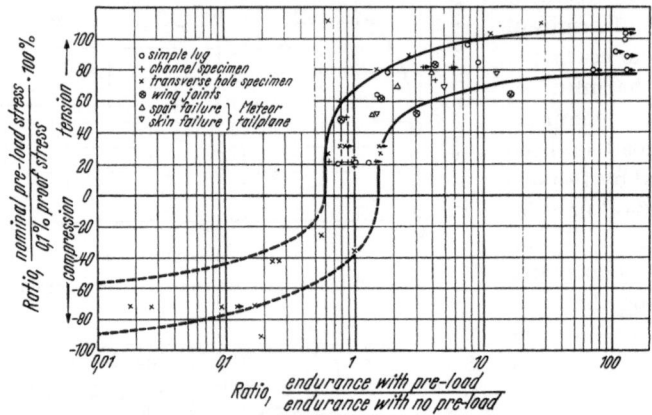

Fig. 5. Effect of pre-load on ratios of endurance.

tensile pre-loads have a marked beneficial effect on fatigue life, and that compressive pre-loads are harmful. Pre-loads in compression have been restricted to transverse hole specimens, because spar boom specimens would fail by buckling, and also lugs would not produce residual stresses at the section of failure.

## b. Batch of high pre-loads

The marked effect of a single pre-load on fatigue has suggested that a number of other high load combinations might be worth investigation. Two such cases have received attention so far, namely a batch of high pre-loads, and high loads applied periodically during the fatigue test.

The channel section boom described above was subjected to ten tensile pre-loads of a magnitude equivalent to half the 0.1% proof stress (16.5 tsi), with the load returning to the mean of the fatigue cycle after each application. In the subsequent fatigue test at stresses of $7.1 \pm 2.74$ tsi, an endurance of 246,000 cycles was obtained. This compares with a geometric mean endurance of 82,000 cycles obtained from tests on eight booms not given pre-loads, when the individual maximum was 125,000 cycles. The ten pre-loads have thus produced a threefold increase in endurance, whereas the same improvement with a single pre-load would only have been obtained with a load of about $^3/_4$ of the proof stress.

A similar test on a Meteor tailplane which had been given ten pre-loads of relatively small magnitude (equivalent to 42% of 0.1% proof

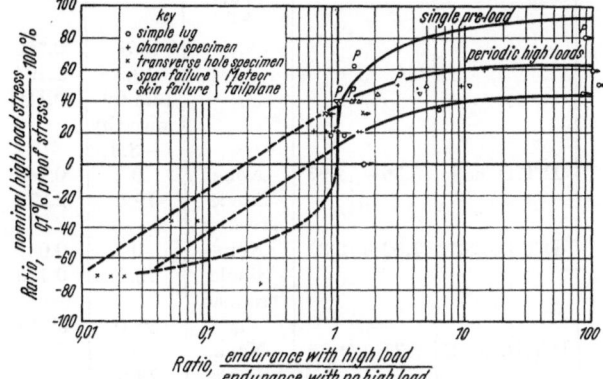

Note: letter 'P' near a point denotes that specimen had received ten pre-loads, all other points represent specimens which were subjected to periodic high loads during fatigue test.

Fig. 6. Effect of ten pre-loads and of periodic high loads on endurance ratio.

stress) increased the endurance from 850,000 cycles to 1,110,000 cycles. Also a few tests on a lug specimen have confirmed the beneficial effect of ten pre-loads. Results are given in table 2 and plotted in fig. 6.

Table 2. *Results of tests on structural elements.*
All specimens tested in fluctuating tension, except for Meteor tailplanes which were tested in bending at resonance.

| Type of specimen | Material | Nominal fatigue stresses, tsi | Type of high load | Magnitude of high load tsi | Endurance, $10^6$ cycles | Ratio of endurances (high load/ no high load) |
|---|---|---|---|---|---|---|
| Boom of channel section | D.T.D. 363 | 7.1 ± 2.74 | None | 0 | 0.079* | 1 |
| ,, | ,, | ,, | Single pre-load | 16.8 | 0.069 | 0.87 |
| ,, | ,, | ,, | ,, | 20.2 | 0.062 | 0.79 |
| ,, | ,, | ,, | ,, | 24.4 | 0.343 | 4.34 |
| ,, | ,, | ,, | ,, | 26.9 | 0.455 u | 5.63+ |
| ,, | ,, | ,, | ,, | ,, | 0.267 u | 3.36+ |
| ,, | ,, | ,, | 10 pre-loads | 16.5 | 0.246 | 3.12 |

* Geometric mean values. For transverse hole specimens (1/4 in. diameter hole in 0.9 in. wide section) endurances in millions without high loads were 6.1, 6.2 u and 12.1 u; with 10 tsi periodic compression 0.386 and 0.633, and with 20 tsi periodic compression 0.101, 0.130 and 0.165.

*Table 2 (Forts.)*

| Type of specimen | Material | Nominal fatigue stresses, tsi | Type of high load | Magnitude of high load tsi | Endurance, $10^6$ cycles | Ratio of endurances (high load/ no high load) |
|---|---|---|---|---|---|---|
| Boom of channel section | D.T.D. 363 | $7.1 \pm 2.74$ | Periodic loads | 13.2 | 0.114 | 1.44 |
| ,, | ,, | ,, | ,, | 16.5 | 0.769 | 9.7 |
| ,, | ,, | ,, | ,, | 19.8 | 1.194 | 15 |
| ,, | ,, | ,, | ,, | 16.5 followed by $-3.3$ | 0.119 | 1.50 |
| Joint A | D.T.D. 683 | $5.36 \pm 1.97$ | None | 0 | 0.145 | 1 |
| ,, | ,, | ,, | Single pre-load | 19.5 | 2.370 | 16.4 |
| Joint B | D.T.D. 683 | $7.82 \pm 2.37$ | None | 0 | 0.087 | 1 |
| ,, | ,, | ,, | Single pre-load | 19.0 | 0.130 | 1.50 |
| ,, | ,, | ,, | ,, | 25.0 | 0.375 | 4.3 |
| Joint C | D.T.D. 364B | $6.35 \pm 1.85$ | None | 0 | 0.580 | 1 |
| ,, | ,, | ,, | Single pre-load | 13.5 | 0.464 | 0.80 |
| ,, | ,, | ,, | ,, | 14.8 | 1.79 | 3.09 |
| Meteor Tailplane | B.S. 2 L40 | $5.70 \pm 1.71$ | None | 0 | 0.850 | 1 |
| ,, | ,, | ,, | Single pre-load | 11.4 | 1.29 | 1.52 |
| ,, | ,, | ,, | ,, | 15.2 | 1.82 | 2.15 |
| ,, | ,, | ,, | ,, | 17.1 | 3.50 | 4.12 |
| ,, | ,, | ,, | 10 pre-loads | 9.1 | 1.11 | 1.31 |
| ,, | ,, | ,, | Periodic loads | 9.1 | 1.14 | 1.34 |
| ,, | ,, | ,, | ,, | 10.2 | 1.76 | 2.08 |
| ,, | ,, | ,, | ,, | 11.4 | 4.17 | 4.9 |
| Simple lugs | D.T.D. 364 B | $6 \pm 2.2$ | None | 0 | 0.124* | 1 |
| ,, | ,, | ,, | 10 pre-loads | 17.7 | 0.155 | 1.25 |
| ,, | ,, | $6 \pm 2.2$ | 10 pre-loads | 22.1 | 10.6 u | 85+ |
| ,, | ,, | | | | | |
| ,, | ,, | ,, | Periodic loads | 10.0 | 0.738 | 6.3 |
| ,, | ,, | ,, | ,, | 12.0 | 9.0 u | 73+ |
| ,, | ,, | ,, | ,, | 14.0 | 11.0 u** | 94+ |
| ,, | ,, | ,, | ,, | 16.6 | 11.0 u** | 94+ |
| Transverse hole specimens | D.T.D. 364 B | $9 \pm 3.5$ | None | 0 | 7.7+ | 1.0 |
| ,, | ,, | ,, | Periodic loads | $-10$ | 0.494* | 0.064 |
| ,, | ,, | ,, | ,, | $-20$ | 0.130* | 0.017 |

** Tests continued with stresses increased to $6 \pm 4.24$ tsi (no further over-loads applied), giving failure in 145,000 and 131,000 cycles, respectively.

## c. Periodic high loads

Periodic high loads of a given amount were applied at intervals during the fatigue test, with the load returning to the mean of the fatigue test after each application. The intervals of high loading were as follows: —

At commencement of test, and every 20,000 cycles to 500,000 cycles.
Then every 50,000 cycles to 1,000,000 cycles.
Then every 100,000 cycles to 2,000,000 cycles.
Then every 200,000 cycles to 4,000,000 cycles.
Then test continued to failure without further overloads.

Tests on simple lugs have shown that a spectacular increase in life can be obtained by applying periodic tensile overloads of only moderate intensity, equivalent to about half the 0.1% proof stress. As shown in table 2, the life was improved from a mean of 124,000 cycles to non-failure in 11,000,000 cycles.

Tests on both channel section booms and Meteor tailplanes showed similar trends due to periodic tensile overloads and results for all tests are given in table 2 and fig. 6. It will be observed that the effect of periodically reducing the mean load to zero has not been ascertained, but may well be harmful.

Tests using periodic overloads in compression were carried out on D. T. D. 364 B flat plates containing a $1/4$ in. diameter transverse hole. With nominal fatigue stresses of $9 \pm 3.5$ tsi, specimens not overloaded failed at a geometric mean endurance of over 7.7 million cycles, those given 10 tsi periodic overloads failed in 494,000 cycles, whilst those given 20 tsi overloads failed in only 130,000 cycles. The last result compares with a mean endurance of 325,000 obtained for a 20 tsi single pre-load.

## 4. Conclusions

The improvement in life due to occasional tensile loads in excess of about half the proof stress demonstrates that the cumulative damage rule is not even qualitatively correct for such cases. With compressive loads the large reduction in life that can be obtained in practice compares with the extremely small reduction that would be indicated by this rule. The cumulative damage rule is therefore entirely unsatisfactory for the type of loading considered.

For tensile loads of given magnitude, periodic overloading produced greatest improvement in the endurance, then ten pre-loads, and lastly a single pre-load produced least improvement. The beneficial effect undoubtedly becomes less when the fatigue stresses are comparatively high, due to fading of the residual stresses during the fatigue test.

7*

There are two possible explanations why tensile periodic loading is most effective. Residual stresses may fade during the fatigue test, but may be restored to their original level by the repeated application of high load, so ensuring that a beneficial stress distribution is always maintained. Alternatively, fatigue cracks may form during the early stages of a fatigue test, and the subsequent application of a high load might produce residual compressive stresses at the crack extremities, so preventing or retarding further progression.

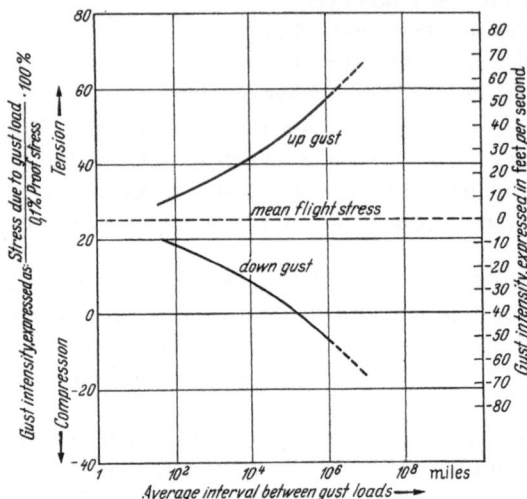

Fig. 7. Results showing average interval between gust loads which exceed the intensity shown.

The question as to whether the life of air-craft is affected by high loads may be assessed for average civil air-craft conditions by inter-preting the gust data as-certained by Taylor to stresses, fig. 7. The ordi-nate shows the stress in wing bottom spar booms due to a gust which equals or exceeds a given value, and is expressed as a fraction of the 0.1% proof stress, and the abscissa gives the frequency, as assessed by the miles flown per high load. This data, when combined by means of the cumulative damage rule with a representative fatigue curve for aircraft wing joints, shows that the average joint will fail at 8 million miles of flight. Dividing by a typical test endurance[1] gives the equi-valent miles flown per fatigue cycle, and this has a value of 42 miles per cycle, assuming no safety factors are included.

Fig. 7 shows that the highest single load likely to be encountered during an entire aircraft life of say 5 million miles is 64% of the 0.1% proof stress in tension, and 14% in compression. The tensile load if occurring at the beginning of service use would about double the life, whilst the compressive load is unlikely to have an effect. Thus a small increase in aircraft life is probable, depending on the severity and time of occurrence of the greatest gust.

For periodic overloading, the high loads were applied at intervals of

---

[1] As obtained when the alternating stress corresponds to a 10 ft per second gust at cruising speed, as suggested by Walker [5].

20,000 cycles for the first half million. This represents a high load applied once every $20,000 \times 42 = 840,000$ miles, and from fig. 7 it is seen that this load is equivalent to 57% of the proof stress. Now fig. 6 indicates that a periodic load of this magnitude produces a very substantial increase in life. Thus the strange fact is demonstrated that the larger positive gusts should actually increase the aircraft life by a considerable amount.

Stresses due to severe down gusts are small and are not expected to influence life. Of greater importance are the compressive stresses due to landing or taxying, since they occur very frequently — for a flight of 840 miles the compressive stresses are applied once every 20 fatigue cycles — they may therefore drastically reduce life.

The combined effect to tensile and compressive high loads is not known. The single result for a channel section boom shown in table 2 suggests that the beneficial effect of a tensile load is lost if immediately followed by a small compressive load. For aircraft, it may well be that the improvement in life due to tensile high loads from gusts is nullified completely by the compressive loads from landing and taxying.

High loads could be applied deliberately to aircraft by flight manoeuvres in order to increase life. However the fatigue results show that a single pre-load would probably be of too high a magnitude for this to be done with safety. Multiple pre-loading would require smaller loads, and is therefore a possibility, although more practical data is required. Periodic overloading applied at long intervals during an aircraft's use appears to offer the most promising method of improvement. Only moderate loads, equivalent to about half the proof stress or say a 2 to 2.5 $g$ load, applied once every 100,000 to 1,000,000 miles may well be all that is necessary to ensure a reasonable aircraft life. True, the gusts themselves produce loads of this magnitude and frequency, but as one cannot guarantee their presence to order, there appears to be an advantage in deliberately applying loads. Such a procedure would probably be used to reduce the risk of occasional compressive loads in causing premature catastrophic fatigue failure, rather than that a general improvement in life of aircraft should be attempted.

This paper covers only some of the many high loads cases of obvious importance; there is need for tests on other combinations of high load, both tensile and compressive, before the overall picture can be fully appreciated.

The author wishes to express his appreciation to the Chief Scientist, British Ministry of Supply, who has kindly given permission for this paper to be presented at the Colloquium, and also to his colleagues, particularly Mr. G. M. NORRIS, who have carried out most of the experimental work.

## Bibliography

[1] TEED, P. L.: Aeroplane **82**, 787 (1952).
[2] FORREST, G.: J. Inst. Metals **72**, 1—17 (1946); also: J. ROY. aeronaut. Soc. **58**, 261—276 (1954).
[3] ROSENTHAL, D., and G. SINES: Proc. ASTM **51**, 593—610 (1951) (Discussion by Templin).
[4] KERRY, F. A., J. NICHOLS and K. VINCENT: Saunders-Roe Ltd Rep. (England) SR/S/762 (1952).
[5] WALKER, P. B.: J. ROY. aeronaut. Soc., **57**, 12 (1953).

## Discussion

J. SCHIJVE: Tests on notched specimens performed at N.L.L. and described by PLANTEMA in his paper have a complementary character to the tests of HEYWOOD. The test results are in good agreement with the comprehensive results shown by HEYWOOD.

According to HEYWOOD the considerable increase of fatigue life should be attributed to the decrease of the mean stress, as the pre-stressing gives a residual stress distribution with a negative stress $- S_m$ in the root of the notch. In the fatigue test the stress amplitude will be $\pm k_t \cdot S_{\text{nom}}$. As soon as $(-S_m - k_t S_{\text{nom}})$ exceeds the compression yield stress, plastic yielding occurs and the effect is a raising of the mean stress towards zero.

In our tests the pre-stressing occurred at much lower stresses than HEYWOOD used. $(k_t \cdot S_{\text{pre}})$ was of the order of the yield stress. For riveted joints it turned out that one such load cycle did not strengthen the specimen, while a number of pre-stress load cycles did strengthen the specimen. Also simply notched specimens were considerably strengthened by a number of pre-stress load cycles. For both types of specimens the test stress was somewhat above the endurance limit $(N \approx 10^6)$. A reversal of stress gives a reversal of deformation. For the negative loading the deformation will not always occur on the same slip planes as for the positive loading. So an essential difference in strain hardening between a monotonous deformation and an alternating deformation may exist. From this point of view we explored the results of our tests.

In agreement with HEYWOOD's tests a considerable increase of the fatigue life is possible. It remains questionable whether the results of test programmes using such different orders of pre-stress can be explained in the same way.

R. B. HEYWOOD: The author is grateful to SCHIJVE for pointing out the qualitative agreement between PLANTEMA's and his own results as to the effect of high loads on fatigue. The suggestion advanced by SCHIJVE that behaviour is due to strain hardening is of considerable interest. With tensile or compressive pre-loads, it is of course conceivable that slip and therefore strain hardening would occur on different planes of crystals, but it seems improbable that the one should be extremely beneficial whereas the other should be extremely harmful. Moreover the tests on plain specimens reported in table 1 show that tensile strain hardening is actually harmful, but tests on notched specimens are found to benefit by tensile pre-loads. These opposite trends in behaviour suggest that another effect, namely the residual stress effect as reported in the paper, has a greater influence on behaviour than the strain hardening effect.

# Modifications de texture cristalline produites par des efforts alternés

Par

**R. Jacquesson**

Avec 5 figures

## Première partie

L'étude des perturbations cristallines apportées par un cycle, avec des charges très faibles suppose un moyen d'exploration très puissant: nous avons entrepris [1] des essais en utilisant la méthode de focalisation des Rayons X de Guinier-Thénevin qui permet d'apprécier des variations d'orientation cristalline de l'ordre de la minute d'angle, le matériau employé étant un monocristal d'Al raffiné (99,99) soumis à des tractions ondulées. Un cristal idéal parfait donnerait une raie de focalisation très fine, de largeur comparable à celle de la source linéaire de Rayons X. Toute désorientation dans le réseau se traduit par un élargissement de la raie obtenue; inversement on peut dire que toute diminution de la largeur indique que les plans réticulaires se rapprochent d'une orientation commune et, qu'à ce point de vue, le cristal devient plus parfait.

1. — Pendant la mise en charge, la tache de focalisation augmente de largeur progressivement. Il y a donc une désorganisation du cristal qui peut s'interpréter soit par des courbures du réseau cristallin, soit par la formation d'un très grand nombre de blocs très petits, d'orientation variant très peu d'un bloc à l'autre, tant que la déformation est très faible.

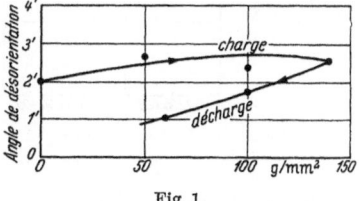

Fig. 1.

Pendant la décharge, la largeur des taches diminue et, pour une même déformation, est plus petite que pendant la mise en charge. Au retour à une charge nulle, le cristal parait plus parfait qu'au départ. C'est ce que la montre fig. 1.

2. — À la température des essais, une traction déclenche une restauration qui évolue spontanément, mais lentement avec le temps. Nous en donnerons deux exemples:

Un cristal d'aluminium a été intentionnellement tordu puis ramené à sa forme initiale. Il en est résulté une distorsion résiduelle de l'ordre de 2° qui s'est stabilisée. L'éprouvette a été ensuite soumise à des contraintes de 300 et 600 g/mm². Le fond d'astérisme ne change pas mais la partie très irradiée qui correspond à une désorganisation de 30' initialement diminue de largeur jusqu'à une désorganisation de 20'. L'éprouvette a été laissée au repos, sans charge, pendant 6 heures et la tache de focalisation a profondément changé d'aspect. Il s'est formé des blocs distincts de désorganisation réduite (12') bien visible sur un fond d'astérisme devenu très faible[1].

De nouveaux cycles de 0 à 600 g/mm² ont été appliqué et on observe une dispersion régulière des cristallites, le fond continu occupant la position qu'il avait dans l'éprouvette initiale.

Le deuxième exemple très curieux est au contraire relatif à un cristal initialement très peu désorienté: Un cristal de désorientation de 3' est chargé progressivement jusqu'à 400 g/mm². Corrélativement, on observe un élargissement des taches de focalisation. Déchargé et abandonné à lui-même pendant 6 heures, il ne donne plus qu'une raie de largeur voisine à 1'. Rechargé à nouveau jusqu'à 700 g/mm² il ne manifeste plus aucune désorganisation, les taches restant toujours aussi fines. Tout se passe comme si sa résistance mécanique était considérablement augmentée. Nous avons peut-être là un exemple très simple d'understressing et un aperçu du mécanisme de ce phénomène. C'est aussi un exemple qui

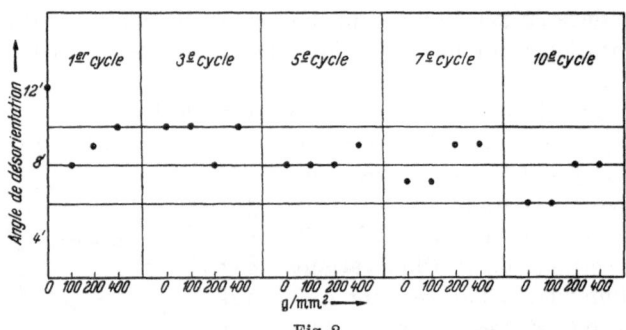

Fig. 2.

expliquerait le rôle bienfaisant des pauses sur la valeur de la limite d'endurance, quand ces pauses interviennent avant que le métal soit trop désorganisé par les alternances précédant cette période de repos.

Cette restauration est encore très sensible lorsque des cycles successifs d'efforts sont parcourus très lentement (fig. 2). Peut-être est-elle en partie la cause de la diminution des taches pendant la phase de la décharge qui,

---

[1] Les angles indiqués dans ce paragraphe mesurent les variations d'orientation des particules cristallines comprises dans le volume irradié par le faisceau X, soit dans 80 mm³ environ de métal.

par suite du temps nécessaire aux prises de clichés, survient assez long-temps après la mise en charge et est d'assez longue durée.

## Deuxième partie

Ces expériences montrent qu'une déformation faible peut déclencher une restauration spontanée qui, sans elle, ne se ferait pas à la température des essais, c'est-à-dire un retour du métal vers un état plus stable et, par suite, plus parfait. C'est ce qu'avaient déjà montré des mesures de capacité d'amortissement de fils préalablement tendus [2]. Des expérien-ces de natures diverses nous ayant montré qu'à tempéra-ture élevée des déformations pouvaient, non plus produire une simple restauration intra-granulaire, mais provoquer un grossissement des grains qui, sans elles, ne se manifesterait pas avec une même intensité, nous avons cherché à mettre ce phénomène en évidence sur des éprouvettes plates de fer soumises à des torsions alter-nées, dans une atmosphère neutre. Une bande de tôle

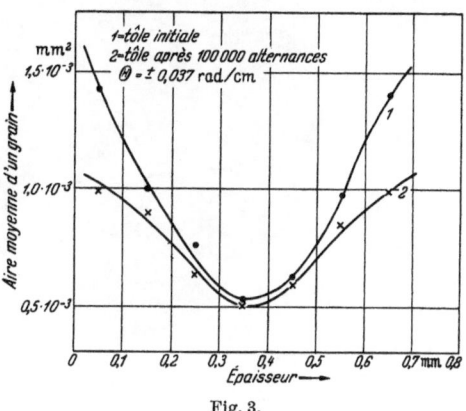

Fig. 3.

identique à celle travaillée était placée, comme témoin, à la même tempé-rature, pendant le même temps.

Je n'indiquerai que les résultats d'une seule série de mesures.[1] La tôle soumise à des efforts alternés avait été préalablement recuite 1 h à 925°C, donc parfaitement stabilisée. Un dénombrement des grains en fonction de l'épaisseur a donné la répartition figurée sur la courbe 1 de la fig. 3. Soumise à des contraintes $\tau = \pm 18$ kg/mm² à la température de 450°C, en atmosphère d'argon, elle a donné au bout de 100.000 alternances (c'est-à-dire après 22 minutes d'essai) la répartition de la courbe 2. Il y a donc un grossissement bien systématique du grain, d'autant plus grand que la contrainte qui croît avec la distance à l'axe est elle-même plus grande. Ce grossissement est bien marqué parce que les déformations à la surface sont largement dans la phase plastique. Il est faible pour des déformations ne dépassant pas la limite élastique. La fig. 4 montre des grains ayant considérablement grossis par rapport à ceux qui sont d'origine (Acier 18—8, 500°C, $10^5$ alternances, $\tau = 18$ kg/mm²).

On voit donc que ce phénomène de recristallisation peut avoir une certaine influence sur la tenue des métaux vibrant à des températures

---

[1] en collaboration avec M. DE FOUQUET.

élevées. On peut prévoir une suite de transformations cristallines en chaîne: une déformation un peu trop forte entraine immédiatement un grossissement du grain, d'où un adoucissement du métal qui, par suite,

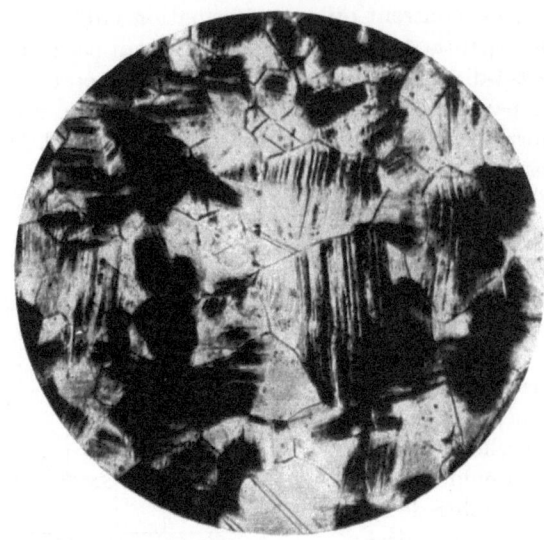

Fig. 4. × 350.

se déforme davantage, provoquant une recristallisation plus rapide, etc. . . ., d'où finalement une rupture assez brutale du métal.

Mais ce grossissement rapide des grains, quand ils sont en phase plastique, peut présenter un autre intérêt: c'est un phénomène général

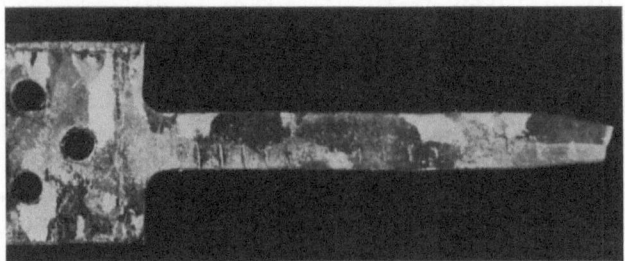

Fig. 5. × 0,8.

accompagnant une déformation plastique ayant absorbé une énergie suffisante, et recevant par unité de temps une puissance mécanique convenable: nous l'avons trouvé en effet en fin de déformation par étirement rapide de l'aluminium à 250°C et du fer et de l'acier au-dessus de 800° C, la transformation cristalline se faisant alors en des durées de l'ordre de la minute.

La macrophoto (fig. 5) à faible grossissement est celle d'une éprouvette d'aluminium initialement microcristallin, étirée en 2 minutes jusqu'à la rupture. On distingue de larges plages de structure paraissant homogène par les ondulations régulièrement disposées qui les parcourent et par leur aspect uniforme après attaque aux réactifs métallographiques. On constate, à grossissement plus élevé, un aspect tourmenté de la zone de séparation entre les plages.

La vitesse anormalement grande d'accroissement des grains à la température des expériences, le fait même que les grains grossissent dans une texture stabilisée à une température beaucoup plus élevée, l'aspect des joints entre plages différentes montrent que ce phénomène est profondément différent de celui qui nous sert pour préparer des monocristaux après un écrouissage critique. Dans cette méthode de préparation, on apporte au métal une énergie de déformation faible qui suffit à faire déclencher, à partir de «germes» d'énergie de déformation particulièrement élevée, la formation *lente* d'une texture étendue d'orientation totalement différente de celles des microcristaux initiaux.

Au contraire, le grossissement que nous considérons se produit pendant l'apport continuel d'énergie (cycles d'efforts ou énergie de déformation par traction).

Dans l'état actuel des recherches, nous ne savons pas s'il y a germination puis croissance, mais les observations semblent plutôt faire croire qu'il s'agirait d'une réorganisation intragranulaire se produisant dans quelques grains particulièrement travaillés et qui déborderait sur les grains contigus.

Nous sommes donc enclins à imaginer une sorte de transformation en chaîne finissant par atteindre une vitesse considérable pour la température mesurée du métal (très peu supérieure à celle du four où il est placé pour les essais de traction ou de déformation alternée). Cette transformation serait entretenue et activée par l'apport extérieur continuel d'énergie mécanique, et propagée sous l'influence de l'agitation thermique et de la diffusion des défauts de texture (dislocations, vacuoles plus ou moins importantes).

Une description mécanique des déplacements atomiques produits pendant cette transformation cristalline rapide est probablement impossible actuellement, mais on peut entrevoir un schéma thermodynamique simplifié. On peut supposer que dans un cristal (de masse unité par exemple), les perturbations de texture produites par une déformation plastique ne puissent se produire qu'en un nombre limité $N$ de positions distinctes ou plutôt d'éléments de volume très exigus. Ces zones de défauts réticulaires sont également des zones de concentration d'énergie, l'aspect cristallographique et l'aspect énergétique traduisant le même fait.

Un travail mécanique $\Delta W$ apporté au cristal pendant une phase de déformation plastique $\Delta x$ se décompose en $n$ fractions que nous supposerons de valeur égale $w$, (on a $\Delta W = n\,w$) qui vont se fixer au hasard dans les $N$ positions possibles, les unes dans des positions encore non occupées, les autres dans des positions déja pourvues d'un nombre entier de ces éléments d'énergie.

Pour que l'un de ces points d'accumulation, d'énergie additionelle $pw$, devienne instable, il faut, comme on l'admet généralement, que son énergie totale soit supérieure à une certaine valeur.

Le retour à l'état stable de l'un de ces points s'accompagnera d'une libération d'énergie et, corrélativement, d'une évacuation par diffusion des défauts qui arriveront dans les centres d'accumulation voisins, lesquels continuent par ailleurs à être alimentés en grains d'énergie $W$ du fait que la déformation se poursuit. Ce double apport d'énergie va amener ces centres en état d'instabilité et le processus va s'amplifier si les régions envahies sont déjà proches du point de saturation en élément $w$.

Il semble intuitif de prévoir qu'un tel mécanisme étant déclenché, il ne s'arrêtera pas aux joints de grains si son énergie est suffisante. D'autre part, la texture restante après le passage de cette avalanche sera relativement stable tant que les apports d'énergie extérieurs ne l'auront pas à nouveau mis en état d'évolution rapide. Ce sera une texture qui pourra paraître homogène macroscopiquement, mais qui, par suite de la rapidité du phénomène, présentera de grosses variations locales.

Une théorie thermodynamique, encore bien schématique, permet cependant de retrouver certaines particularités du phénomène.

Partons d'un métal en équilibre thermodynamique dont l'énergie libre $F_0$ est par suite minima. Parvenu à un certain stade de la déformation, nous lui avons fourni une énergie $W$ mécanique d'une manière quelconque. L'accroissement d'énergie libre est:

$$F_1 = W - T\,S$$

$S$ étant la variation d'entropie qui peut être calculée à partir de la formule de Boltzmann

$$S = k \log p$$

$p$ étant le nombre de distribution discernables.

Or nous avons à disposer $n$ particules d'énergie $\left(n = \dfrac{W}{w}\right)$ dans $N$ positions distinctes. Une formule classique donne le nombre $p$ désiré:

$$p = \frac{(n + N - 1)!}{n!\,(N - 1)!}$$

d'ou:

$$S = k \log \frac{(n + N - 1)!}{n!\,(N - 1)!}$$

et en employant la formule de Stirling et négligeant l'unité devant $N$:

$$S = k\,[(n + N) \log (n + N) - n \log n - N \log N]$$

D'où pour l'énergie libre ($F_0 =$ énergie libre initiale)

$$F = F_1 + F_0$$
$$F = W - TS + F_0$$
$$= nw - kT\,[(n + N) \log (n + N) - n \log n - N \log N] + F_0$$

dont la dérivée par rapport à $n$ s'écrit:

$$\frac{\mathrm{d}F}{\mathrm{d}n} = w - kT \log \frac{n + N}{n}$$

Cette dérivée est négative pour $n$ petit (log $\dfrac{n + N}{n}$ étant grand) et est positive si $n$ est grand, la limite du logarithme étant nulle.

L'énergie libre diminue donc par apport d'une faible énergie $nw$, passe par un minimum pour $n = n_s$ et devient positive. A partir de ce moment le métal devient instable et tend à évoluer spontanément. La valeur seuil $W_s$ a pour valeur:

$$W_s = wn_s = \frac{N\,w}{e^{\frac{w}{kT}} - 1}$$

Si on admet une valeur constante pour $w$ quelle que soit la température — ce qui n'est pas certain — on voit que $W_s$ est d'autant plus petit que $T$ est plus faible. Mais intervient la rapidité de diffusion des défauts. À une température trop basse, la migration est presque nulle et le métal reste en état métastable. Supposons donc la température suffisamment élevée et précisons, autant que possible, les conditions pour que l'avalanche se produise. Il est clair que si, à partir du seuil $W_s$, le métal ne reçoit plus d'apport d'énergie mécanique de l'extérieur, les évolutions de la texture vont faire diminuer l'énergie libre et le phénomène s'arrêtera. Il en sera autrement si le métal reçoit par unité de temps autant et, a fortiori, plus d'énergie que n'en dissipent ces évolutions.

La distribution des $n$ particules élémentaires en $N$ positions distinctes étant faite au hasard, les positions sont garnies de 0, 1, 2 . . . . . ou $p$ de ces particules. Supposons, en négligeant l'énergie thermique dans ces calculs élémentaires, que les régions d'accumulations sont susceptibles d'évoluer quand l'énergie mécanique emmagasinée devient égale à $pw$, cette quantité jouant le rôle de «chaleur d'activation». Nous savons que le nombre $N'$ de ces régions d'énergie potentielle égale ou supérieure à $pw$ est égale à:

$$N' = N\,e^{-\frac{p\,w}{k\,T}}$$

Leur évolution vers un état plus stable va libérer par seconde $q$ éléments d'énergie $w$ dont une fraction $\alpha q$ se dissipera probablement par ondes thermiques alors que, sous forme de défauts diffusant dans la masse, les $q\,(1-\alpha)$ éléments restants iront alimenter les centres voisins. On peut poser, comme il est usuel de le faire, que $q$ est proportionnel au nombre de centres évoluant. L'énergie dissipée sous forme d'ondes thermiques est donc, par seconde:

$$\alpha\,q = \alpha\,AN' = \alpha\,ANe^{-\frac{p\,w}{k\,T}}$$

Pour que la transformation ne s'éteigne pas, il faut donc fournir au métal une puissance mécanique égale ou supérieure à $w\alpha q$

$$W_1 \geq w\,\alpha\,ANe^{-\frac{p\,w}{k\,T}}$$

Si on opère par traction

$$W = f\frac{\mathrm{d}\,l}{\mathrm{d}\,t} = f\,V$$

($V$ vitesse d'étirement, $f$ force fournie) et par cycle

$$W_1 = m \cdot \text{fréquence} = m \cdot v$$

$m$ étant le travail mécanique absorbé par cycle. On voit donc qu'il y a un *seuil* de travail à fournir par unité de temps pour que les phénomènes étudiés se produisent. C'est bien ce que paraissent donner nos premiers essais.

En définitive, nous supposons une analogie entre l'apport de «quanta» d'énergie mécanique $W$ et l'apport, jusqu'ici envisagé uniquement, de quanta d'énergie sous forme thermique. Dans cet exposé, notre attention a été surtout portée vers l'aspect cristallographique mis en évidence par des grossissements de grains, mais la théorie peut être beaucoup plus générale: si l'apport d'énergie mécanique joue le rôle équivalent a l'énergie thermique, des transformations quelconques, accélérées par une augmentation de température, auront lieu à température plus basse quand elles se feront pendant une déformation, à condition que les seuils que nous avons mis en évidence soient dépassés et que la température soit cependant suffisante pour la propagation du phénomène.

## Bibliographie

[1] Caisso, J.: Dr. diss., Poitiers 1955.
[2] Jacquesson, R.: Dr. diss., Paris 1943.

## Discussion

R. Cazaud: Autrefois, avant même que l'on eut fait des observations micrographiques sur le phénomène de la fatigue, on avait supposé, d'après l'observation de cassures de pieces rompues en service que la fatigue cristallisait l'acier et le rendait fragile. Les observations que nous apporte M. Jacquesson montrent que pour l'aluminium ordinaire, cette idée n'aurait pas été absolument fausse et il faut féliciter M. JACQUESSON d'avoir montré à l'aide de la radiocristallographie que les phénomènes obeissent à des schémas très simples.

P. LAURENT: L'étude de M. JACQUESSON fait apparaître les modifications qui se produisent dans un métal quand on inverse le sens de la déformation et le caractère fondamental de ces essais est incontestable; toutefois l'extrapolation aux phénomènes de fatigue doit, à mon avis, n'être faite qu'avec prudence car il a été montré, dans le cas de Al et $Fe_\alpha$, notamment, que le mécanisme de la déformation lors de cycles parcourus lentement comme l'a fait M. JACQUESSON dans la 1. partie de son étude n'était pas le même que pour des cycles parcourus aux vitesses usuelles des essais de fatigue.

L. LOCATI demande si l'on a mésuré la progression, dans le temps, de la diminution de largeur de la tache qu'on a observé après six heures.

R. JACQUESSON: La diminution spontanée de la largeur des taches se fait progressivement dans le temps, d'abord très rapidement puis très lentement. Des mesures précises ne sont pas possibles: Les bords sont trop flous s'il s'agit de taches étendues et quand les bords restent à peu près nets, la largeur de la tache est faible et ses variations peu accessibles. Il serait intéressant cependant de pouvoir trouver une loi d'évolution de la texture, mais les nombres obtenus laisseraient dans la détermination de cette loi trop d'arbitraire.

# Fatigue of steels at constant strain amplitude and elevated temperature

By

## A. Johansson

With 10 figures

## 1. Introduction

From an engineering point of view fatigue at elevated temperatures is of importance under two rather different conditions. One involves vibration stresses or other high frequency stresses generally superimposed on a fairly steady mean stress. This is the type of fatigue which may occur for instance in a vibrating gas turbine blade. The complications compared with fatigue at ordinary temperatures are the influence of the temperature and of a time factor. The time has some influence already for zero mean stress as the fatigue strength to some extent depends on the frequency, i. e. on the total testing time. With increased mean stress in relation to the alternating stress the time becomes more and more important until creep alone determines the strength.

Another type of fatigue of importance for service at elevated temperatures is caused by a limited number of stress cycles of high amplitude. The high stresses are repeated only at intervals, for instance each time a high temperature machinery is started. This type of fatigue is therefore generally connected with heat shocks and the stresses are caused by uneven temperature distribution and thermal expansion. Thin sections are heated faster than thicker sections and restrictions in the heat flow may cause steep temperature gradients. Sectional changes, causing such restrictions in the heat flow are very often at the same time stress raisers due to their geometrical form. The natural stress concentration at such points is therefore still more pronounced when combined with temperature gradients. Local plastic flow may occur already at low general stress levels. It is not always possible to avoid such stress raisers in the design of high temperature machinery and it is therefore important to know the stresses or strains which may be allowed for a limitid number of cycles without risk for fatigue fracture. For this type of fatigue therefore another part of the endurance diagram is of interest than when designing with regard to high frequency fatigue and endurance limit.

## 2. Testing method

A number of different testing methods has been used for the testing of different materials at conditions corresponding to this second type of fatigue at elevated temperature. As mentioned above the high stress or strain peaks are generally combined with temperature shocks. Most of the previous testing therefore was carried out in apparatus designed to give such heat and stress shocks. The test results have been valuable for a comparison of different materials under specific test conditions but the actual variations in stress, strain and temperature have often been very complicated and therefore insufficiently known. In the literature there are however descriptions of some arrangements which allow a good control of these factors.

It was considered desirable to separate the different variables as far as possible without complicating the testing equipment too much. The fatigue testing machine was therefore designed for constant temperature and constant strain amplitude during each test. When testing in the plastic region a constant strain amplitude gives much more stable conditions than for instance a constant stress amplitude or a constant bending moment. It should also be pointed out that if the loading is caused by thermal expansions and uneven temperature distribution the result is a certain change in total strain more than a certain stress.

If the total strain amplitude is kept constant the relation between the elastic and plastic strain amplitude will change during the test. In order to follow this change it is necessary to measure the force needed to give the strain amplitude and to follow the variation of this force during the test. This variation is caused by a number of factors including strain hardening, Bauschinger effect, creep and metallurgical changes at elevated temperatures. Obviously also the growth of cracks changes the force amplitude.

In order to obtain some information about the influence of creep the maximum strain is kept constant for a great part of each period and the relaxation is measured.

## 3. Machine design

Fig. 1 shows the principle of the machine. A round conical test piece is fixed at its lower end to the frame of the machine. The upper end of the specimen is connected to a rod. The other end of this rod is coupled to an air servo motor. The movement of the rod is limited by two adjustable stops. The position of these stops thus determines the amplitude of the upper end of the test specimen.

The force required to bend the test pieces between the two limit positions is measured with the strain gauge dynamometer which is a part of the rod. The end of the apparatus containing the test specimens is placed in the furnace but all measuring and regulating devices are placed outside the furnace at sufficient distance to avoid disturbance from the temperature in the furnace.

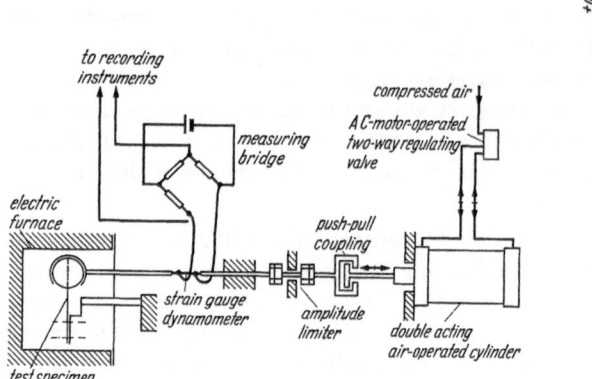

Fig. 1. Schematic diagram of test apparatus.          Fig. 2. Test specimen.

The air valve of the servo motor is controlled by a cam which is turned by a gear motor at a speed of 0.5 r/min.

Fig. 2 shows the test specimen. As usual a conical test length is used in order to get a uniform strain and stress distribution near the section with the highest stress.

Three specimens are tested simultaneously. The temperature is controlled with thermocouples. The strain amplitude is the same for all three specimens, but the load may be different and can be measured separately for each specimen.

The working of the machine is as follows. The end with the test specimens is placed in the furnace and heated to the testing temperature

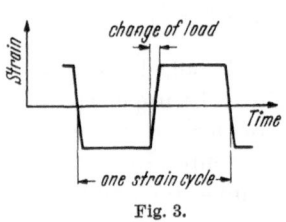

Fig. 3.

without load on the specimens. The stops on the connecting rod are adjusted to the desired amplitude. The motor driving the cam is started and air is admitted to the valve of the servo motor. The air valve alternatively admits air to the two sides of the piston. The speed of the piston when moving from one position to the other can be varied between wide limits by changing the throttling in the air pipes. The movement of the piston is in principle as shown in fig. 3. This therefore also represents the change in strain in the test specimens. The force or stress diagram may be somewhat different due to relaxation during the constant strain periods.

## 4. Test material

Test results are given for three different steels. They are an austenitic 18/8 chromium-nickel steel, a 13% chromium steel and a low alloy chromium-molybdenum steel with 3% Cr, 0.4% Mo. The analysis is given in table 1. The type of steel and their properties differ and it was

*Table 1*

|  | 18-8 Cr-Ni steel A | 18-8 Cr-Ni steel B | 13% Cr steel A | Cr-Mo steel A; B |
|---|---|---|---|---|
| C % | 0.08 | 0.10 | 0.17 | 0.25 |
| Si % | 0.17 | 0.15 | 0.24 | 0.35 |
| Mn % | 0.46 | 0.58 | 0.32 | 0.59 |
| P % | 0.032 | 0.031 | 0.026 | — |
| S % | 0.016 | 0.016 | 0.018 | — |
| Cr % | 17.48 | 17.95 | 13.8 | 2.98 |
| Ni % | 8.75 | 7.95 | 0.26 | 0.40 |
| Mo % | — | — | — | 0.39 |

hoped that a comparison might indicate common influences caused by the fatigue testing.

The mechanical properties at room temperature are given in table 2.

*Table 2*

| Test material | | Yield point kg/mm² | Tensile strength kg/mm² | Reduction of area per cent | Elongation L = 5d per cent | Impact resistance kgm/cm² Charpy |
|---|---|---|---|---|---|---|
| 18-8 Cr-Ni steel; A, | 20° C | 24.1 | 76.3 | 74.3 | 74.8 | 17.9 |
| 18-8 Cr-Ni steel; B, | 20° C | 27.2 | 71.8 | 80.8 | 79.2 | 19.2 |
|  | 300° C | 14.8 | 53.0 | 70.5 | 47.4 | — |
|  | 500° C | 14.5 | 49.4 | 65.7 | 44.8 | — |
| 13% Cr steel; A, | 20° C | 35.7 | 53.8 | 70.8 | 33.2 | 9.75 |
| Cr-Mo steel; A, | 20° C | 64.5 | 79.3 | 75.2 | 22.4 | 17.7 |
| Cr-Mo steel; B, | 20° C | 70.75 | 85.5 | 73.7 | 20.5 | 16.6 |
|  | 300° C | 62.1 | 75.5 | 70.7 | 18.2 | — |
|  | 500° C | 51.1 | 54.9 | 81.7 | 21.0 | — |

Figures from short time tensile tests on the austenitic 18/8 steel and the low alloy steel at 300 and 500° C are also included in the table.

8*

## 5. Discussion of test results

Tests were made at 20, 300 and 500° C. Each steel was tested at four strain levels at each temperature, generally at 2, 4, 6 and 7.5 mm deformation amplitude, corresponding to 0.51, 1.02, 1.52 and 1.91% maximum strain amplitude. As already mentioned the specimens were tested in reversed plane bending with zero mean stress.

Fig. 4 shows the results of the tests on the 18/8 Cr-Ni steel. The number of cycles for fracture at each temperature is given as a function

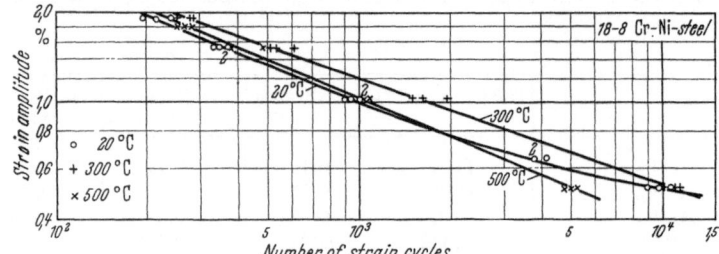

Fig. 4. Variation of cycles to failure with strain amplitude. 18/8 Cr-Ni-steel.

of the strain amplitude. Each point in the diagram represents a single test. Generally three tests were made at each temperature and each strain amplitude. The scatter between tests run at identical conditions is small and check tests made after long intervals have confirmed that the reproducibility is good. As a rule, however, the standard deviation

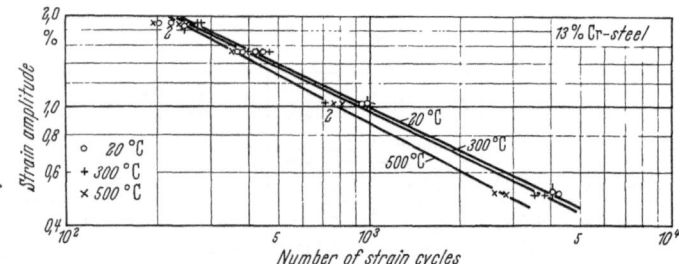

Fig. 5. Variation of cycles to failure with strain amplitude. 13% Cr-steel.

is reduced when the stress level is increased in fatigue tests and it is therefore natural that the scatter should be small in these tests.

The difference between the three temperatures is not very great. The 300° line falls somewhat above the 20° and 500° lines.

Fig. 5 is the corresponding diagram for the 13% Cr steel. In this case the difference between the different temperatures is still smaller than for the 18/8 steel.

The results for the Cr-Mo steel are shown in fig. 6. Here the tests at 500° C show considerably lower strength than those at 20° and 300° C. This steel, however, scaled very much during the tests at 500° C. The brittle scale cracked during the continuously repeated deformation of the test piece. The cracks in the scale no doubt acted as notches and this may be one reason for the low fatigue strength in this case. The metallographic examination of the broken test pieces also showed a general oxidation of the fatigue cracks. They had the general appearance of corrosion fatigue cracks.

The test results for the three materials may also be compared at each temperature. At 20° C there is little difference between the steels.

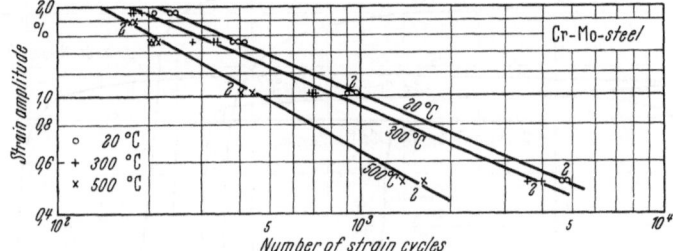

Fig. 6. Variation of cycles to failure with strain amplitude. 3 °/₀ Cr, 0.4 °/₀ Mo-steel.

The curve for the 18/8 Cr-Ni-steel at this temperature is an exception with regard to its form. The tests on 18/8 at other temperatures and all tests on other materials fall on straight lines when plotted in the log strain amplitude versus log cycles for failure diagram. 18/8 steel at 20° C however gives a line which is slightly curved corresponding to increased number of cycles for failure at low amplitudes. An explanation for this difference has not been found.

The fatigue limit for steels tested in air at room temperature increases with increased tensile strength approximately in direct proportion. This is obviously not the case for fatigue at high strain amplitudes.

The curves at room temperature may be compared with the ordinary tensile properties in table 2. The yield points vary from about 25 to 70 kg/mm² and the tensile strength from 54 to 85 kg/mm². In spite of these wide differences the fatigue strength in the range covered by the tests is very near the same.

Similar results are reported in the literature. GROSS and STOUT [4] have tested a number of pressure vessel steels in bending at constant strain amplitudes and show in diagrams the relative strain ranges which give fracture in 5,000, 20,000 and 100,000 cycles. In this connection the results at 5,000 cycles are of most interest. An increase of tensile strength

from 42 to 91 kg/mm² and of yield point from 27 to 86 kg/mm² did not
increase the allowable strain amplitude for a fatigue life of 5,000 cycles.
Actually there is instead some reduction in fatigue life with increased
tensile strength. This result was obtained both for smooth test pieces and
for notched as well as for welded test pieces. Tests on two materials at
343° C showed the same tendency. The material in this investigation is
more limited but also more varied and seems to confirm that the allowable strain range for failure after a given number of strain cycles is fairly

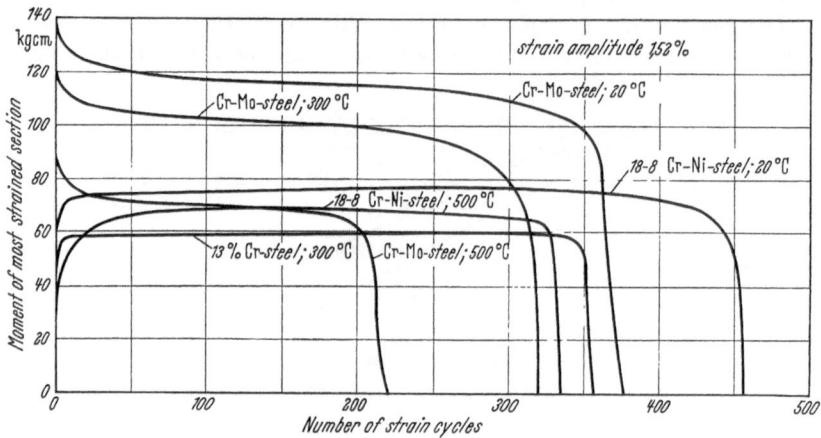

Fig. 7. Variation of load with number of strain cycles.

independent of the tensile strength and does not vary much with temperature if increased scaling does not occur.

It was pointed out that the differences between the tensile properties
of the materials at room temperature are not reflected in the number
of cycles for fatigue at a given strain amplitude. A comparison of the
elastic forces during the testing is therefore of interest. Fig. 7 is a summary of some of the force measurements given as bending moment in
the most strained section of the test piece. The strain amplitude is
1.52% for all tests in the diagram. It is obvious that both the magnitude
of the elastic forces and their variation during the test is very different
for different materials and temperatures. In the 18/8 Cr-Ni steel the
strain hardening dominates and the originally low moment is soon
increased considerably to a value which is fairly constant until it begins
to fall due to the formation of cracks. The 13% Cr steel follows a similar
curve but with less pronounced strain hardening. The Cr-Mo steel on the
other hand shows an opposite behaviour. The originally high bending
moment during the first cycles falls off but it still remains high compared
with the two other materials. Anyhow the differences between the

actual stresses during the fatigue test are not as big as the differences between their yield points. It should be pointed out that in fig. 7 the scale for the number of cycles is linear. In a logarithmic scale as in other diagrams the end points of the curves are not very different.

Fig. 8 shows the relaxation which takes place during the constant strain part of the cycle. It is of course different for different materials and temperatures, but in some cases it has been quite appreciable. The influence of a considerable high temperature creep is therefore included in some of the test results.

The present tests are not sufficient to show if this creep has any significant influence apart from the increase of the plastic portion of the total strain. At high strain amplitudes, where the plastic deformation dominates, this influence should be small. The low frequency of the tests reported here seems to have given a lower number of cycles for failure than some other similar tests. A few tests with varying frequency have indicated lowered strength at low frequency [1], [4]. This reduction is however not limited to high temperatures and it is therefore probable that other factors than creep are the reason.

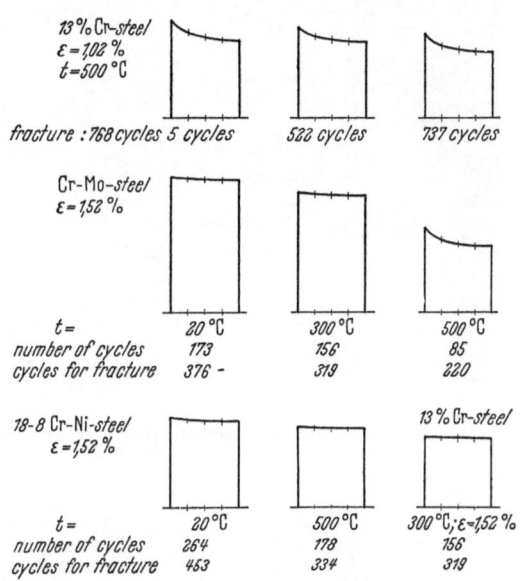

Fig. 8.

Load variation and relaxation during constant strain period.

## 6. Metallographic observations

One or two metallographic observations seem to be of a more general interest.

The first refers to structural changes in 18/8 Cr-Ni steel during tests at 500° C. The steel is not stabilized with columbium or titanium against carbide precipitation. Sections through broken test pieces showed a very great increase in the precipitation at grain boundaries when going from the neutral axis in the center to the strained surfaces. The difference can be seen in fig. 9. This shows very definitely the great influence of repeated straining on the precipitation of carbides at the grain boundaries.

A. JOHANSSON

It may be expected that also other metallurgical changes are accelerated by repeated straining in particular at high temperatures.

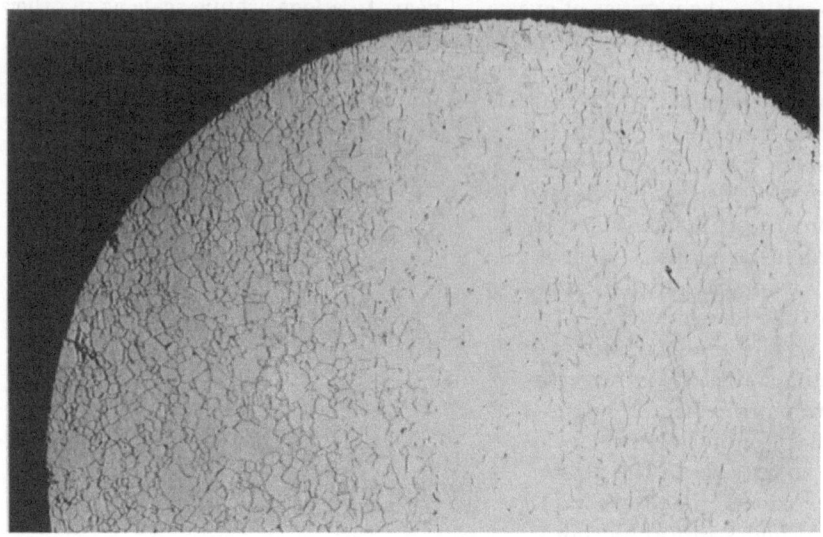

Fig. 9. Acceleration of carbide precipitation due to repeated straining. 18/8 Cr-Ni-steel. 500° C. Strain amplitude ± 1 %. × 30.

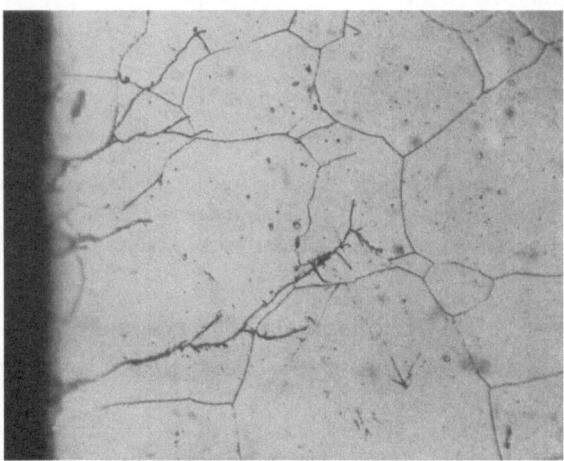

Fig. 10. Fatigue cracks in 18/8 Cr-Ni-steel. 500° C. Strain amplitude ± 1 %. × 300.

The precipitation at the grain boundaries has not caused inter-granular cracking. Fig. 10 shows the typical transgranular path of the fatigue cracks.

Another observation is that the cracks formed at high strain amplitudes have a tendency to become branched. This may occur already at room temperature, but it is particularly the case at higher temperatures.

There is also a tendency for the number of small cracks at the surface to increase at increased temperature.

## 7. Conclusions

The following conclusions seem to be allowed for fatigue in the plastic range and the temperatures covered by the tests.

a) The strain amplitude largely determines the number of cycles for failure. The allowable strain amplitude for a given life is not very different for materials with widely varying tensile properties and in particular it does not follow the tensile strength or yield point.

b) The number of cycles for failure at a certain strain amplitude is about the same from room temperature and up to 500° C if the scaling resistance is sufficient at the higher temperatures. It must be taken into account that the scaling at repeated plastic deformation may be considerable more severe than at static conditions.

c) For a given total strain amplitude the elastic stresses during fatigue may be very different and yet the number of cycles for failure be about the same.

d) With increased temperature there is a tendency for the cracks to become branched.

e) Repeated straining accelerated the carbide precipitation at the grain boundaries when 18/8 Cr-Ni steel was tested at 500° C.

This investigation was made in the Laboratory of the STAL Steam Turbine Company, Finspong, Sweden. Most of the testing and design work was carried out by L.-E. KARLSSON and the author wishes to thank him and other members of the laboratory staff.

### Bibliography

[1] COFFIN JR., L. F.: ASME Ann. Meet. New York, Pap. 53-A-76 (1953).
[2] COFFIN JR., L. F.: ASTM spec. techn. Publ. 165, 31 (1954).
[3] TÖR, S. S., J. M. RUZEK and R. D. STOUT: Weld. J. Res. Suppl. 31, 238—246 (1952).
[4] GROSS, J. H. and R. D. STOUT: Weld. J. Res. Suppl. 34, 161 (1955).
[5] OROWAN, E.: Weld. J. Res. Suppl. 31, 273—282 (1952).
[6] THIELSCH, H.: Weld. Res. Council Bull. 10 (1952).

## Discussion

I. ODING pointed out that plastic strain may be very ununiformly distributed across the gauge length of a test piece.

A. JOHANSSON: Local strain measurements with electric resistance strain gauges of gauge length 6.3 and 3.2 mm, respectively, revealed no such inhomogeneities. The tests were made in bending and therefore the conditions are favourable with regard to uniform strain.

C. E. PHILLIPS: Would the same results have been obtained with rectangular test pieces ?

A. JOHANSSON: Yes, such tests have also been made and have given consistent results.

R. E. PETERSON: Some tests of the kind described by the author were made by TRUMPLER of Westinghouse. A typical diagram is shown in the accompanying figure, the ordinate being strain amplitude in per cent of cold yield strain.

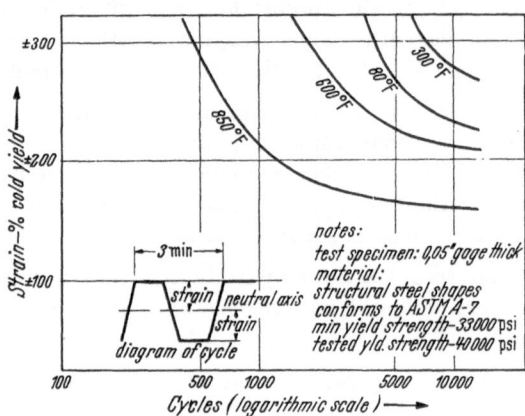

# Une définition theorique de la limite de fatigue

Par

## A. Kammerer

L'étude expérimentale des propriétés mécaniques des matières dites «plastiques» montre qu'elles ne sont pas «élastiques» au sens que l'on donne à ce mot en général:

a) il existe un frottement intérieur ayant les caractéristiques de la viscosité; en effet, la déformation limite d'un solide soumis à un système de charges fixes, n'est atteinte qu'au bout d'un temps théoriquement infini (fluage); de même, après suppression des forces, ce solide reprend sa forme et ses dimensions initiales après un temps théoriquement infini (relaxation);

b) la déformation limite pour un système de charge donné, n'est pas proportionnelle aux forces: elle croît plus rapidement; la loi de Hooke n'est donc pas vérifiée.

On peut compléter les équations classiques de l'élasticité par des termes correspondant à la viscosité et rendre compte ainsi des résultats expérimentaux, déformation instantanée, fluage, relaxation, variation de la limite du domaine élastique avec la vitesse de mise en charge . . . .

Dans cette note, nous négligerons la viscosité, c'est-à-dire que nous considérerons qu'elle est suffisamment faible pour que l'on puisse admettre qu'à chaque instant la déformation réelle est sensiblement égale à la déformation limite correspondant à la valeur que prennent les forces appliquées à cet instant. Nous indiquerons sommairement à la fin de cette note «l'influence de la viscosité».

Les relations entre les contraintes et les éléments de la déformation peuvent être établies à partir du potentiel élastique $U$ dont nous admettons l'existence puisque nous négligeons la viscosité.

Nous noterons: $c^{ij}$ les six composantes du tenseur des contraintes par rapport à trois axes rectilignes orthogonaux (les contraintes normales correspondent à $i=j$, les cisaillements, à $i \neq j$), $e^{ij}$ celles du tenseur des déformations ($e^{ii}$ sont les allongements unitaires et $2e^{ij}$ les glissements ou distorsions); les indices $i$ et $j$ prennent les valeurs 1, 2, 3; d'autre part:

$$e^{ij} = e^{ji} \qquad\qquad c^{ij} = c^{ji}$$

Le potentiel $U$, fonction des six variables $e^{ij}$, étant développé en série, le terme constant peut être considéré comme nul; les termes du premier ordre le sont également, si les tenseurs des contraintes et des déformations s'annulent en même temps; les termes du second degré correspondent à la loi de Hooke suivant laquelle on considère comme négligeables les termes de degré supérieur à deux.

Une approximation meilleure consiste à conserver les termes du troisième degré. En tenant compte de l'isotropie et des relations

$$c^{ij} = \frac{\partial U}{\partial e^{ij}}$$

on est amené à considérer en plus des coefficients classiques $E$ (module d'Young) et $\nu$ (coefficient de Poisson), trois autres coefficients $a_1 a_2 a_3$ caractérisant la matière au point de vue mécanique.

Nous nous limiterons, pour l'instant, aux systèmes élastiques uniformes dans lesquels le tenseur des contraintes est identique en chaque point; les axes de coordonnées $ox^i$ étant dirigés suivant les contraintes principales $c^i$, on a

$$c^{ij} = 0 \text{ pour } i \neq j$$

$$c^{ii} = c^i = f^i (e^i \, e^j \, e^l) = \frac{E\,[(1-2\nu)\,e^i + \nu\,\Theta]}{(1+\nu)\,(1-2\nu)} + (a_2 - a_1)\,(e^i)^2 -$$

$$- a_2\,(\Theta)^2 + (2a_2 - a_3)\cdot\frac{e^1\,e^2\,e^3}{e^i} \tag{1}$$

$\Theta = \sum e^i$ étant la dilatation cubique, $e^i$ les allongements principaux $(i = 1, 2, 3)$.

Les relations (1) différentiées conduisent à

$$\mathrm{d}\,c^i = \sum_j \frac{\partial c^i}{\partial e^j}\,\mathrm{d}\,e^j \tag{2}$$

pour $j = i$

$$\frac{\partial c^i}{\partial e^i} = \frac{E\,(1-\nu)}{(1+\nu)\,(1-2\nu)} - 2a_1\,e^i - 2a_2\,(e^j + e^l)$$

pour $j \neq i$ avec $l \neq j$, $l \neq i$:

$$\frac{\partial c^i}{\partial e^j} = \frac{E\,\nu}{(1+\nu)\,(1-2\nu)} - 2a_2\,(e^i + e^j) - a^3\,e^l$$

On en déduit facilement le Jacobien:

$$\triangle = \left| \frac{\partial c^i}{\partial e^j} \right| \quad (i, j = 1, 2, 3,)$$

On peut tirer des relations (2) les expressions inverses donnant les $\mathrm{d}e^i$ en fonction des $\mathrm{d}c^j$; elles seront de la forme

$$\mathrm{d}e^{\,i} = \frac{\sum_j A_i^j\,\mathrm{d}c^j}{\triangle}$$

les $A_j^i$ étant des fonctions du second degré des $e^1\,e^2\,e^3$.

Pour un état élastique uniforme, caractérisé par les trois allongements principaux $e^1$ $e^2$ $e^3$ et les trois contraintes principales que l'on en déduit par les relations (1), le *module d'élasticité instantané* $E^i$ suivant la direction $ox^i$ est défini par le rapport de la variation infiniment petite $dc^i$ de la contrainte principale $c^i$ à la variation correspondante $de^i$ de l'allongement principal $e^i$ les contraintes $c^j$ et $c^l$ étant maintenus constantes:

$$E^i = \left(\frac{dc^i}{de^i}\right)_i = \frac{\triangle}{A^i_i} = \frac{\triangle}{\frac{\partial c^j}{\partial e^j} \cdot \frac{\partial c^l}{\partial e^l} - \frac{\partial c^j}{\partial e^l} \cdot \frac{\partial c^l}{\partial e^j}} \tag{3}$$

Pour $e^i = c^i = 0$ (état initial) $E^i$ se reduit bien à $E$ quel que soit $i$.

Par contre, lorsque les $e^i$ et, parsuite, les $c^i$, sont différents de zéro, les trois modules $E^i$ ont, en général, des valeurs différentes, de telle sorte que le solide est devenu anisotrope pour les propriétés élastiques; ce résultat est en accord avec la biréfringence optique des matières transparentes sous contraintes.

Remarques. a) Ces résultats ont été établis en ne considérant que les termes du premier et du second degrés dans les expressions des contraintes; on vérifie très facilement qu'ils restent vrais quelles que soient les fonctions $c^i = f^i$ $(e^i \, e^j \, e^l)$ pourvu que ces fonctions soient symétriques par rapport aux variables $e^j \, e^l$:

$$f^i\left(e^i e^j e^l\right) = f^i\left(e^i e^l e^j\right) \tag{4}$$

cette symétrie traduisant l'isotropie initiale du solide libre.

b) Si les trois allongements principaux $e^i$ sont égaux, la matière reste isotrope, car les modules $E^i$ ont alors une valeur commune d'ailleurs différente de $E$ et calculable par (3) dans laquelle on écrit $e^1 = e^2 = e^3$.

Il en est ainsi lorsque le solide subit une variation de température provoquant une dilatation, telle que les trois allongements unitaires $e^i$ sont égaux; l'expérience confirme bien la variation du module d'élasticité sous l'action d'une variation de température.

c) Lorsque les coefficients $a_1$ $a_2$ $a_3$ satisfont aux relations

$$a_2 = a_1 \quad 2a_1 = a_3$$

les termes du second ordre dans (1) ne dépendent que de $\Theta$; il en est de même pour les dérivés $\partial c^i / \partial e^j$ et par suite des modules $E^i$. Le solide reste donc isotrope dans ce cas. L'expérience montre que certaines matières plastiques transparentes ne présentent sous charge qu'une biréfringence optique extrêmement faible.

Considérons un état élastique, $c^i$, $e^i$, pour lequel l'un des modules principaux $E^j$ s'annule: à une augmentation infiniment petite $dc^j$ de la contrainte principale $c^j$ correspondra une augmentation infiniment grande de l'allongement principal $e^j$ puisque $E^j = (dc^j/de^j)_j$ est nul; cet état correspond donc à une instabilité de l'équilibre élastique; cette instabilité définit la limite du domaine de stabilité qui contient l'origine.

Or, les relations (3) montrent que les trois modules $E^j$ s'annulent avec $\triangle$; l'équation

$$\triangle (e^1 e^2 e^3) = 0 \tag{5}$$

représente donc, dans le système de coordonnées $e^i$, la surface $S$ limitant le volume où l'état élastique est stable et réversible; le point figuratif de cet état $(e^i)$ ne peut franchir la surface $S$ où les déformations augmentent indéfiniment pour une variation infiniment petite des contraintes.

La surface $S$ coupe la droite $D$ d'équation:

$$e^1 = e^2 = e^3$$

en deux points de coordonnées:

$$\frac{E}{(1 + v)(2 a_1 - a_3)} \text{ et } \frac{E}{2(1 - 2v) \cdot (a_1 + 6 a_2 + a_3)}$$

Le premier, $F$, est un point singulier tel, que toutes les sections de $S$ par des plans contenant la droite $D$, présentent en $F$ un point de rebroussement de tangente $D$.

En éliminant les $e^i$ entre les équations (1) et (5), on formera l'équation de la surface $S'$ transformée de $S$ dans le système de coordonnées des $c^i$.

Il existe sur la droite $D'$ d'équation $c^1 = c^2 = c^3$ un point $F'$ ayant les mêmes propriétés que $F$.

La surface $S'$ possède les propriétés suivantes:

a) $F'$ se trouve du côté des tractions; il correspond donc à la décohésion;

b) la surface $S'$ ne coupe pas la droite $D'$ dans la région de l'espace où $c^1$ $c^2$ et $c^3$ sont négatives; il n'y a pas de limite pour la compression hydrostatique;

c) l'existence d'un point singulier en $F'$ se conserve quelle que soit la fonction $c^i = f^i (e^i\, e^j\, e^l)$ pourvu que la relation (4) soit satisfaite.

d) l'intersection de $S'$ avec les axes de coordonnées donne les limites de traction simple (côté positif des axes) et de compression simple; ces deux limites peuvent être égales en valeur absolue ou différentes suivant les valeurs relatives de $a_1\, a_2\, a_3$; les points correspondant au cisaillement pur se trouvent dans chaque plan de coordonnées, à l'intersection de $S'$ avec les droites

$$c^i = 0, c^j = c^l \qquad (l \neq j \neq i \neq l, i = 1, 2, 3)$$

On retrouve ainsi la surface caractéristique, limite du domaine élastique, avec toutes les propriétés que l'expérience met en évidence. Les limites de ce domaine dépendraient donc, en première approximation, de trois constantes $a_1\, a_2\, a_3$ lorsque le solide est isotrope à l'état initial.

Les surfaces représentant dans le système de coordonnées $c^i$, les conditions de MOHR-CAQUOT ou de VON MISES sont des cas particuliers de cette surface; elles correspondent à des valeurs particulières des coefficients $a_1\ a_2\ a_3$ qui varient, bien entendu, d'une matière à une autre.

Si la viscosité n'est pas négligeable, elle a pour effet d'augmenter la valeur de la contrainte limite lorsque la vitesse de mise en charge croît.

Plus généralement, la surface $S'$, définie précédemment correspond à une vitesse de mise en charge infiniment petite; la vitesse $V$ étant déterminée par les relations:

$$c^i = K^i\ Vt \qquad (i = 1, 2, 3)$$

où $t$ est le temps, on peut montrer que les surfaces limites du domaine élastique dépendent du paramètre $V$ et sont telles que la surface $S'_{V_1}$ enveloppe entièrement la surface $S'_{V_2}$ pour:

$$V_1 > V_2$$

Lorsque le système élastique n'est pas uniforme, les limites ne sont plus les mêmes. Si l'on considère, par exemple, la flexion à moment constant dans laquelle il n'existe qu'une seule contrainte principale non nulle variant d'un point à un autre, les équations générales conduisent, pour la limite de la réversibilité (viscosité nulle) à une valeur supérieure à celle de l'état uniforme correspondant à la flexion c'est-à-dire, de la traction ou de la compression simple, dans lesquelles une seule contrainte principale est également différente de zéro.

Les équations (1) montrent aussi que la ligne neutre dans une éprouvette de section rectangulaire n'est plus située à mi-hauteur. Tous ces résultats sont vérifiés par l'expérience.

Considérons maintenant un système élastique uniforme déterminé par les trois contraintes principales

$$c^i = h^i(t) \qquad (i = 1, 2, 3) \tag{6}$$

$h^i(t)$ étant des fonctions périodiques du temps $t$. Par extension des résultats précédents on peut définir la limite du domaine de stabilité, c'est-à-dire tel que l'essai peut être poursuivi indéfiniment par la condition suivant laquelle une variation infiniment petite du temps $dt$ provoque une variation non infiniment petite de la déformation; or, les équations (1) dans lesquelles on tient compte des relations (6) donnent par différentiation:

$$\frac{\partial h^i}{\partial t}\, dt = \sum_j \frac{\partial f^i}{\partial e^j} \cdot \mathrm{d}\,e^j \qquad (i, j, = 1, 2, 3)$$

On en tire:

$$\mathrm{d}\,e^j = \frac{F^j}{\triangle}\,\mathrm{d}\,t$$

avec

$$\triangle = \left| \frac{\partial f^i}{\partial e^j} \right|, \quad F^j \text{ étant des fonctions des } h^i \text{ et des } \frac{\partial f^i}{\partial e^j}$$

Les de$^j$ augmentent indéfiniment quel que soit d$t$ lorsque $\triangle$ s'annule, c'est-à-dire sur les surfaces $S$ ou $S'$.

Par suite, la condition de sécurité consiste à écrire que le point figuratif de l'état élastique (6) doit, à chaque instant de la période, rester à l'intérieur de la surface $S'$.

Si la fonction $h$ se réduit à un *sinus* ou un *cosinus*, le lieu du point figuratif, dans le système de coordonnées $c^i$, est un segment de droite dont les extrémités sont symétriques par rapport à l'origine.

Supposons que la fonction $h$ renferme en outre une constante, $h^2$ et $h^3$ étant nuls:

$$c^1 = c' + c'' \sin \omega t, \quad c^2 = c^3 = 0$$

La valeur moyenne $c'$ est positive ou négative, tandis que l'amplitude $c''$ est essentiellement positive; le point figuratif se déplace sur l'axe $oc^1$ et doit être limité, pour que la stabilité soit assurée, à l'un au moins des deux points représentant les limites de traction et de compression simples, auxquelles on rattache ainsi la limite de fatigue; si l'on étudie la variation de l'amplitude $c''$ en fonction de la contrainte moyenne $c'$ on est amené à tracer un diagramme qui ne diffère des résultats expérimentaux que par la relation:

$$c' + c'' = \text{limite de traction simple lorsque } c' > 0$$
$$c' - c'' = \text{limite de compression simple lorsque } c' < 0$$

L'expérience semble en effet indiquer que $(c'+c'')$ dans le premier cas, de même que $-(c'-c'')$ dans le second, croissent avec $|c'|$.

Les seconds membres des relations (1) peuvent être complétés par des termes correspondant au frottement intérieur considéré comme visqueux: pour le premier degré, ces termes sont de la forme:

$$\lambda' \frac{d\Theta}{dt} + 2\mu' \frac{de^i}{dt}$$

Pour certaines valeurs particulières des coefficients $a_1 \ a_2 \ a_3$ on peut discuter entièrement l'équation différentielle obtenu lorsque

$$c^1 = c' + c'' \sin \omega t, \quad c^2 = c^3 = 0$$

(traction-compression). On arrive aux résultats suivants qui confirment les conclusions précédentes:

pour les faibles valeurs de $c''$, la solution de l'équation différentielle en $e^1$ est une fonction du temps qui a pour limite une fonction périodique de période $T = 2\pi/\omega$ et d'amplitude constante;

pour les fortes valeurs de $c''$ au contraire, $e^1$ est une fonction périodique du temps dont l'amplitude croît et augmente indéfiniment lorsque le temps prend une valeur particulière. L'augmentation de l'amplitude de $e^1$ correspond à une augmentation de l'énergie dissipée par le frottement intérieur: la température de l'éprouvette augmente donc également.

L'expérience confirme bien ces conclusions.

. En résumé, les raisonnements que nous avons exposés rattachent directement la limite d'endurance à la limite élastique de l'essai statique correspondant à l'essai de fatigue considéré: traction ou compression simples pour la traction-compression, flexion simple pour la flexion alternée ou rotative . . .

Par suite, les propriétés de la limite de fatigue doivent être analogues à celles de la limite élastique: elle varie avec le nature du système élastique (uniforme ou non uniforme, . . .) avec la forme de la section d'une éprouvette de flexion alternée, . . . comme on peut le vérifier.

On peut tirer une conséquence importante de cette extension de la théorie de l'élasticité:

la connaissance de la fonction exacte exprimant les $c^i$ à l'aide des $e^j$ ou, en première approximation, des trois coefficients $a_1$ $a_2$ $a_3$, détermine la surface limite $S'$ et, par suite, la limite de fatigue d'un système uniforme où les contraintes principales sont des fonctions périodiques du temps,

ces résultats peuvent également être étendus aux systèmes élastiques non uniformes à l'aide des équations générales de l'élasticité.

Les coefficients $a_1$ $a_2$ $a_3$ pourraient être déterminés soit par des expériences directes, soit à partir de trois limites correspondant à trois systèmes uniformes différents. Des mesures de cette nature sont actuellement en cours.

Tout ce qui précède concerne les solides isotropes et homogènes à l'état libre. Les métaux ne rentrent pas dans cette catégorie; pour leur appliquer les raisonnements précédents il conviendrait d'abord pour un cristal cubique par exemple, de partir des expression de $c^i$ renfermant trois coefficients au lieu de deux ($E$, $\nu$) pour les termes linéaires et cinq coefficients au lieu de trois ($a_1$ $a_2$ $a_3$) pour les termes du second degré.

Il faudrait ensuite tenir compte de la répartition et des orientations des cristaux élémentaires dans le solide.

La limite de fatigue expérimentale de traction-compression (valeur moyenne nulle) par exemple n'est pas égale, comme l'indiquent les raisonnements précédents, à la limite élastique de traction ou de compression simple; elle lui est, en général, notablement inférieure. Pour tenter d'expliquer cette divergence on peut faire les deux remarques suivantes:

a) la limite élastique statique, déterminée par un essai normalisé, diminue lorsque la vitesse de mise en charge décroît: sa détermination précise à l'aide d'extensomètres, avec une vitesse très faible, donne des valeurs beaucoup plus basses que les valeurs classiques;

b) lorsque, dans un essai de fatigue les contraintes se rapprochent de la limite; le dégagement de chaleur dû au frottement intérieur, provoque une augmentation de température qui, par la dilatation qu'elle produit, diminue la limite de fatigue comme l'étude de la surface $S$ le montre immédiatement.

## Discussion

F. GATTO : Je crois qu'il est nécessaire d'introduire l'équation d'état du matériau pour tenir compte du fait que quand les termes du second ordre deviennent sensibles, les déformations auront le caractère des déformations thermoélastiques.

A. KAMMERER: On peut admettre des déformations adiabatiques ou isothermes et ainsi obtenir de relations univoques entre contraintes et déformations.

F. ODQVIST: Dans le cas des contraintes uniaxiales la théorie de l'Auteur peut s'interpréter comme dans la figure (trait plein).

A. KAMMERER: Oui.

F. ODQVIST: Alors il me semble que l'application de la belle théorie de l'Auteur sera limitée aux phénomènes avec des relations univoques entre contraintes et déformations, c'est à dire à la mise en charges monotone. Pour les phénomènes reversibles au delà du domaine de la loi de Hooke et aussi pour les essais de fatigue il faut admettre une courbe qui se rende compte de l'hysterese (voir la figure, courbe pointillée).

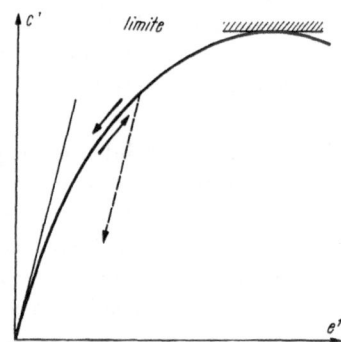

A. KAMMERER: La théorie exposée permet d'établir, même en l'absence de frottement intérieur, la notion de limite du *domaine des déformations réversibles*, celles-ci n'étant jamais parfaitement linéaires.

Ce frottement, lorsqu'il a les caractères de la viscosité, *modifie* les limites de la réversibilité qui n'existe alors, comme en thermodynamique, que pour les déformations infiniment lentes.

Suivent les forces appliquées (lentement croissantes, périodiques, . . . . . , uniformes, . . . .) et la nature des matières (isotropes, anisotropes, cristallinnes, amorphes, multicristallinnes, . . . .) les phénomènes qui apparaissent à la limite ainsi définie, varient : rupture, déformation permanente par glissement, . . . . .

# Effect of geometric size on notch fatigue

By

**P. Kuhn**

With 12 figures

## 1. Introduction

It has been known for about 25 years that the stress concentration produced by a notch on a fatigue specimen is less severe than predicted by the theory of elasticity. It has also been known for a long time that the factor of stress concentration increases with the absolute size of the specimen. Many tests on notch effect may be found in the literature, but a mass of uncorrelated test data is of little use to a designer; moreover, unless some correlation is effected, research on notch effects is rather aimless and inefficient. In order to alleviate this situation, a method for estimating the effect of varying geometric size of notch has been developed for steels and for strong aluminum alloys and is presented in this paper.

## 2. Definitions

Fig. 1 shows the $S$-$N$ curves for an unnotched and a notched specimen of the same material, subjected to completely reversed cyclic loading. The nominal stresses carried by these specimens are designated $S_A$ and $S_B$; the ratio $S_A/S_B$ is called the fatigue factor $K_F$. In this paper, attention is confined to factors $K_F$ determined in the neighbourhood of the endurance limit.

The condition that the material must be the same is intended to imply not only the same chemical composition, but identical histories of hot work, cold work,

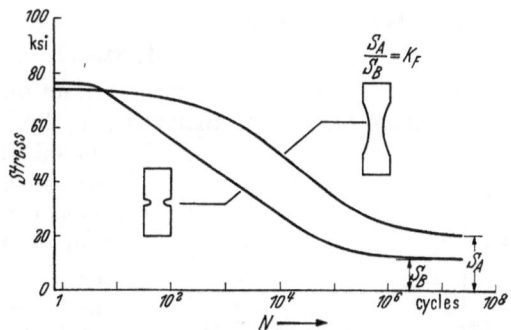

Fig. 1. Typical $S$-$N$ curves for aluminum alloys. $R = -1$.
($R$ = ratio of minimum to maximum stress).

and heat treatment. The term "geometric size effect" was chosen to emphasize this assumption that no metallurgical size effects are present.

## 3. Basis of method

Engineering alloys have a granular structure. When viewed on a scale commensurate with the size of the grains, they are neither homogeneous nor isotropic, and consequently the conventional theory of elasticity cannot be expected to be valid on such a scale. In his book "Kerbspannungslehre", H. NEUBER proposed a mathematical formulation of these ideas by introducing the concept of a "building block". With the aid of this concept, he arrived at the formula which reads, after some changes in symbols

$$K_N = 1 + \frac{K_T - 1}{1 + \frac{\pi}{\pi - \omega} \sqrt{\frac{A}{r}}}$$

The factor $K_N$ is the effective factor of stress concentration; the subscript $N$ stands for NEUBER in our notation. The factor $K_T$ is the theoretical factor obtained by the theory of elasticity or some equivalent method, such as photoelastic tests. The quantities $r$ and $\omega$ are the root radius and the flank angle of the notch. The quantity $A$, finally (denoted $\varrho'$ by NEUBER), is a "materials constant" which we have chosen to call the NEUBER constant.

NEUBER himself evaluated the constant for a few materials by the analysis of static tests. However, the constant is obviously not a directly measurable materials property in the usual sense of the word; it is a somewhat artificial concept, and there is no a priori reason to believe that the constant applicable to static tests must also apply to fatigue tests. The contribution made in this paper, then, consists in the determination of the constant for fatigue loading for a large number of materials and in establishing a correlation between these constants for steels. In principle, this determination is a simple task, but in practice, it is a rather tedious one.

## 4. Steels

A large number of notch-fatigue tests on steel specimens found in the literature have been analyzed [1]. From this analysis, it was concluded that the NEUBER constant for steels could be represented by the curve shown in fig. 2 as a function of the tensile strength of the material. The tests analysed were made on a large variety of steels, it might be mentioned, however, that no tests on austenitic stainless steels were available.

Some typical comparisons for systematic test series on rotating beams

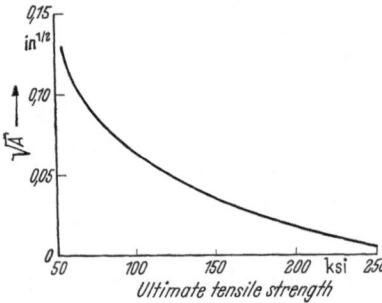

Fig. 2. Neuber constant, $A$.

with notches are shown in fig. 3, where factors are plotted against diameter of test specimen in inches. The full lines show the theoretical factors, the dotted lines the NEUBER factors, and the circles show the experimental fatigue factors. For the two top sketches, the specimens

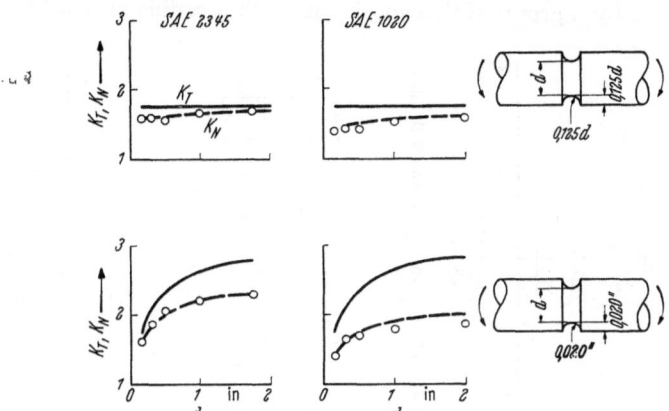

Fig. 3. Calculated and experimental fatigue factors for rotating beams with grooves.

in each series are geometrically similar; thus, the factor $K_T$ is constant. For the two bottom sketches, the groove is of fixed dimensions while the diameter of the specimen varies; thus, $K_T$ is not constant. The agreement between the NEUBER factors $K_N$ and the fatigue factors $K_F$ is very good in all cases here. Fig. 4 shows similar comparisons for shafts with shoulders.

The agreement between the NEUBER factor and the fatigue factor for all the tests analyzed is shown in fig. 5 to 8. In these figures, the ratio $K_N/K_F$ is plotted against the notch radius. The choice of the root radius

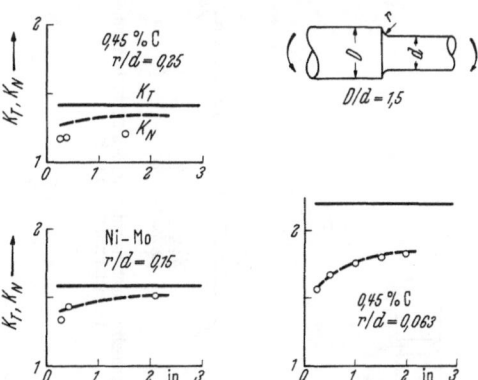

Fig. 4. Calculated and experimental fatigue factors for rotating beams with fillets.

as ordinate has no special significance except that for small radii, the accuracy of measurement is obviously more questionable[1]. A ratio

---

[1] Editors' remark: In figures 5 through 11 other parameters than notch radius, such as absolute size, may vary within wide limits.

$K_N/K_F$ equal to unity would indicate a perfect prediction. Vertical lines have been drawn to define a scatter band of $\pm$ 10 per cent.

Fig. 5 shows the results for groóved rotating beams. Most of the points fall within the $\pm$ 10 per cent scatter band, the only large deviations being caused by a group of five specimens with a radius of 0.002 inch.

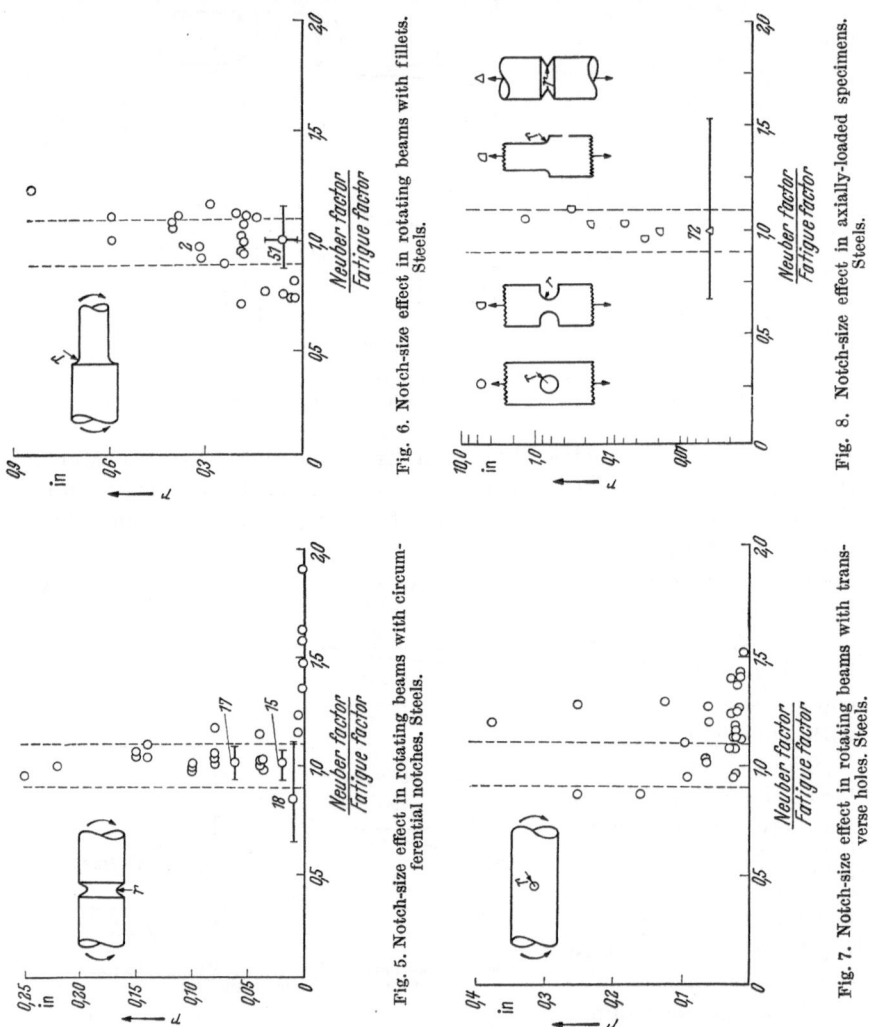

Fig. 5. Notch-size effect in rotating beams with circumferential notches. Steels.

Fig. 6. Notch-size effect in rotating beams with fillets. Steels.

Fig. 7. Notch-size effect in rotating beams with transverse holes. Steels.

Fig. 8. Notch-size effect in axially-loaded specimens. Steels.

Fig. 6 shows the results for shouldered shafts.

Fig. 7 shows the results for shafts with transverse holes. It may be remarked that some of the scatter can probably be attributed to the fact that the theoretical factor $K_T$ for this configuration is only roughly estimated, because no theoretical solution is known.

Fig. 8 shows the results for axially loaded specimens. The line at the bottom indicates the scatter range for a group of 72 tests, with the symbol indicating the average of the group. The radius for these specimens is fairly small (0.004 inch) and of unknown accuracy.

## 5. Aluminum alloys

An early attempt to determine the NEUBER constant for aluminum alloys was made utilizing rotating beam tests found in the literature. The amount of information was much less than for steels, and large inconsistencies were noted. Inconsistencies continue to be troublesome to this day; the experiences with aluminum alloys will therefore be described in some detail.

Attention was directed next to tests on sheet material (24 S-T and 75 S-T) under axial loading, for which three investigations had been conducted either as contract work for the NACA or by the NACA itself. The three investigations were:

1. An investigation conducted by the National Bureau of Standards, using central-hole specimens [2].

2. An investigation conducted by the Battelle Memorial Institute using central-hole specimens as well as specimens with edge notches and filleted shoulders [3].

3. An investigation conducted in the NACA Laboratory using central-hole specimens.

The material for the first investigation came from several batches, and the specimens were not polished to simulate actual service conditions. The material for the second and the third investigation came from one single batch of material, produced under close control. All specimens for these two investigations were electro-polished by the Battelle Memorial Institute, which has done a large amount of work in the development of electro-polishing. The second investigation was intended chiefly to develop the fatigue diagrams; the third investigation concentrated on size effect.

Two conclusions were drawn from the analysis of these three investigations:

1. There was no difference between unpolished and electro-polished sheet specimens.

2. The NEUBER constant was about the same for 24 S-T and for 75 S-T material. A value of $A = 0.02$ inch was found to give a reasonable

fit for both materials if some consideration was given to the rotating beam data to be discussed later.

Fig. 9 shows the agreement achieved. Almost 90 per cent of the points fall within the ± 10 per cent scatter band; the remaining 10 per cent fall to the right of the band, indicating a conservative prediction. In-

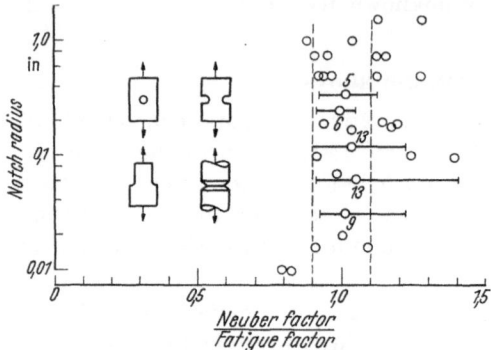

Fig. 9. Notch-size effect in fatigue of axially-loaded specimens 24 S-T and 75 S-T.

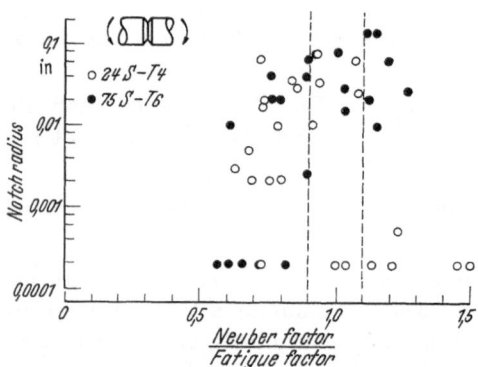

Fig. 10. Notch-size effect in fatigue of rotating beam specimens 24 S-T 4 and 75 S-T 6.

cluded in the figure are five points for cylindrical (round) specimens from two other investigations [4].

Fig. 10 shows the results of evaluating the avais lable rotating beam test on 24 S-T and 75 S-T [5] and [6], using the NEUBER constant of 0.02 inch. In this figure, different symbols are used for the two materials. It is evident that when all points are considered, there is no systematic difference between the two materials. A comparison with the preceding figure for axial loading on sheet material shows two differences:

1. There is more scatter in the rotating beam tests.

2. A considerable number of points fall to the left of the ± 10 per cent band, indicating unconservative predictions.

Qualitatively, both differences might be explained by differences in surface finish of the unnotched specimens. Most of the unnotched rotating beams were hand-polished. Hand-polishing is known to increase the fatigue strength, but gives also highly variable results. Increased fatigue strength of the unnotched specimens results in higher values of the fatigue factor $K_F$, and thus in lower values of the ratio $K_N/K_F$.

Fig. 11 shows the results for rotating beams of aluminum alloys other than 24 S-T and 75 S-T and includes American as well as British alloys [6] and [7]. The results are similar to those for the first two alloys, indicating that within the rather wide scatter no significant differences between the alloys are apparent, and the same NEUBER constant may be used.

For the steels, the NEUBER constant was found to be dependent on the tensile strength. Within the test range covered, the tensile strengths of the steels varied by a factor of five. On the aluminum alloys, the strength varies only by a factor of 1.5 if the two weakest alloys (53 S and 61 S) are excluded. This relatively small spread in strength together with the larger scatter explains why one value of the NEUBER constant appears to be reasonably adequate to describe the size effect of quite a number of aluminum alloys. The two weakest alloys, which have only about half the strength of the strongest ones, should probably be considered separately and assigned a larger value of the NEUBER constant. This change would move the three most extreme points in fig. 11 (at $r = 0.0001$ inch) to the left and thus reduce the scatter.

Fig. 12 shows the results of a recent test series on sheet specimens with very sharp V-notches under axial loading. The 1/2-inch wide specimen represents rough-

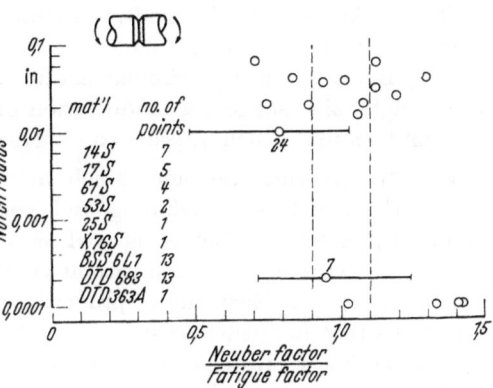

Fig. 11. Notch-size effect in fatigue of rotating beam specimens. Aluminum alloys.

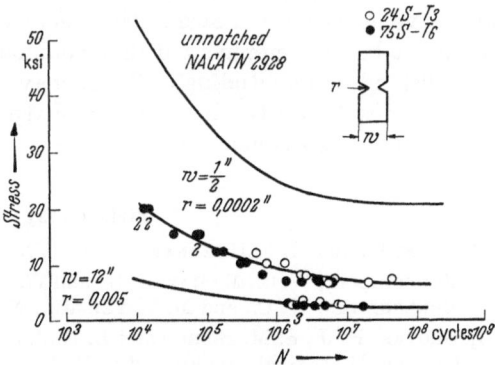

Fig. 12. Axial load fatigue tests of sheet specimens with sharp notches. $R = -1$.

ly the longitudinal section of a standard-size rotating beam; the 12-inch wide specimen has a geometrically similar notch configuration. The notch configuration is that used as standard by the Aluminum Company of America and has a theoretical factor of about 27 in this two-dimensional version. The $S$-$N$ curve for the unnotched sheet shown on top was used to calculate the curves for the two types of notched specimens. It is evident that the calculated curves are in excellent agreement with the test results for both sizes and both materials.

## 6. Concluding remarks

The figures shown demonstrate that the effect of changes in geometric size can be predicted with fair accuracy. If the accuracy of prediction is to be improved, a number of items entering into the problem must be studied in more detail.

On the theoretical side, mention should be made of the lack of exact solutions for the theoretical factors, for instance, for the V-notch and for the circular hole in a circular shaft. An exact solution for the V-notch might also suggest a modification of the factor $\pi/(\pi-\omega)$ in the NEUBER formula, which appears to exaggerate the effect of flank angle.

On the experimental side, much more knowledge is needed concerning the effects of machining and polishing. Improper machining conditions, such as a chattering tool or a dull tool, can produce very high surface stresses, and the second condition at least is not always readily recognized. Even under proper machining conditions, there are indications that high surface stresses might be generated at the bottom of a groove due to restraint of flow. Not enough is known about what constitutes proper machining conditions. Hand polishing is an uncontrolled process, and mechanical polishing may not be much better. Electro-polishing is at present an art as much as a science, and the arts have never been known to be amenable to scientific control. Finally, it cannot be over-emphasized that nominally identical operations, such as polishing or longitudinal milling, may produce quantitatively quite different results on the bottom of a sharp notch and on the surface of an unnotched specimen.

### Bibliography

[1] KUHN, P., and H. F. HARDRATH: NACA TN 2805, (1952).
[2] BRUEGGEMAN, W. C., M. MAYER, JR. and W. H. SMITH: NACA TN 955 (1944).
   BRUEGGEMAN, W. C., and M. MAYER, JR.: NACA TN 1611 (1948).
[3] GROVER, H. J., S. M. BISHOP and L. R. JACKSSON: NACA TN 2324, (1951).
   GROVER, H. J., S. M. BISHOP and L. R. JACKSSON: NACA TN 2389 (1951).
   GROVER, H. J., S. M. BISHOP and L. R. JACKSSON: NACA TN 2390 (1951.
   GROVER, H. J., W. S. HYLER and L. R. JACKSSON: NACA TN 2639 (1952).
[4] LAZAN, B. J., and A. A. BLATHERWICK: Univ. Minnesota, Dec. 1952.
   WÅLLGREN, G.: FFA Medd. (Aeronaut. Res. Inst. Rep.) (Stockholm) No. 48 (1953).
[5] MAC GREGOR, C. W., and N. GROSSMAN: NACA TN 2812 (1952).
   HYLER, W. S.: R. A. LEWIS and H. J. GROVER: NACA TN 3191 (1954).
   FOUND, G. H.: Proc. ASTM, 46, 715 (1946).
   MANN, J. Y.: Aeronaut. Res. Lab. (Australia) SM 147 (1950).
   MOORE, H. F.: Air Force Techn. Rep. 5726 (Dayton) (1948).
   TEMPLIN, R. L., F. M. HOWELL and E. C. HARTMAN: Product Engrng, 21, 126—130 (1950).

[6] HOWELL, F. M.: Aluminum Res. Lab. M. T. Rep. 9—49—1 (New Kensington) (1949).

BENNETT, J. A., and J. G. WEINBERG: J. Res. nat. Bur. Stand., 52, 235—245 (1954).

DERVISHYAN, A. O.: Dr. diss., California Inst. Techn. (1952).

[7] DOLAN, T. J.: NACA TN 852 (1942).

War Metallurgy Committee, Office Sc. Res. Devel. 3579 (April 1944).

TAYLOR, W. J., and N. J. F. GUNN: Roy. Aircr. Establ. Rep. Met. 42 (1950).

GUNN, N. J. F.: Roy. Aircr. Establ. Rep. Met. 163 (1952).

## Discussion

G. V. UZHIK remarked that elastic stress distribution at points of stress concentration in fatigue tests could be relied upon for stress concentration factors up to 4 ... 5, as shown by tests in the USSR.

P. KUHN: The scatter in fatigue tests is so great that significant deviations from elastic stresses could not be detected for stress concentration factors smaller than 4 ... 5.

R. E. PETERSON: From the standpoint of design application, the Author has put forth a useful idea in relating the material constant with the tensile strength. Some designers like to work with notch sensitivity $q = (K_F - 1)/(K_T - 1)$ KUHN's results can be put in the form shown in fig. 1. We have used a somewhat

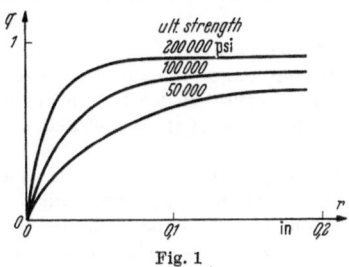

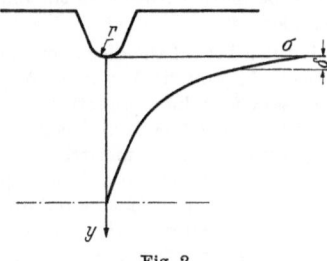

Fig. 1                                    Fig. 2

different approach based on failure at a distance $\delta$ beneath the surface, see fig. 2. This leads to the equation

$$q = \frac{1}{1 + \dfrac{K_{t'}}{K_{t'} - 1} \cdot \dfrac{C\delta}{r}}$$

where $C = \dfrac{d\sigma}{dy}$, stress gradient, $K_{t'} = m\,K_T$ ($m$ = Mises factor). Assuming average values of $K_{t'}$ and $C$ and constant $\delta$, we obtain

$$q = \frac{1}{1 + \dfrac{a}{r}}$$

One can also utilize a material factor similar to that of KUHN to make up a "$q$ vs. $r$" design chart.

An interesting feature of the above approach is that it indicates that notch specimens of fixed shape should give higher $q$ values in torsion than in bending. This is primarily due to a lower stress gradient in torsion.

R. B. Heywood: The determination of notch sensitivity involves the measurement of many quantities, some of which cannot be measured accurately. Kuhn is to be congratulated in obtaining the general trends in notch sensitivity, particularly in its relationship to tensile strength, from the mass of data which is not always consistent.

It can be shown that Neuber's equation for the technical factor, whilst giving good agreement with observed trends for most shapes and sizes of notch, is nevertheless unsatisfactory in two cases. Thus Neuber's correction for included angle of a V-notch is open to doubt, and the reduction in strength due to extremely small notches appears to be too great. These difficulties can be overcome and the same trends obtained for other conditions by use of a formula that has been suggested by me (Engineering, **179**, 146—148, 1955).

$$K_N = \frac{K_T}{1 + 2\sqrt{\dfrac{a}{r}\dfrac{K_T - 1}{K_T}}}$$

where $r$ is the root radius of notch, and $a$ is the material notch length, determining notch insensitivity.

Kuhn has shown that for reversed loading the two aluminium alloys 24 S-T and 75 S-T have approximately the same notch sensitivity. It would be interesting to have Kuhn's views as to whether the sensitivity would be the same in fluctuating tension, when one might expect the higher proof stress material 75 S-T to be more sensitive to the effect of mean load, and so to have the greater notch sensitivity.

P. Kuhn: Two of the discussers mentioned other procedures for estimating the size effect. In any field where sweeping simplifying assumptions and empiricism are necessary to achieve practical results, it is only natural that a number of methods will be developed, and it is quite possible for some of these methods to be very evenly matched in merits.

With regard to Heywood's last question, I should like to point out that the paper deals only with factors obtained in the region of the endurance limit, i. e., cycle numbers well over 10 million. In this region, I would expect the difference between 24S-T and 75S-T due to higher proof stress to be so small as to be overshadowed by scatter.

# Les travaux récents de l'Institut de Recherches Métallurgiques de Sarrebruck dans le domaine de la fatigue

**P. Laurent**

Avec 6 figures

Nous nous proposons, dans cette communication, de rapporter brièvement les travaux actuellement en cours à Sarrebruck.

## 1. Application des méthodes statistiques à la fatigue
(H. Bühler et W. Schreiber)

Les essais de fatigue présentent une dispersion considérable, contrairement aux essais statiques; essayées dans les mêmes conditions, des éprouvettes apparemment identiques peuvent supporter un nombre de répétition des efforts variant de 1 à 10. Ainsi que l'a proposé Freudenthal [1], le logarithme du nombre d'alternances $N$ qui provoque la

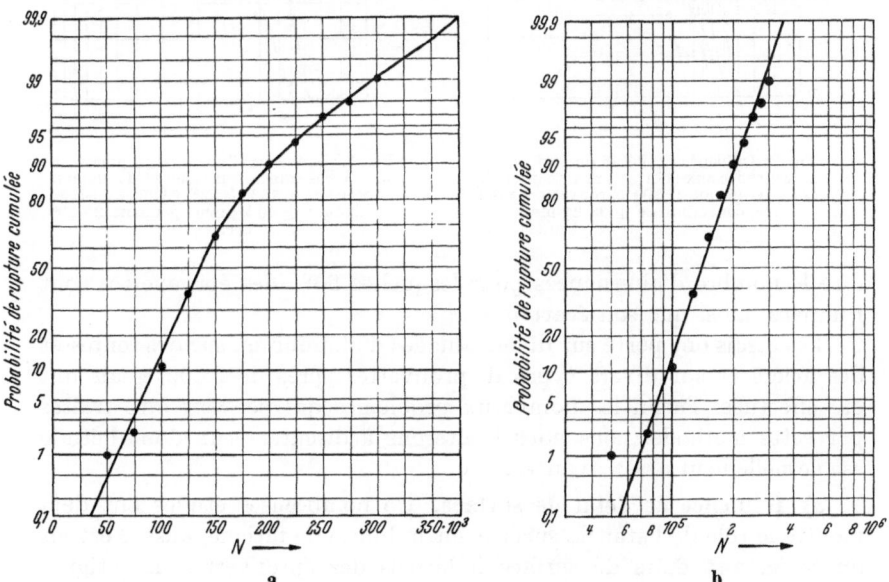

Fig. 1. Répartition du nombre d'alternances avant rupture pour des éprouvettes de flexion rotative polies en travers. Sur la figure a, le nombre d'alternances est porté en abscisse, tandis que son logarithme est porté en b. (Acier C 35, lot de 100 éprouvettes essayées pour ± 38 kg/mm²)

rupture dans des conditions données, présente une répartition de Gauss, comme on le vérifie aisément en utilisant des diagrammes de probabilité.

La fig. 1 montre la répartition de $N$ et de log $N$ pour un acier à 0,3% C (St 50—11) en flexion rotative pour une contrainte maximum de 38 kg/mm²; en réalité, pour obtenir une droite, Bühler et Schreiber ont porté, non pas log $N$, mais: log $(N + N_0)$ où $N_0$ est petit par rapport à $N$. De ce diagramme, on peut déduire la «vie» moyenne $N_{1/2}$ c'est-à-

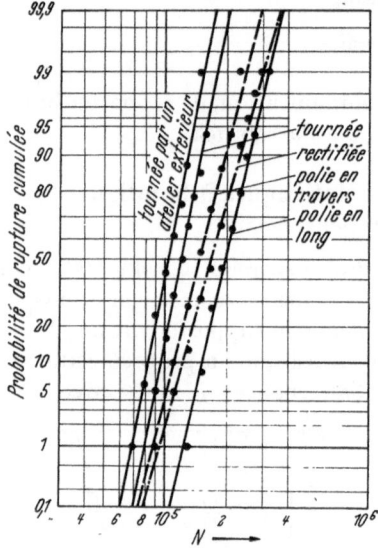

Fig. 2. Influence de l'état de surface sur la résistance aux efforts de flexion alternée (Acier C 45, lot de 100 éprouvettes) pour une contrainte de ± 38 kg/mm².

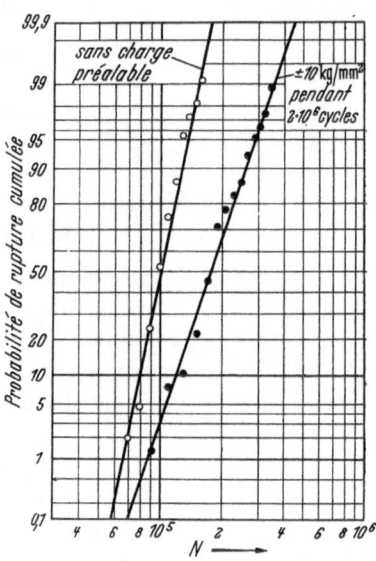

Fig. 3. Influence d'une charge préalable sur la résistance aux efforts de flexion alternée de ± 19 kg/mm². (Alliage Al-Mn; précharge: ± 10 kg/mm² pendant 2 · 10⁶ cycles).

dire le nombre d'alternances pour lesquelles 50% des éprouvettes sont rompues, ainsi que son écart probable.

Les essais ont porté sur divers alliages d'aluminium, sur des fontes et des aciers et sur divers types d'éprouvettes; près de 6.000 essais ont été effectués. Parmi les nombreux problèmes qui peuvent être traités par cette méthode, nous nous limiterons à discuter ceux dont l'étude est actuellement assez avancée.

a) **Influence de l'état de surface.** De nombreuses études ont déjà montré le rôle de l'état de surface sur la limite de fatigue, aussi s'est-on limité ici aux états de surface habituels des éprouvettes de fatigue. La fig. 2 montre que les éprouvettes polies longitudinalement ont, toutes choses égales par ailleurs, une «vie» plus longue que celles polies transversalement ou rectifiées. L'influence des conditions d'usinage est particulièrement nette sur deux séries d'éprouvettes préparées l'une par l'atelier de l'Institut et l'autre dans un atelier d'usinage extérieur.

**b) Restauration.** Il est admis qu'une pause dans les essais de fatigue prolonge la vie des éprouvettes, c'est-à-dire qu'il y a restauration des propriétés pendant le repos. Pour confirmer ce résultat, un lot d'éprouvettes en acier Ni-Cr traité (f = 40 kg/mm²) a été maintenu 14 jours au repos après 150.000 alternances à + 46 kg/mm²; il n'a pas été constaté de différence entre ce lot et un lot identique non restauré.

**c) Understressing.** On sait que la limite de fatigue d'un métal est élevée quand il a été soumis à des efforts répétés inférieurs à la limite de fatigue. Considérons un lot de 100 éprouvettes en alliage d'aluminium soumis à + 10 kg/mm²; après 2.000.000 d'alternances, 20 sont rompues et les 80 restantes sont soumises à + 19 kg/mm². La vie moyenne de ces 80 éprouvettes est supérieure à celle d'un lot de 100 éprouvettes soumises directement à + 19 kg/mm²; on peut même vérifier que si l'on élimine les 20 éprouvettes les moins bonnes de ce dernier lot, la vie moyenne des 80 éprouvettes restantes est plus courte que celle des éprouvettes soumises initialement à 10 kg/mm². Donc, les efforts répétés améliorent le métal vis-à-vis des contraintes plus élevées, contrairement à l'hypothèse émise par EPREMIAN et MEHL (fig. 3) [2].

**d) Dispersion.** Quand la contrainte maximum augmente, la dispersion a tendance à diminuer, mais cet effet est plutôt faible et l'on peut admettre qu'il existe une dispersion caractéristique de l'alliage étudié. Pour illustrer cette notion de dispersion caractéristique, prenons l'exemple d'une éprouvette de flexions alternées type Schenk, percée d'un petit trou de 1 mm de diamètre. La vie moyenne dépend de la position du trou comme le montre la fig. 4, tandis que la dispersion reste constante.

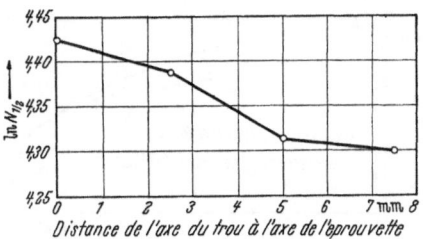

Fig. 4. Influence sur la vie moyenne $N_{1/2}$ des éprouvettes de flexion alternée de la position d'un trou de 1 mm perpendiculaire au plan de l'éprouvette.

Nous venons d'indiquer que la dispersion est caractéristique du matériau et il semble logique de relier cette dispersion à celle d'autres caractéristiques, notamment la dureté. BÜHLER et SCHREIBER ont ainsi pu établir que, dans certains cas, une partie de la dispersion peut être reliée à une hétérogénéité de la dureté du lot étudié; dans d'autres cas, il n'en est pas ainsi. La dispersion n'a pu non plus être reliée à des variations dans l'état de surface ou dans la forme des éprouvettes, probablement par suite du soin apporté à l'usinage. Il existe donc une dispersion intrinsèque du métal et Bühler et Schreiber ont vérifié que, pour deux lots possédant la même dispersion, il y avait identité dans la nature et la répartition d'inclusions, confirmant ainsi les conclusions de Fotiadi [3].

## 2. Influence du grain sur la limite de fatigue du fer Armco
### (H. Hendus et G. Kraus)

L'effet des dimensions des cristaux est bien connu sur les propriétés plastiques, mais par contre, peu d'auteurs ont étudié le cas de la limite de fatigue; aussi, ce fut le but de ce travail en se limitant au cas du fer Armco.

Les essais ont été effectués sur une machine de flexions alternées du type Schenk utilisant des éprouvettes plates d'une section de $20 \times 3$ mm²; ces éprouvettes ont été préparées à partir de barres de fer Armco (C 0,03; N 0,003; Mn 0,035; P 0,02; S 0,035; Cu 0,06) de 30 mm de diamètre; ces barres ont été forgées pour obtenir une section rectangulaire de $35 \times 7$ mm², puis usinées à une épaisseur de 3 mm. Les éprouvettes ont été ensuite recuites pendant 2 heures dans l'hydrogène purifié et sec à 950° C et l'hydrogène dissous a été éliminé par un maintien de 8 jours à l'ambiante, suivi d'un chauffage d'une heure dans le vide à $10^{-2}$ mm pendant une heure. Après des écrouissages variés, les éprouvettes ont été recristallisées par recuit pendant 24 heures à 870° C dans l'hydrogène, puis l'hydrogène a été éliminé comme précédemment. Les éprouvettes à grains plus fins ont été obtenues par refroidissement à différentes vitesses dans le domaine $\gamma$ - $\alpha$ sans écrouissage préalable.

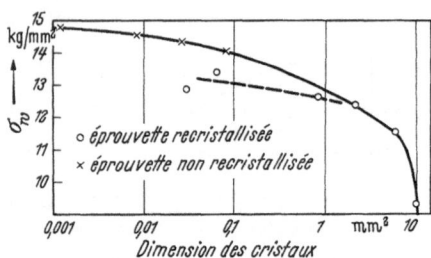

Fig. 5. Influence de la dimension des cristaux sur la limite de fatigue en flexion alternée du fer Armco.

Après ces traitements, le grain de chaque éprouvette était uniforme et variait selon les cas de $6 \cdot 10^{-2}$ mm² à 10 mm².

La fig. 5 montre la variation de la limite de fatigue avec la dimension des cristaux; elle diminue régulièrement quand le grain augmente, comme l'ont observé notamment Sinclair et Craig dans le cas du laiton $\alpha$, ref. [4]. Quand les cristaux ont des dimensions de l'ordre de l'épaisseur de l'éprouvette, la limite de fatigue décroît brusquement, tandis que le caractère de la fissure se modifie:

a) Pour les grains inférieurs à 10 mm², la fissure est, comme il est normal avec le fer, transcristalline et, en moyenne, parallèle à l'axe de flexion. La fissure principale est souvent accompagnée d'autres moins importantes; ces fissures ont parfois en surface un parcours rectiligne dans un cristal donné, mais en profondeur, elles présentent un parcours moins régulier. Il n'a pas été possible d'identifier le plan cristallin de ces fissures, mais ce n'est pas le plan (100) de clivage classique du $Fe_\alpha$. De plus, on observe dans certains cristaux des précipités en plaquettes parallèles à (110) qui se redissolvent entre 420 et 450° C. Une analyse précise de ce constituant n'a pu être faite, mais son orientation laisse penser qu'il pourrait s'agir de carbure hexagonal.

b) Pour les cristaux de l'ordre de l'épaisseur de l'éprouvette, la fissure principale est intercristalline, mais quand l'orientation du joint qui suit la fissure n'est plus parallèle à l'axe de flexion, elle peut dans certains cas devenir transcristalline, tandis que, dans d'autres, elle s'arrête et de fortes déformations locales apparaissent dans les cristaux à l'extrémité de la fissure.

### 3. Application des mesures magnétiques à la fatigue

(P. Laurent et A. Kovacs)

Dans la plupart des essais de fatigue, la répartition des contraintes est hétérogène et celles-ci sont en général maximum à la surface. Dans ces conditions, les modifications pouvant se produire dans le métal sont limitées à un petit volume, aussi est-il difficile de les déceler; on peut espérer que, dans un essai de fatigue en traction répétée, où toute l'éprouvette est soumise aux mêmes contraintes, ces modifications sont plus accessibles.

Pour nos mesures, l'éprouvette à étudier constituait le noyau métallique d'une bobine dont nous mesurions la variation des caractéristiques. Cette variation était mesurée par un pont d'impédance alimenté par un courant de 8.000 Hz; ce pont étant initialement équilibré en phase et en amplitude, le déséquilibre du pont en cours d'expérience est dû aux modifications de l'éprouvette. La mesure en haute fréquence des caractéristiques de la bobine a l'avantage de limiter le flux d'induction aux couches superficielles de l'éprouvette où s'amorcent les fissures de fatigue.

Pour une éprouvette donnée, on peut alors tracer la courbe donnant l'induction de la bobine, c'est-à-dire la perméabilité de l'éprouvette en fonction de la contrainte statique régnant sur l'éprouvette. Si l'éprouvette est soumise à des efforts répétés, son induction varie, aussi la bobine est-elle le siège d'une force électromotrice induite ayant la fréquence de vibration qui empêche d'équilibrer le pont de mesure. Cette force électromotrice est $e = K \dfrac{\mathrm{d}B}{\mathrm{d}t}$ où $K$ est une constante. Si nous intégrons cette force électromotrice, nous obtenons une différence de potentiel:

$$V = \int_0^t e\, \mathrm{d}t = K B\,(t)$$

Pour étudier la variation de $B$ au cours d'un cycle de contraintes, il suffit de relier $V$ aux plaques verticales d'un oscillographe cathodique, tandis qu'un potentiel proportionnel à la contrainte sur l'éprouvette est appliqué aux plaques horizontales. Dans ces conditions, on obtient sur l'écran de l'oscillographe une courbe fermée représentant les variations de l'induction en fonction de la contrainte au cours de chaque cycle.

Sauf avis contraire, nous limiterons cet exposé au cas d'un acier Ni-Cr à 0,3% C trempé et revenu, donc à structure sorbitique homogène.

a) Au cours de nos essais, l'éprouvette sollicitée en traction-compression fait partie d'un système mécanique qui vibre à sa fréquence de résonance; toute modification du module de l'éprouvette se traduit alors par une variation de la fréquence.

Quand l'amplitude de la contrainte croît, on observe une diminution progressive du module de quelques pourcents. Au-dessus de la limite de fatigue, à contrainte constante, la variation du module est inférieure aux erreurs d'expérience (0,25%) pendant 80% de la vie de l'éprouvette; le module diminue ensuite, probablement quand les premières fissures de fatigue apparaissent; au-dessous de la limite de fatigue, pour une contrainte donnée, aucune variation du module n'a pu être observée. Remarquons que, dans les essais de fatigue en flexion rotative, on constate une variation importante de la flèche que l'on interprète comme une variation du module [5]. La variation de flèche dans le cas d'un état de contraintes hétérogènes est ainsi due, non à une variation du module, mais à l'apparition de contraintes internes.

b) Peut-on déceler une différence entre une éprouvette ayant subi un grand nombre d'alternances et une éprouvette non vibrée? Dans tous les cas étudiés, nous avons trouvé une différence entre les éprouvettes vibrées et non vibrées.

c) Au cours d'un cycle de contrainte, le cycle d'hystérésis induction-contrainte enregistré à l'oscillographe, comme nous l'avons indiqué, dépend des conditions d'essai. On remarque qu'à la limite de fatigue (+ 38 kg/mm²), le cycle d'hystérésis ne change pas, tandis qu'à 39 kg/mm², il s'ouvre progressivement.

d) Si l'on arrête un essai de fatigue, on constate que l'induction de l'éprouvette varie au cours du temps; il y a un trainage (Nachwirkungseffekt) analogue au trainage magnétique. Adoptons comme amplitude du trainage la valeur qu'il prend trois minutes après suppression des vibrations; l'amplitude du trainage dépend des conditions d'essais (fig. 6), mais au-dessus de la limite de fatigue, il croît quand le nombre d'alternances des contraintes augmente. Signalons que nous avons fréquemment observé des grands sauts de BARKHAUSEN pendant ce trainage.

e) Nous avons indiqué dans l'étude statistique de la fatigue que l'understressing correspondait à une réalité physique; nous avons effectivement observé que, pour l'acier Ni-Cr revenu à 600° C (f = + 43 kg/mm²) le trainage n'est pas le même quand l'éprouvette est essayée directement à cette charge ou quand elle a été soumise auparavant à un grand nombre d'alternances à une charge plus faible.

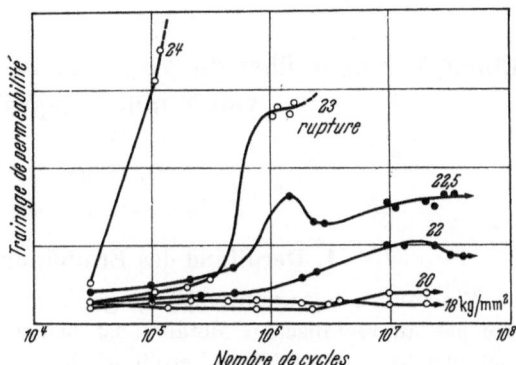

Fig. 6. Influence du nombre de cycles sur le trainage après arrêt de l'essai de fatigue (acier de cémentation au carbone normalisé).

### Bibliographie

[1] FREUDENTHAL, A. M.: ASTM spec. Rep. No 121, 3 (1952).
[2] EPREMIAN, E. et R. F. MEHL: ASTM spec. Rep. No 137, 58 (1953).
[3] FOTIADI: Rev. Métall. 44, 12 (1947).
[4] SINCLAIR et CRAIG: Trans. Amer. Soc. Metals 44, 929 (1952).
[5] LAZAN: Trans. Amer. Soc. Metals 42, 499 (1950).

### Discussion

F. A. McCLINTOCK: It is interesting to note the relatively low values of $\sigma_{\log_{10} N}$ (= 0.08 to 0.15) obtained by the author. This is further evidence that the variability in fatigue life is not excessive if careful experimental work is carried out.

Regarding the inter-crystalline fractures, could these be caused by possible inclusions in the grain boundaries? Such embrittlement of Armco iron has previously been found by the writer and a British worker (see F. A. McCLINTOCK, Fatigue Tests on Single Crystals of Ingot Iron, Proc. 1st Nat. Cong. App. Mech., Chicago 1951).

# Einige Versuche über die Vorgänge in der Oberflächenschicht von Ermüdungsproben

Von

## O. Lißner

Mit 4 Abbildungen

## 1. Der Stand des Ermüdungsproblems

Eine anerkannte und vollständige Klärung der Ursachen des Dauerbruches an technischen Metallen ist bisher nicht gelungen. Nach der fast gleichzeitig erfolgten Veröffentlichung der Hypothesen von OROWAN [1], DEHLINGER [2] und AFANASIEW [3] um 1940 hatte sich die Forschung von neuen Versuchen zur Erklärung der physikalischen Probleme bei der Ermüdung abgewandt, da offenbar mit den damals bekannten Mitteln und Vorstellungen die als wesentlich erkannte „kritische Deformationsgrenze" nicht einwandfrei zu definieren und experimentell zu beweisen war. Zusammenstellungen, wie die von BOAS [4], weisen auf den Mangel an Beweiskraft in den genannten Erklärungsversuchen hin. Es wird heute versucht, diese Hypothesen mit Hilfe der Versetzungstheorie besser zu unterbauen, doch sind ja gerade hier erhebliche experimentelle Schwierigkeiten zu erwarten, wenn es gilt, Ansammlungen von Versetzungen u. ä. nachzuweisen.

Seit den obengenannten Veröffentlichungen war man zu statistischen Methoden übergegangen, und es sind in wertvollen Arbeiten [5], [6] Formeln zur Berechnung der Dauerfestigkeit mit Hilfe statistisch gewonnener Parameter für bestimmte Werkstoffe und Konstruktionsteile entwickelt worden. Die Frage nach den physikalischen Ursachen des Dauerbruchs wurde aber damit in einer gewissen Resignation nicht mehr gestellt.

Erst in allerjüngster Zeit sind neue Ansätze zur Lösung des Ermüdungsproblems gemacht worden. Ganz neue Wege geht dabei die Hypothese von SCHAUB und LIEDTKE [7], die die Grundlage für die vorliegende Untersuchung bildet. Sie sei im folgenden nur kurz umrissen, da sie außerdem noch in einem Vortrag dieses Kolloquiums vom Autor selbst behandelt werden soll.

## 2. Schaubs Ermüdungshypothese

Die neue Hypothese von SCHAUB fordert, daß zwei Voraussetzungen zur Einleitung eines Dauerbruches erfüllt sein müssen, wovon die eine mit den älteren Hypothesen die allgemein anerkannte Tatsache gemeinsam hat, daß eine Gleitverformung im Werkstoff auftreten muß. Die zweite Forderung verlangt eine Reaktion der durch Gleitverformung aktivierten Oberflächenatome mit dem umgebenden Medium, in erster Linie dem Luftsauerstoff. Diese Forderung baut auf den von KRAMER [8], PEPPERHOFF [9] und CHURCHILL [10] beschriebenen Beobachtungen über reaktionskinetische Vorgänge in Metalloberflächen auf.

KRAMER [8] hatte eine Elektronenemission an kaltverformten Metalloberflächen mit dem Spitzenzähler gemessen, während PEPPERHOFF [9] eine Schwärzung von fotografischen Schichten durch einen sekundären Vorgang bei der Chemosorption von Sauerstoff an der bearbeiteten Metalloberfläche erhielt. Übereinstimmend mit Ergebnissen von CHURCHILL [10] gelangten dann SCHAUB und LIEDTKE [7] auf Grund eigener Versuche zu der Vorstellung, daß die Schwärzung der fotografischen Schicht auf einer Bildung von $H_2O_2$ beruht, die gleichzeitig mit der Chemosorption des Sauerstoffs in der Metalloberfläche abläuft. Die Chemosorption macht außerdem genügend Energie für die Austrittsarbeit der Elektronen aus der Metalloberfläche frei. SCHAUB und LIEDTKE beschreiben diesen Vorgang durch folgende Reaktionsgleichung:

$$Me + O_2 + H_2O = MeO + H_2O_2,$$

worin MeO den Zustand des vom Metall chemosorbierten Sauerstoffs bedeutet.

Mit Hilfe der geschilderten physikalischen Vorgänge wurde dann von SCHAUB und LIEDTKE folgende Arbeitshypothese für den Ermüdungsvorgang aufgestellt:

Örtliche Gleitvorgänge ergeben bei Wechselbeanspruchung eine ständige Aktivierung von Metallatomen an der Oberfläche, die schließlich zur Zerstörung der metallischen Bindung führen und damit den Dauerbruch einleiten. Erst nachdem der Anriß mit dem Fortschreiten dieses Prozesses eine genügende Ausdehnung erlangt hat, werden Kerbwirkung und angelegte Spannung zu den bestimmenden Faktoren für das Fortschreiten des Dauerbruchs.

## 3. Versuchsplanung

In einem Sonderausschuß des Schwedischen Nationalkomitees für Mechanik und des Jernkontorets wurde eine experimentelle Nachprüfung der SCHAUBschen Hypothese beschlossen. Von SCHAUB selbst wurden Versuche an Stahlstäben vorgeschlagen, wovon ein Teil bei einer gewissen Wechselspannung direkt bis zum Ermüdungsbruch und ein anderer Teil nach der halben Laufzeit, die in den erstgenannten Versuchen bestimmt worden war, leicht (etwa 0,1 mm) überdreht und dann bei der gleichen Wechselspannung weiter bis zum Bruch belastet werden sollte. Eine Erhöhung der Bruchlastwechselzahl an überdrehten Stäben würde als erster Beweis für eine Oberflächenreaktion gedeutet werden können. Dem Verfasser wurde die Planung und Durchführung der Versuche übertragen.

Von vornherein mußte bei einer Untersuchung an Stäben, deren Oberfläche eine so wesentliche Bedeutung zugemessen wurde, eine sorgfältige Bearbeitung vorgesehen werden. Es wurde deshalb ein elektrolytisches Polieren des hochbeanspruchten Teiles der Probestäbe gewählt.

Außerdem mußte aber auch Rücksicht auf Erholungs- und Alterungserscheinungen während der für das Abdrehen erforderlichen Unterbrechung des Laufes der Probe genommen werden. Arbeiten von KÖRBER und HEMPEL [11] sowie von SINCLAIR [12] hatten gezeigt, daß Ruhepausen eine Erhöhung der Bruchlastwechselzahl und der Dauerfestigkeit durch Alterung oder Trainieren hervorrufen können. KARIUS [13], [14] sowie DAEVES, GEROLD und SCHULZ [15] hatten zwar Alterungserscheinungen als Ursache einer erhöhten Lebensdauer von Ermüdungsproben abgelehnt, jedoch hatten sie ebenfalls höhere Lebensdauer erhalten und diese mit Erholungseffekten erklärt. Es wurden deshalb noch eine Anzahl Proben geprüft, bei denen eine Ruhepause von 24 Stunden nach der halben Bruchlastwechselzahl (der ersten Serie) eingeschaltet wurde. Gleichzeitig wurden drei einfache Kohlenstoffstähle und ein vergüteter Cr-Ni-Stahl als Versuchsmaterial gewählt, um die Frage zu klären, ob es sich bei der Erhöhung der Gesamtlebensdauer durch Ruhepausen um Alterung oder Erholung handelte. Der Vergütungsstahl konnte als völlig alterungssicher angesehen werden, während die Kohlenstoffstähle mehr oder weniger deutliche Alterungserscheinungen zeigen mußten. Um die möglichen Alterungs- und Erholungsvorgänge möglichst vollständig ablaufen zu lassen, wurden die Proben während der Ruhepausen einer Temperatur von 100° C ausgesetzt.

Als Belastungsart wurde umlaufende Biegung gewählt. Die Höhe der Spannung für die Umlaufbiegeversuche wurde so bestimmt, daß die mittlere Bruchlastwechselzahl der direkt bis zum Bruch belasteten Stäbe etwa 300.000 betragen sollte. Mit Hilfe einiger Stichprobenversuche wurde diese Spannung nach der Wöhler-Methode bestimmt. Bei dieser Spannung, die etwa 25% über der Dauerfestigkeit der Werkstoffe liegen dürfte, konnte außerdem angenommen werden, daß eine tiefergehende Schädigung nicht vor dem Ablauf der halben Bruchlastwechselzahl eingetreten sein kann. Die „Schadenslinie" dürfte erst bei 70 bis 80% der gesamten Lastwechselzahl überschritten werden.

## 4. Versuchswerkstoffe, Probenherstellung und Versuchsprogramm

Die Versuchswerkstoffe, drei Kohlenstoffstähle und ein Cr-Ni-Vergütungsstahl, standen als Rundstangen von etwa 20 mm Durchmesser zur Verfügung. Sie wurden in Rohlinge mit Stablänge aufgeteilt und vor der Bearbeitung wärmebehandelt, um größte Gleichmäßigkeit im Versuchswerkstoff zu erhalten. Die Kohlenstoffstähle wurden normalgeglüht und der Cr-Ni-Stahl vergütet. Die Tab. 1 gibt die Ausgangsdimension, die Zusammensetzung, die Wärmebehandlung und die nach dieser erhaltenen Festigkeitswerte an. Außerdem wurde die Härte an allen Stäben nach der Wärmebehandlung bestimmt. Die Grenzwerte der Härte sind ebenfalls in Tab. 1 wiedergegeben.

Tabelle 1. *Eigenschaften der Versuchswerkstoffe*

| Bezeichnung | Werkstoff-Art | Rohstangen-Durchmesser mm | Zusammensetzung in % | | | | | | | | | Wärmebehandlung | Festigkeitswerte | | | | |
|---|---|---|---|---|---|---|---|---|---|---|---|---|---|---|---|---|---|
| | | | C | Si | Mn | P | S | Ni | Cr | Mo | N | | $\sigma_S$ kg/mm² | $\sigma_B$ kg/mm² | $\delta_6$ % | $\psi$ % | $H_B$ kg/mm² |
| A | St 37.12 | 22 | 0,10 | Spur | 0,57 | 0,048 | 0,047 | — | — | — | 0,015 | Normalisieren 1 h 900° C, Luftabkühlung | 22,7 / 23,4 / 23,4 | 38,3 / 41,2 / 41,2 | 41 / 36 / 38 | 68 / 66 / 67 | 90 bis 115 |
| B | St 60.11 | 19 | 0,48 | 0,24 | 0,33 | 0,006 | 0,036 | — | — | — | — | Normalisieren 1 h 830° C Luftabkühlung | 36,9 / 37,6 / 37,6 | 63,8 / 63,2 / 62,8 | 27 / 29 / 27 | 47 / 45 / 47 | 170 bis 184 |
| C | 0,3% C | 20 | 0,27 | Spur | 0,60 | 0,033 | 0,014 | — | — | — | 0,011 | Normalisieren 1 h 900° C, Luftabkühlung | 42,7 / 42,7 / 42,1 | 57,2 / 56,7 / 56,1 | 29 / 30 / 30 | 55 / 55 / 57 | 158 bis 170 |
| D | VCN 35 | 20 | 0,46 | 0,30 | 0,51 | 0,024 | 0,009 | 2,83 | 0,74 | Spur | — | Härten: 850° C, Öl Anlassen: ½ h 500° C, Öl | 118,5 / 122,2 / 120,1 | 127,8 / 130,0 / 129,5 | 15 / 14 / 14 | 48 / 51 / 51 | 330 bis 365 |

Die Probestabform geht aus Abb. 1 hervor. Die Prüfmaschine war eine schwedische Alpha-Maschine für umlaufende Biegung, die bei einseitiger Einspannung des Stabes eine dreieckförmige Momentenfläche ergibt; sie hatte eine Umdrehungszahl von 3.000 pro Minute.

Die Probestücke wurden nach der Wärmebehandlung fertigbearbeitet, geschliffen und über eine Länge von etwa 40 mm im Gebiet des größten Biegemomentes elektrolytpoliert. Etwa 10 bis 20 μ der Oberflächenschicht wurden durch das elektrolytische Polieren abgeätzt.

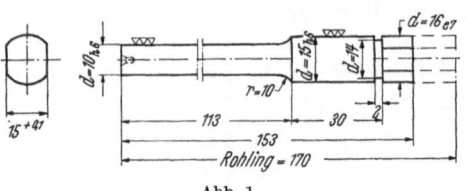

Abb. 1.

Die Stäbe, die nach der Hälfte der Laufzeit abgedreht wurden, erhielten im Gebiet des größten Biegemoments einen 0,2 mm kleineren Durchmesser durch das Abdrehen, worauf die Oberfläche erneut elektrolytisch poliert wurde.

Für die Vorversuche zur Bestimmung der geeigneten Spannungsstufe wurden etwa vier bis sieben Stäbe verwendet. Die Hauptversuche wurden mit je neun Stäben von jedem Werkstoff durchgeführt. Das Versuchsprogramm zeigt untenstehendes Schema, wozu zu ergänzen ist, daß mit den Kohlenstoffstählen noch eine vierte Serie mit wiederholten Ruhepausen nach jedem 60.000. Lastwechsel gefahren wurde.

*Schema für das Versuchsprogramm:*

| 1. Serie | 2. Serie | 3. Serie | 4. Serie (nur Kohlenstoffstähle) |
|---|---|---|---|
| 9 Stäbe bis zum Bruch belastet. Bestimmung der mittleren Bruchlastwechselzahl. | 9 Stäbe bis zu 50% der mittleren Bruchlastwechselzahl von Serie 1. | 9 Stäbe wie Serie 2. | 6—9 Stäbe mit Ruhepause sowie gleichzeitigem Anlassen 24 Stunden bei 100° C nach jedem 60.000. Lastwechsel. Bestimmung der Gesamtbruchlastwechselzahl. |
| | Ruhepause mit Anlassen 24 Stunden bei 100° C. | Abdrehen einer Schicht von 0,1 mm Dicke, darauf Elektrolytpolieren. | |
| | Bestimmung der Restlebenslänge. | Bestimmung der Restlebenslänge. | |

## 5. Versuchsergebnisse

Die Wöhler-Kurven zur Bestimmung der geeigneten Spannungsstufen für die Hauptversuche sind in Abb. 2 zusammengestellt. Folgende Wechsel-

spannungen wurden für die vier
Versuchswerkstoffe gewählt:

| Werkstoff | Wechselspannung für etwa 300.000 Lastwechsel bis zum Bruch |
|---|---|
| A | ± 26 kg/mm² |
| B | ± 27,5 „ |
| C | ± 33 „ |
| D | ± 58 „ |

Die Hauptversuche gaben
mit diesen Wechselspannungen
die Ergebnisse nach Tab. 2.
Außerdem sind die Ergebnisse
in Schaubildern für die Gesamt-
lebenslänge (Abb. 3) und für die
Restlebenslänge (Abb. 4) dargestellt worden.

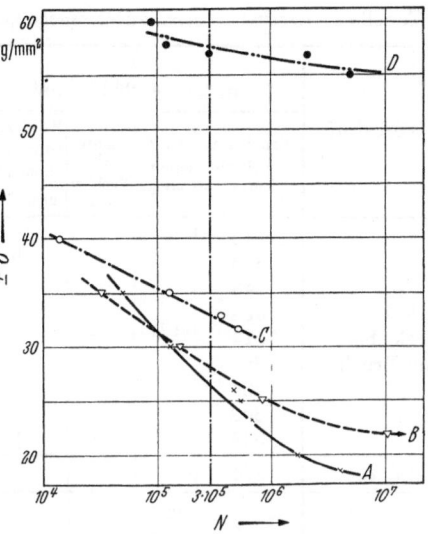

Abb. 2. Wöhler-Kurven der vier untersuchten
Stähle (Rotierende Biegung).

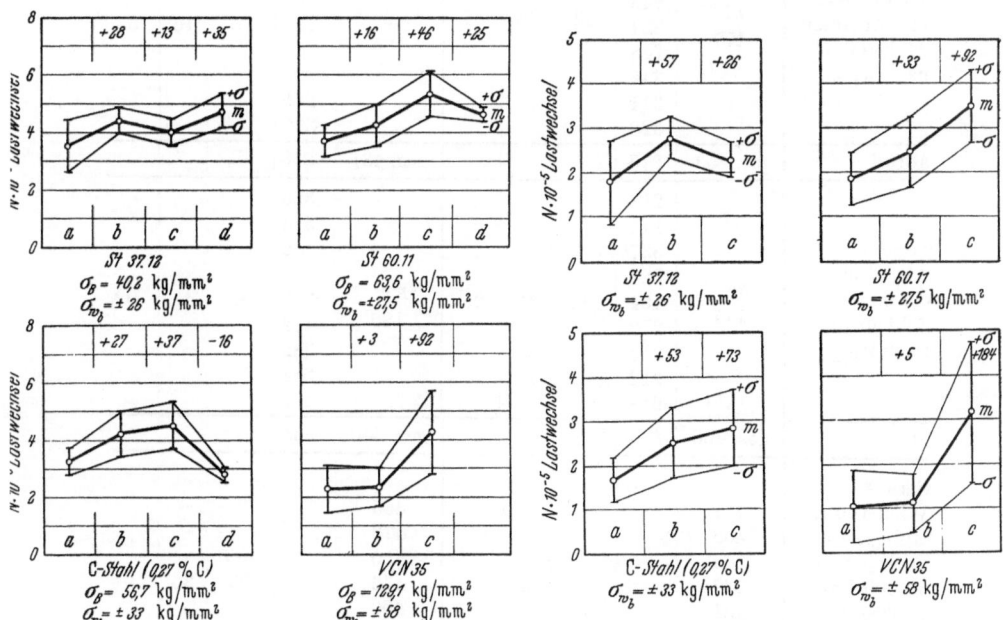

Abb. 3.
Prozentualer Oberflächeneinfluß bei Dauerbiegeversuchen.
  a direkt bis zum Bruch
  b 1 Ruhepause 24 h bei 100° C
  c abgedreht
  d Ruhepausen nach jeder 60. 000. U.

Abb. 4.
Prozentualer Oberflächeneinfluß bei Dauerbiegeversuchen. Restlebenslänge.
  a direkt bis zum Bruch
  b 1 Ruhepause 24 h 100° C
  c abgedreht

Tabelle 2. *Ergebnisse der Dauerversuche mit umlaufender Biegung* $n = N \cdot 10^{-3}$

| Werkstoff | A $\sigma_{Wb} = \pm\, 26\ \mathrm{kg/mm^2}$ | | | | | B $\sigma_{Wb} = \pm\, 27{,}5\ \mathrm{kg/mm^2}$ | | | | |
|---|---|---|---|---|---|---|---|---|---|---|
| | Bruchlast-wechsel-zahl | Rest-lebens-länge | Mittl. quadr. Ab-weichg. $\sigma \pm$ | Proz. Änderung der Lebenslänge ges. | Restl. | Bruchlast-wechsel-zahl | Rest-lebens-länge | Mittl. quadr. Ab-weichg. $\sigma \pm$ | Proz. Änderung der Lebenslänge ges. | Restl. |
| Serie 1 Direkt bis zum Bruch | 445 316 243 398 514 357 234 303 378 | (177) | 92 | | | 476 358 437 393 401 343 306 290 338 | (186) | 60 | | |
| Mittel $n_B$ | 354 | | | | | 371 | | | | |
| Serie 2 1 Ruhepause mit Anlassen 24 h 100°C nach $n_{B/2}$. | $n_{B/2} = 177$ | 231 235 224 243 324 248 342 311 328 | 43 | 28 | 57 | $n_{B/2} = 185$ | 256 213 131 161 286 308 226 249 377 | 75 | 16 | 33 |
| Mittel | ges. 453 | 276 | | | | ges. 431 | 246 | | | |
| Serie 3 Abgedreht, 0,1 mm Schichtdicke nach $n_{B/2}$. | $n_{B/2} = 177$ | 218 141 337 224 164 272 215 212 218 | 43 | 13 | 26 | $n_{B/2} = 185$ | 326 346 152 417 393 412 382 364 402 | 82 | 46 | 92 |
| Mittel | ges. 400 | 223 | | | | ges. 540 | 355 | | | |
| Serie 4 Wiederholte Ruhepausen nach jedem 60.000. Last-wechsel mit Anlassen 24 h 100° C | 437 468 584 537 421 433 475 | — | 60 | 35 | — | 455 473 456 472 500 432 | | 23 | 25 | — |
| Mittel | ges. 479 | | | | | ges. 465 | | | | |

*Tabelle 2 (Forts.)*

| Werkstoff | C $\sigma_{Wb} = \pm 33\ \text{kg/mm}^2$ | | | | | D $\sigma_{Wb} = \pm 58\ \text{kg/mm}^2$ | | | | |
|---|---|---|---|---|---|---|---|---|---|---|
| | Bruchlast-wechsel-zahl | Rest-lebens-länge | Mittl. quadr. Ab-weichg. $\sigma \pm$ | Proz. Ände-rung der Le-benslänge ges. | Restl. | Bruchlast-wechsel-zahl | Rest-lebens-länge | Mittl. quadr. Ab-weichg. $\sigma \pm$ | Proz. Ände-rung der Le-benslänge ges. | Restl. |
| Serie 1 Direkt bis zum Bruch | 363 317 397 294 280 360 248 348 350 | (168) | 47 | | | 116 366 240 303 233 117 235 197 | (111) | 85 | | |
| Mittel $n_B$ | 328 | | | | | 226 | | | | |
| Serie 2 1 Ruhepause mit Anlassen 24 h 100° C nach $n_{B/2}$. | $n_{B/2} =$ 160 | 305 306 328 302 253 226 81 202 293 | 77 | 27 | 53 | $n_{B/2} =$ 115 | 95 244 40 45 98 165 76 140 150 | 65 | 3 | 5 |
| Mittel | ges. 415 | 251 | | | | ges. 232 | 117 | | | |
| Serie 3 Abgedreht 0,1 mm Schichtdicke nach $n_{B/2}$. | $n_{B/2} =$ 160 | 298 299 148 306 341 321 373 320 379 | 84 | 37 | 73 | $n_{B/2} =$ 115 | 245 651 235 211 487 173 350 318 313 | 154 | 92 | 184 |
| Mittel | ges. 448 | 284 | | | | ges. 435 | 322 | | | |
| Serie 4 Wiederholte Ruhepausen nach jedem 60.000. Last-wechsel mit Anlassen 24 h 100° C | 249 274 323 295 259 300 267 246 263 | | 26 | -16 | — | — | — | — | — | — |
| Mittel | ges. 275 | | | | | | | | | |

Zur Tab. 2 ist noch zu bemerken, daß für die Serien 2 und 3, d. h. mit einer Ruhepause und mit Abdrehen einer 0,1 mm dicken Schicht, nur die Einzelwerte der „Restlebenslänge" angegeben wurden. Unter Restlebenslänge sei hier die Lastwechselzahl nach der Unterbrechung bis zum Bruch verstanden. In den Spalten für die Mittelwerte der Bruchlastwechselzahlen sind aber auch die Gesamtlebenslängen angegeben. Außerdem wurden die mittlere quadratische Abweichung und die prozentualen Änderungen der Gesamt- und der Restlebenslänge eingetragen.

In den Schaubildern der Gesamtlebenslängen (Abb. 3) und der Restlebenslängen (Abb. 4) wurden die prozentualen Änderungen über jeder Spalte für die einzelnen Versuchsserien angegeben. Aus den Schaubildern geht hervor, daß eine Ruhepause eine Erhöhung der Bruchlastwechselzahl nur bei den Kohlenstoffstählen ergab, während dies beim Vergütungsstahl nicht der Fall war. Die wiederholten Ruhepausen führten bei den Stählen A und B zu einer noch etwas größeren Erhöhung der Bruchlastwechselzahl, während beim Stahl C eine Erniedrigung mit 16% erfolgte. Eine Erklärung für dieses Verhalten des Stahles C kann nicht gegeben werden, doch wird diese Frage weiter unten noch diskutiert werden.

Das Abdrehen der 0,1-mm-Schicht führte in allen Fällen zu einer beträchtlichen Erhöhung der Bruchlastwechselzahl. Vor allem sind die Zahlen der prozentualen Erhöhung für die Restlebenslänge zu betrachten, die sich wie folgt ergaben:

Für Stahl A: 26%
,, ,, B: 92%
,, ,, C: 73%
,, ,, D: 184%

## 6. Diskussion der Versuchsergebnisse

Ganz allgemein können aus den Versuchsergebnissen folgende Schlüsse gezogen werden, die auch trotz der ziemlich großen Streuungen gelten:

a) Ruhepausen ergeben eine Erhöhung der Bruchlastwechselzahlen, wenn es sich um Werkstoffe handelt, die alterungsfähig sind.

b) Nicht alternde Werkstoffe erfahren keine Veränderung der Ermüdungseigenschaften, wie das Beispiel des Vergütungsstahles zeigt.

c) Das Entfernen einer dünnen Oberflächenschicht genügt, um eine wesentliche Erhöhung der Bruchlastwechselzahlen zu erreichen.

Von diesen Regeln macht nur noch der Versuch mit wiederholten Ruhepausen an Stahl C eine Ausnahme. Eine Erklärung mit Hilfe der neuen SCHAUBschen Hypothese wäre denkbar, wenn man annehmen will, daß die reaktionskinetischen Vorgänge während der Ruhepausen weiter ablaufen und schließlich sogar die Alterungsvorgänge überwiegen.

Dagegen spricht auch nicht die Erhöhung der Bruchlastwechselzahl nach nur einer Ruhepause, doch ist nicht recht einzusehen, warum die zwei anderen Kohlenstoffstähle ein wesentlich abweichendes Ergebnis brachten. Ein Versuchsfehler konnte nachträglich nicht nachgewiesen werden, doch bleibt ein solcher Verdacht nach wie vor bestehen.

Die Versuche mit den während der Pause überdrehten Stäben zeigen dagegen ein völlig eindeutiges Ergebnis, das auf jeden Fall als Beleg für die hervorragende Bedeutung der Metalloberfläche und der Vorgänge in dieser angesehen werden kann. Beim Cr-Ni-Vergütungsstahl ist die Erhöhung des Mittelwertes mit 184% so groß, daß diese nicht allein physikalisch erklärt werden kann. Vielmehr zeigte dieser Werkstoff die größten Streuungen, und um diese mehr auszugleichen, wäre eine wesentlich größere Zahl von Probestäben notwendig gewesen. Die Tendenz kann aber zur Genüge aus den Ergebnissen abgelesen werden.

Nach Abschluß der hier vorgelegten Versuche ist kürzlich eine Notiz in „Engineering" von THOMPSON [16] erschienen, der von ähnlichen Ergebnissen berichtet. THOMPSON erhielt nämlich an Kupferstäben, von denen nach je 25% der Bruchlastwechselzahl von direkt bis zum Bruch belasteten Proben Schichten von 10 bis 20 $\mu$ elektrolytisch abgeätzt wurden, eine 125% größere Laufzeit, ohne daß Ansätze zu Ermüdungsrissen zu erkennen waren. Er zieht daraus den Schluß, daß man den Einfluß des Luftsauerstoffs näher untersuchen müsse. Die Ergebnisse von THOMPSON deuten also in die gleiche Richtung wie die hier vorgetragenen und können als weitere Stütze für die SCHAUBsche Hypothese angesehen werden.

Eine gewisse Kritik kann natürlich gegen die hier angewandte Versuchsausführung mit Umlaufbiegung gerichtet werden, da Biegung eine inhomogene Belastung mit der höchsten Spannung in der Oberflächenschicht der Proben ergibt. Die ersten und größten Verformungen treten daher in dieser auf, doch dürfte auch unter Berücksichtigung der Stützwirkung durch die im Innern der Probe liegenden, weniger beanspruchten Schichten eine Überspannung von etwa 25% eine Gleitverformung in wesentlich dickerer Schicht ergeben, als sie durch das Abdrehen von 0,1 mm entfernt wurde.

Weitere Versuche sind daher auch mit wechselnder Zug-Druck-Beanspruchung geplant. Außerdem sollen auch andere Werkstoffe wie Kupfer und Aluminium untersucht werden. Schließlich muß noch das umgebende Medium variiert werden, was bedeutet, daß Versuche in neutralen sowie in stärker angreifenden Stoffen ausgeführt werden müssen.

Mit den hier vorgelegten Ergebnissen ist zunächst nur ein Schritt getan, um einen neuen Versuch zur Klärung des Ermüdungsproblems zu wagen, doch glauben wir, daß diese Ergebnisse uns dazu berechtigen,

auf dem eingeschlagenen und durch SCHAUBS Hypothese aufgezeigten
Wege fortzusetzen. Es ist jedoch klar, daß noch sehr viel Arbeit zu
leisten ist, bevor diese Hypothese wirklich als bewiesen angesehen werden kann.

### Literaturverzeichnis

[1] OROWAN, E.: Proc. Roy. Soc. (A), 171, 79—105 (1939).
[2] DEHLINGER, U.: Z. Metallk., 32, 199 (1940).
[3] AFANASIEW, N. N., Zhur. Techn. Fiziki, 10, 1553 (1940).
[4] BOAS, W.: Symp. Failure of Metals by Fatigue, Melbourne, 28—39 (1947).
[5] WEIBULL, W.: KTH Handl. (Trans. Roy. Inst. Tech.) (Stockholm) Nr. 27
    (1949).
[6] EPREMIAN, E., und R. F. MEHL: Carnegie Inst. Techn., June 1952.
[7] SCHAUB, C., und W. LIEDTKE: Z. Metallk. 44, 570—572 (1953).
[8] KRAMER, J.: Der metallische Zustand, Göttingen 1950.
[9] PEPPERHOFF, W.: Z. Metallk. 43, 402—403 (1952).
[10] CHURCHILL, J. R.: Trans. electrochem. Soc. 76, 341 (1939).
[11] KÖRBER, F., und M. HEMPEL: Mitt. K.-Wilh.-Inst. Eisenforsch. 17, 247—257
    (1935).
[12] SINCLAIR, G. M.: Proc. ASTM 52, 743—751 (1952).
[13] KARIUS, A., E. GEROLD und E. H. SCHULZ: Arch. Eisenhüttenw. 18, 113—124
    (1944—45).
[14] KARIUS, A.: Metallwirtsch., 23, 419—434 (1944).
[15] DAEVES, K., E. GEROLD und E. H. SCHULZ: Stahl u. Eisen, 60, 100—103 (1944).
[16] THOMPSON, N.: Engineering 178, (1954, Dec. 3).

### Diskussion

I. A. ODING berichtete über ähnliche Versuche, die in der Sowjet-Union ausgeführt worden sind, bei denen aber keine Ruhepausen eingeschaltet waren. Eine
bestimmte Erhöhung der Lebensdauer wurde dabei beobachtet. Auch wurden
Parallelversuche zur Bestimmung der Wöhlerkurve in Luft- und Wasserstoffatmosphäre mit Hilfe von je 20 Probestäben ausgeführt. Die Wechselfestigkeit wurde
dabei dieselbe, aber die Bruchflächen sahen verschieden aus.

O. LISSNER: Die Versuche von GOUGH und SOPWITH ergaben bereits vor 20 Jahren
eine Verbesserung der Lebensdauer in Wasserstoffatmosphäre gegenüber in Luft.

L. HIMMEL: It may be of interest to point out that G. C. SMITH and D. R.
HARRIES at Cambridge University have also produced a significant increase in the
mean fatigue life of high purity aluminum merely by stopping the fatigue test at
intervals in order to grind away the surface layers. Specimens which were rested
for equivalent periods, but not reground, failed to exhibit any improvement in
fatigue life. The evidence strongly indicates that the fatigue cracks which eventually cause failure of the material originate in the surface layers and propagate
inward. It is to be expected, therefore, that the removal of the "damaged" surface
layer will result in an increase in fatigue life. On the other hand, once micro-cracks
appear, annealing the specimen should have relatively little effect on the fatigue
life. This has been amply demonstrated by a number of investigators.

J. SCHIJVE: I would like to call your attention to the fact that after removal
of a surface layer the new surface layer need not be fatigued in the same way as
the original one, because a sub-surface layer does not have the same possibilities
of micro-deformation as a surface layer.

W. Weibull emphasized the importance of the surrounding medium for fatigue life and referred to his own paper in this Colloquium, see p. 291.

A. M. Freudenthal: Yes, according to my experience cleaning of the test piece surface with $C\,Cl_4$ gave longer fatigue life than cleaning with $C\,Cl_4 + CH_3OH$.

A. Petrussewitsch referred to his own paper, where Sovjet-Russian investigations of atmospheric influences on fatigue life had been reviewed, see p. 204.

O. Lissner: Aus den verschiedenen Diskussionsbeiträgen geht hervor, daß auch an anderen Stellen gleichartige Beobachtungen gemacht wurden wie bei unseren Versuchen. Auf den Einwand von Herrn Schijve möchte ich besonders erwidern, daß es das Ziel der geplanten Versuche in neutralen Medien sein wird zu beweisen, daß auch die größere Mikrodeformation der Oberflächenschicht nicht allein ausreichend ist, um einen Dauerbruch hervorzurufen.

# Essais de fatigue par flexion avec fréquences superposées

Par

## L. Locati

Avec 9 figures

Les relevés de la sollicitation de fonctionnement sur un grand nombre d'organes mécaniques démontrent combien la réalité est différente des conditions extrêmement simplifiées des essais de fatigue ordinaires, effectués sous effort constant [1].

On peut obtenir des diagrammes de charge pouvant être rapportés au type AA′ (à superposition de fréquence) ou au type BB′ (à modulation d'amplitude) (Fig. 1). Quelques machines de fatigue permettent d'effectuer des essais de type B: par exemple le Vibrophore Amsler (cycles d'amplitude variables avec continuité), le nouveau Pulsator Schenck selon GASSNER (cycles à fréquence et amplitude différentes, appliqués en des temps distincts) [2], la machine à flexion rotative à poids mobile, construite par l'Auteur [3] en modifiant une Schenck «Simplex», etc.

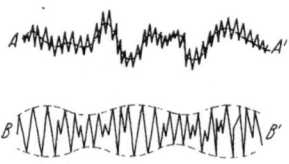

Fig. 1. Superposition de fréquences très différentes (Superposition). Superposition de fréquences très prochaines (Modulation d'amplitude).

Au contraire, on ne dispose, tout au moins d'après ce qu'il nous résulte, d'aucune machine pour la réalisation d'une loi de charge du premier type.

La nécessité d'expérimentation avec ce premier cas (superposition de fréquence) est très ressentie; en effet, tandis que dans le cas d'amplitude modulée, le constructeur peut baser son evaluation sur la théorie du dommage cumulatif (MINER), aucun critère n'a été jusqu'ici proposé pour le cas de fréquences superposées.

Avec un diagramme complexe d'efforts, relevé expérimentalement, même en le simplifiant au maximum, on reste bien perplexe pour décider quelle est l'amplitude réelle du cycle qu'il faut comparer sur le diagramme de Goodman.

Par exemple, tout en réduisant le graphique des sollicitations vérifiées sur un vilebrequin en forme extrêmement schématique A (voir fig. 2), on ne sait pas si pour prévoir la vie de l'éprouvette on doit considérer le matériau assujeti à un cycle idéal compris entre les extrêmes, soit entre 1 et 4 et entre 4 et 7, ou bien à des cycles partiels 1—2, 2—3, 3—4, 4—5, 5—6, 6—7.

Dans un autre exemple, encore plus schématique, nous ne savons pas si le graphique B puisse être équivalent à des cycles entre 1 et 2, 3 et 4 de moindre amplitude.

Dans le but de porter une contribution, même initiale, à cette complexe question, l'Auteur a construit une machine d'essai à même d'imposer à une éprouvette une sollicitation variable; la loi de variation

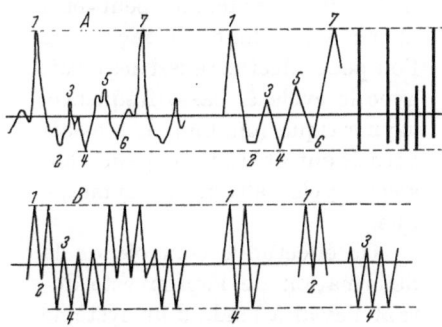

Fig. 2. Schématization de cycles réels.

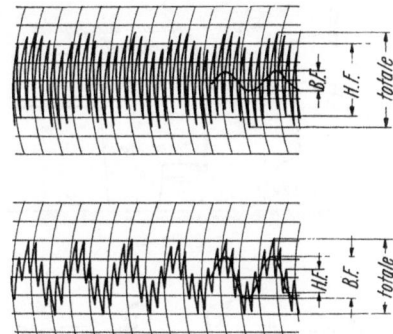

Fig. 3. Lois de contraintes sur la machine.

résulte de la superposition de deux sinusoïdes à amplitude constante, de fréquences très différentes, selon la formule

$$F(t) = A \sin 2\pi\, nt + B \sin 2\pi\, n't$$

où $A$ et $B$ sont des amplitudes constantes et $n$ et $n'$, deux fréquences avec la valeur de $n'$ au moins 3 fois supérieure à $n$.

Dans cette hypothèse, l'allure des sollicitations est simplifiée aux deux graphiques de la fig. 3, dont le premier se rapporte à une superposition d'une grande amplitude à haute fréquence (H. F.) et d'une petite à basse fréquence (B. F.), tandis que le deuxième correspond à une dentelure à haute fréquence sur une grande amplitude à basse fréquence.

Si le rapport des fréquences est suffisamment grand, l'amplitude totale peut être considérée constante et égale à la somme des amplitudes des deux mouvements superposés.

La machine se base sur l'accouplement d'un système bielle-manivelle à basse fréquence, avec un excitateur à haute fréquence constitué par une turbine à air, déséquilibrée; cette machine est résultée fort simple.

La bielle agit sur l'éprouvette par l'intermédiaire d'un organe élastique (2 ressorts à lames) qui, grâce à sa grande flexibilité, n'empêche pas le mouvement de résonnance du système éprouvette-turbine. La machine est montrée schématiquement par la fig. 4 et les éprouvettes par la fig. 5.

La partie à déformation imposée travaille avec une fréquence pouvant être choisie entre 170 et 550 r/min, au moyen d'un variateur de vitesse.

La fréquence du système turbine-éprouvette est, au contraire, de l'ordre de 3.000 r/min et peut-être modifiée par une variation des dimensions de l'éprouvette même. La bielle de la machine peut-être allongée à volonté de façon que l'on peut effectuer aussi des essais avec le cycle à basse fréquence, asymétrique (ondulé). Les essais actuels ont été toutefois effectués sous cycle alternatif symétrique.

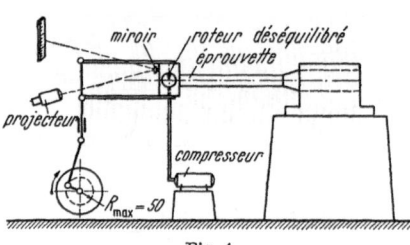

Fig. 4.

On effectue le contrôle de la déformation de l'éprouvette durant l'essai à l'aide d'un système optique, consistant en un appareil projectant une trace lumineuse sur une échelle et dans un miroir relié à la tête de l'éprouvette.

L'étalonnage a été effectué à l'aide d'un extensomètre électrique, et précisément avec deux «strain-gages» collés sur la partie utile.

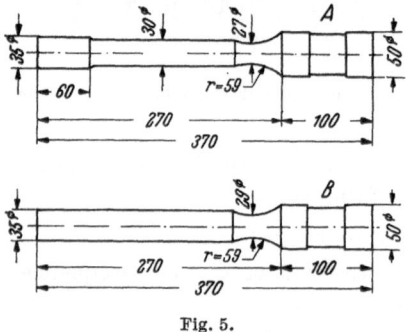

Fig. 5.

Cet étalonnage s'effectue en deux phases distinctes, pour la haute et la basse fréquence, et les coefficients de calcul, qui résultent différents, s'emploient distinctement au cours des essais, durant les opérations de charge de l'éprouvette.

La «sensibilité» de sollicitation est environ de 0,5 kg/mm² pour l'acier et de 0,3 kg/mm² pour le duralumin.

Le rayon de congé de la gorge de l'éprouvette est grand, toutefois il produit un effet de concentration non négligeable, de 15%; cette valeur a été relevée expérimentalement et est en accord avec la littérature. De toute façon, étant donné que l'étalonnage est rapporté à la sollicitation réelle dans la gorge de l'éprouvette mesurée avec l'extensomètre, la concentration d'effort est comprise dans l'expression des résultats.

## 1. Matériaux essayés

Les recherches sont encore en phase préliminaire, et les résultats, pas nombreux, constituent plutôt des exemples de diverses méthodes d'essai.

On a pris jusqu'ici en considération deux matériaux, à savoir:

a) Un acier au charbon C43 ayant la composition suivante:

$$C = 0{,}41\%; \quad Cr = 0{,}48\%; \quad Mn = 0{,}7\%; \quad Si = 0{,}27\%$$

Les éprouvettes sont obtenues de barres laminées de diamètre 60 mm, normalisées à 910° C durant 1 h, refroidissement à 620° C et séjour à cette température durant 1 h 15 min, avec refroidissement successif à l'air.

La résistance, déduite de la dureté, est comprise entre 70 et 72,5 kg/mm². Les caractéristiques mécaniques obtenues sur une éprouvette de traction sont:

```
limite de proportionnalité . . . . . . . .   35 kg/mm²
limite d'écoulement  . . . . . . . . . .   37,2  ,,
résistance à la traction . . . . . . . . .   70,4  ,,
allongement . . . . . . . . . . . . . .   27%
limite de fatigue en H. F. . . . . . . . .   34 kg/mm²
```

b) un alliage léger, type Superdural, de composition:

$$Cu = 4{,}28\%; \quad Si = 0{,}59\%; \quad Mg = 0{,}85\%; \quad Mn = 1{,}08\%; \quad Fe = 0{,}33\%.$$

Ces éprouvettes ont été tirées également d'une barre de diamètre 60 mm, et sont ébauchées, chauffées 3 h à 515° C, trempées dans l'eau froide et vieillies naturellement.

Leurs caractéristiques mécaniques sont les suivantes:

```
dureté Brinell . . . . . . . . . . . . .   140 (± 5)
limite d'élasticité (0,1%) . . . . . . . .   38,5 kg/mm²
résistance à la rupture . . . . . . . . .   59      ,,
allongement . . . . . . . . . . . . . .   16%
limite de fatigue en H. F. (10⁷) . . . . .   19 kg/mm²
```

## 2. Essais sur acier

On a tracé initialement les courbes $S$-$N$ selon la méthode traditionelle, soit à haute fréquence (3.400 r/min), soit à basse fréquence (500 r/min).

Les deux courbes se différencient un peu, et quoique nous soyons généralement habitués à négliger l'influence de la fréquence, il faut, dans ce cas, en tenir compte. Quelques éprouvettes cassées à la fréquence très basse de 180 r/min concordent bien avec la courbe relative à la fréquence de 500 r/min; pour simplifier, dans le présent mémoire, on a jugé que les courbes $S$-$N$ à 500 r/min et 180 r/min, doivent pratiquement coïncider.

Les courbes obtenues sont montrées par la fig. 6 et on peut en déduire les limites de fatigue suivantes:

```
— haute fréquence . . . . . . . . . . .   34 kg/mm²
— basse fréquence . . . . . . . . . . .   32      ,,
```

La différence de 6% concorde avec ce qui a été trouvé par d'autres expérimentateurs [4], [5].

On est ensuite passé aux essais avec superposition de fréquences, qui se sont déroulés initialement suivant le principe de maintenir constante, pour toutes les éprouvettes du groupe, l'amplitude d'efforts à haute fréquence en variant, au contraire, d'une éprouvette à l'autre, l'amplitude à basse fréquence.

Pour cette série d'essais, l'amplitude à haute fréquence fut choisie de valeur élevée, et précisément, égale à la limite de fatigue correspondante, ce qui fait qu'il était naturel d'arriver assez rapidement à la rupture en superposant une amplitude à basse fréquence, même peu importante, comme cela s'est vérifié en effet.

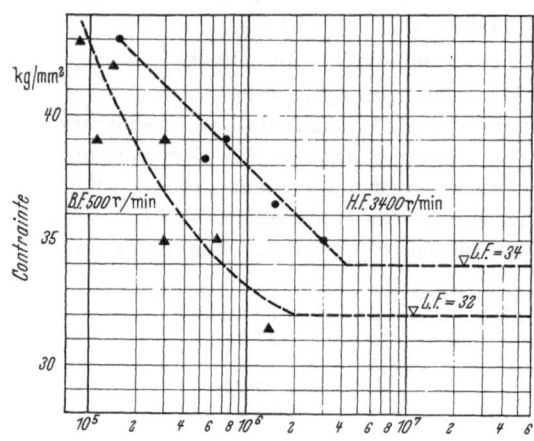

Fig. 6.
Courbe *S-N* (de Wöhler) en haute et basse fréquence.

Dans les essais à deux fréquences superposées, la question particulière d'exprimer la durée de l'éprouvette surgit: elle peut, en effet, être donnée en nombre de cycles à haute fréquence, ou en nombre de cycles à basse fréquence; la question n'est pas essentielle, car on peut passer d'une méthode à l'autre au moyen du rapport des fréquences, mais si l'on ne tient pas compte de ce fait, il est possible de tomber dans des équivoques lors de l'interprétation des résultats.

| Contrainte ± kg/mm² | | | Durée (nombre de cycles) | | |
|---|---|---|---|---|---|
| H. F. | B. F. | Totale | B. F. = 180 r/min | B. F. = 500 r/min | Prévue pour une amplitude totale en H. F. |
| 34 | 0 | 34 | ∞ | ∞ | ∞ |
| 34 | 2 | 36 | 10.200.000 | 1.800.000 | 2.000.000 |
| 34 | 5 | 39 | 1.124.000 | 910.000 | 700.000 |
| 34 | 8 | 42 | 510.000 | 410.000 | 260.000 |

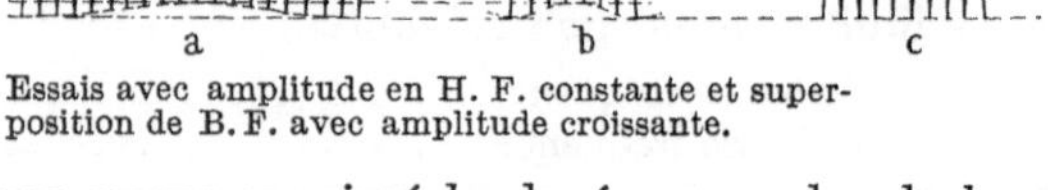

Fig. 7. Essais avec amplitude en H. F. constante et superposition de B. F. avec amplitude croissante.

Dans la fig. 7 nous avons exprimé la durée en cycles de haute fréquence. Chaque nombre est la moyenne logarithmique de deux résultats.

On déduit de la fig. 7 que la superposition d'une basse fréquence réduit la durée au fur et à mesure que son amplitude devient plus importante; toutefois, la durée de l'éprouvette est toujours supérieure à celle que l'on aurait avec une éprouvette soumise à une amplitude totale, à haute fréquence.

L'ensemble et les durées des éprouvettes ne changent pas de façon sensible en passant d'une fréquence de 180 à 500; ce qui porte à conclure que, dans ces essais, la principale détérioration est provoquée par la haute fréquence.

Une autre façon de conduire les essais est celle de maintenir constante la sollicitation *totale* pour toutes les éprouvettes d'une même série, en changeant chaque fois le «dosage» des amplitudes, soit en variant le rapport entre les amplitudes en H. F. et en B. F.

Afin d'obtenir une représentation complète et sûre, beaucoup d'éprouvettes ont été nécessaires, car on doit les expérimenter à *divers niveaux* de sollicitation totale et avec de *différents «dosages»*.

Au tableau 1 sont rassemblées les valeurs obtenues avec 3 différents

Tableau 1. *Acier C43 — Résultats des essais à amplitude totale constante à des différents «dosages» de H. F. et B. F.*

| Sollicitation ± | | | | Durée réelle exprimée en B. F. | | Durée réelle exprimée en H. F. | |
|---|---|---|---|---|---|---|---|
| Totale | H. F. | B. F. | HF—BF °/₀ | essais à 500 r/min | essais à 180 r/min | essais à 500 r/min | essais à 180 r/min |
| 35.5 | 35,5 | 0 | 100—0 | — | — | 2.500.000 | 2.500.000 |
| | 33,5 | 2 | 94—6 | 264.000 | — | 1.800.000 | — |
| | 25 | 10,5 | 70—30 | 290.000 | — | 1.960.000 | — |
| | 18,5 | 17 | 52—48 | 640.000 | — | 4.500.000 | — |
| | 0 | 35,5 | 0—100 | 400.000 | — | — | — |
| 39 | 39 | 0 | 100—0 | — | — | 680.000 | 680.000 |
| | 34 | 5 | 87—13 | 135.000 | — | 930.000 | — |
| | 34 | 5 | 87—13 | — | 59.400 | — | 1.130.000 |
| | 29 | 10 | 75—25 | — | 32.500 | — | 610.000 |
| | 29 | 10 | 75—25 | 85.000 | — | 560.000 | — |
| | 27,5 | 11,5 | 70—30 | 240.000 | — | 1.650.000 | — |
| | 19,5 | 19,5 | 50—50 | 114.000 | — | 780.000 | — |
| | 10,3 | 28,7 | 26—74 | 260.000 | — | 1.800.000 | — |
| | 10 | 29 | 25—75 | — | 119.000 | — | 2.350.000 |
| | 4 | 35 | 10—90 | — | 432.000 | — | 8.200.000 |
| | 0 | 39 | 0—100 | 190.000 | 190.000 | — | — |
| 43 | 43 | 0 | 100—0 | -- | — | 160.000 | 160.000 |
| | 38 | 5 | 88—12 | 45.000 | — | 300.000 | — |
| | 35 | 8 | 81—19 | 60.000 | — | 408.000 | — |
| | 35 | 8 | 81—19 | — | 27.000 | — | 510.000 |
| | 12 | 31 | 28—72 | 75.000 | — | 510.000 | — |
| | 0 | 43 | 0—100 | 100.000 | — | — | — |

niveaux de sollicitation totale: 35,5; 39; 43; la première valeur a été choisie peu au dessu de la limite de fatigue à haute fréquence.

Les essais sont faits par groupes d'éprouvettes sous sollicitation *totale* constante; en réalité, la sollicitation totale devrait varier légèrement et augmenter au fur et à mesure que «l'aliquote H. F.» augmente, en tenant compte que la résistance à la fatigue H. F. est supérieure à celle B. F. Cependant, dans ces essais d'orientation, on a négligé cette précaution, pour simplifier.

L'expression de la durée a été déterminée avec le nombre de cycles à basse fréquence et à haute fréquence; cette double expression est possible en tous cas, en dehors des essais conduits exclusivement en haute fréquence ou bien en basse fréquence.

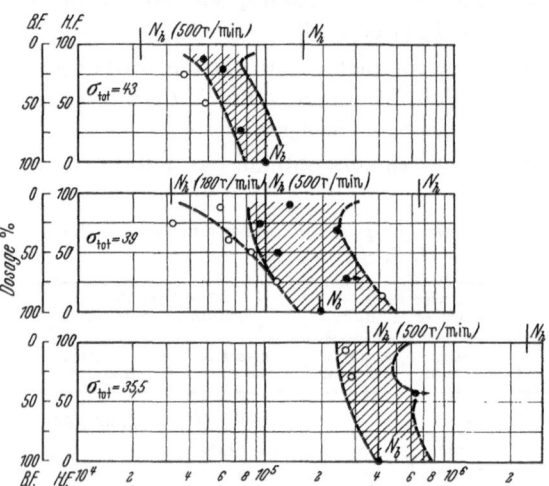

Les valeurs obtenues se prêtent à une représentation tout à fait semblable à celle employée par les métallographes pour représenter les propriétés d'un alliage binaire. Comme on représente sur un axe de coordonnées les «compositions» de l'alliage avec deux échelles complémentaires, on représente de même les divers «dosages» de la sollicitation en H. F. et B. F. Sur l'autre axe des coordonnées, on porte les durées, exprimées en basse fréquence.

Fig. 8. Essais avec amplitude totale constante — acier C 43. Les durées sont exprimées en cycles de B. F.
$N_h$ = durée en pure H. F. à 3.400 r/min
$N_h$ (500 r/min) = $N_h$ : 6,8
$N_h$ (180 r/min) = $N_h$ : 19
$N_b$ = durée en pure B. F. à 500 r/min
• Essais à 500 r/min
○ Essais à 180 r/min

Pour maintenir une certaine analogie avec les courbes de Wöhler, on porte les durées en abscisses, et en ordonnées les divers «dosages» (voir fig. 8). Chaque niveau de sollicitation donne naissance à un graphique distinct, mais tous trois pourraient être groupés en une même représentation à trois dimensions.

Nous avons jugé opportun de rassembler tous les points représentatifs en une unique bande de dispersion, qui, par ailleurs, n'a pas une amplitude beaucoup plus étendue que celle des dispersions normales d'une série homogène.

Pour les trois niveaux de sollicitation, on remarque une réduction de la durée au fur et à mesure que croît le pourcentage d'amplitude en H. F.; cependant, jusqu'à des valeurs de 40% à H. F., la diminution est si faible que la «durée» peut être considérée *pratiquement constante*, à égalité d'amplitude totale; pour des pourcentages de H. F. plus importants que 40%, c'est-à-dire lorsqu'on a une plus grande prévalence de H. F., la durée reste encore presque constante si elle est toujours calculée en cycles de B. F. à 500 r/min, tandis qu'elle se réduit fortement, pour des cycles de 180 r/min.

Ces remarques ont la signification physique suivante: jusqu'à 40% d'amplitude à H. F., cette dernière est pratiquement inactive et la «durée» est uniquement déterminée par les cycles à B. F.

Pour les pourcentages de H. F. au-dessus de 40%, c'est-à-dire au fur et à mesure que l'on se rapproche de la H. F. pure, c'est celle-ci qui commande, et la durée est toujours davantage déterminée par les cycles à H. F. et toujours moins par ceux à B. F.

### 3. Essais sur duralumin

Les essais sur duralumin ont été conduits selon le principe de l'amplitude constante, et, pour le moment, uniquement avec un pourcentage plus élevé de B. F. (de 0 à 40% de H. F.).

On a expérimenté avec trois niveaux de sollicitations: 22, 27 et 32 kg/mm², correspondant à des durées à B. F. pure, d'environ $10^6$, $10^5$ et $5 \cdot 10^4$

Les résultats ont été représentés dans la fig. 9. La réduction non négligeable de la durée, qu'on observe au fur et à mesure qu'une dentelure de H. F. se superpose à la

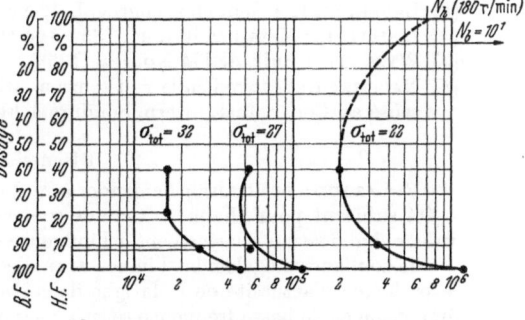

Fig. 9. Essais avec amplitude totale constante — duralumin. Les durées sont exprimés en cycles de B. F. (180 r/min) H.F. de 2.500 r/min.

B. F., correspond à un comportement du materiau différent de celui remarqué sur l'acier.

On a des réductions maxima de durée variables selon des niveaux de sollicitation, mais qui, exprimées en des termes de résistance à la fatigue, correspondent toutes à un abaissement maximum des courbes de Wöhler, d'environ 4 kg/mm², soit 20% sur la limite de fatigue à 10 millions.

Les essais sont en cours de complément dans le champ voisin de la H. F.

## 4. Conclusions

La machine construite fonctionne de façon satisfaisante et commence à donner les premiers résultats.

Pour l'acier C 43 normalisé, à égalité de sollicitation totale, une dentelure de haute fréquence ne réduit pas la durée de façon sensible, jusqu'à ce que son amplitude ne dépasse pas 40% de celle totale; entre cette limite, c'est uniquement la basse fréquence qui est cause du dommage causé par la fatigue.

Pour des amplitudes de H. F. au-delà de 40%, l'effet d'une dentelure à H. F. est sensible, et l'on doit tenir compte des cycles à H. F. plus que de ceux à B. F.

Pour le duralumin, une dentelure à H. F. avec amplitude croissante partant du zéro jusqu'à 40% de la valeur totale, maintenue constante, réduit graduellement la durée calculée à B. F., comme si la résistance du matériau se réduisait jusqu'à 80% par rapport à la valeur initiale.

Dans ce matériau, la H. F., même en petit pourcentage, intervient activement dans la formation du dommage, c'est-à-dire dans le sens d'accélérer la rupture de l'éprouvette.

### Bibliographie

[1] Gabrielli, G.: Aerotecnica (Rom) 22, 429—440 (1942).
[2] Leber, H. K.: Gen. Mot. engrng J. 1, Nr. 8 (1954).
[3] Locati, L.: Metallur. ital. 44, 135—144 (1952).
[4] Wyss, Th.: Bull. ASTM No. 188 (1953).
[5] Nacher: Indicazioni sulla resistenza a fatica di strutture saldate. Mémoire présenté au Congr. Inst. intern. Soudure à Florence 1954, non publiée.

### Discussion

R. Cazaud: Je voudrais demander à M. Locati si le nombre de ses expériences a été suffisant pour chaque niveau de contrainte, pour que les résultats aient une valeur significative relativement à l'influence de la fréquence.

Je soulignerai également l'importance d'essais comme ceux de M. Locati pour le problème d'actualité de la fatigue dans l'aéronautique où les rafales de grande amplitude et de basse fréquence se superposent aux vibrations de faible amplitude et de grande fréquence.

L. Locati: Malheureusement on n'a que deux essais pour chaque point des diagrammes; les expériences vont continuer pour donner une réponse exacte du point de vue statistique.

# Ziele der Ermüdungsforschung in der Schweiz, gezeigt am Beispiel von Dauerversuchen an Schraubenverbindungen[1]

Von

## L. Martinaglia

Mit 4 Abbildungen

In Anbetracht der wenigen Forschungsstellen, die sich in der Schweiz mit Ermüdungsforschung befassen, hat man sich im allgemeinen auf die Untersuchung der *Gestaltfestigkeit* konzentriert, um der Praxis mit unmittelbar verwendbaren Ergebnissen zu dienen. Untersucht wird die Dauerfestigkeit von Maschinenelementen und Verbindungen mit dem Ziel, die wirkliche Gebrauchsfestigkeit zu ermitteln. Dieses Ziel hat zur Untersuchung einer größeren Anzahl von Maschinenelementen, wie Druckgefäßen, Wellen, Schweißverbindungen usw. geführt, wobei immer die wahren Betriebsbeanspruchungen als Prüfbasis dienten. Dies wird am Beispiel der Prüfung von Schraubenverbindungen gezeigt.

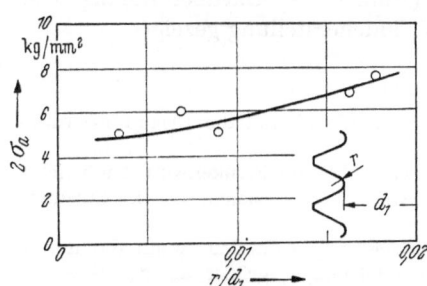

Abb. 1.
Einfluß der Ausrundung im Gewindegrund auf die Zugdauerfestigkeit von Schrauben 38 mm Durchmesser. $2 \cdot \sigma_a$ = Schwellspannung.

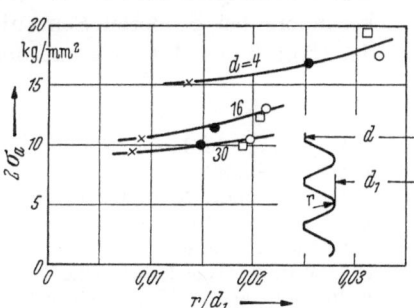

Abb. 2.
Einfluß der Ausrundung im Gewindegrund auf die Zugdauerfestigkeit bei Schrauben von 4, 16 und 30 mm Nenndurchmesser.

Untersucht wurde immer eine Mutterschraubenverbindung mit glattem Dehnschaft und Normmutter. Die im Maschinenbau verwendeten Schrauben werden — von wenigen Sonderfällen abgesehen — zuerst vorgespannt. Im Betrieb kommt dann noch eine zusätzliche schwellende

---

[1] Gedruckt nach dem Vordrucksmanuskript des Verfassers.

Beanspruchung hinzu. Darum wurden alle Schrauben mit einer be-
triebsähnlichen Beanspruchung geprüft: Ermittelt wurde diejenige
Schwellast $2\sigma_a$ die über der statischen Vorspannung hinaus dauernd
ertragen wird.

Im Vortrag werden die Ergebnisse einer Reihe von Dauerversuchen
gezeigt und besprochen, bei denen die verschiedenen Einflüsse auf die

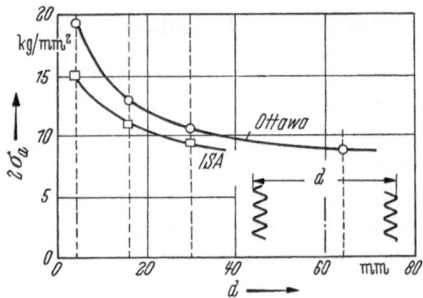

Abb. 3.
Einfluß des Gewindedurchmessers auf die
Dauerzugfestigkeit von Schrauben mit ver-
schiedenen Gewinden.

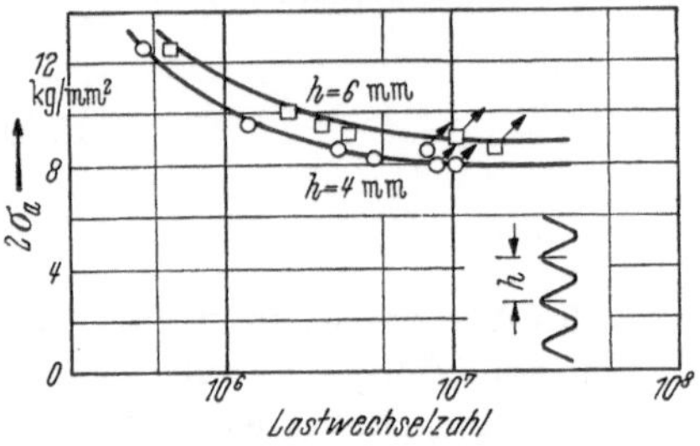

Abb. 4.
Einfluß der Gewindesteigung auf die Dauer-
zugfestigkeit von Schrauben von 64 mm
Durchmesser.

Ermüdungsfestigkeit von Schraubenverbindungen untersucht wurden.
Von überragendem Einfluß ist die Ausrundung des Gewindegrundes
(Abb. 1) und des Schraubendurchmessers (Abb. 2 und 3). Besondere
Untersuchungen galten der Wahl der günstigsten Gewindesteigung,
besonders bei größeren Schrauben (Abb. 4). — Darüber hinaus wird
der Einfluß des Materials und der Gewindeherstellung gezeigt.

### Diskussion

I. A. Oding: Wurde der Einfluß der Formgenauigkeit auf die Ermüdungsfestigkeit kontrolliert?

L. Martinaglia: Nein. Es wurde jedoch versucht, die Flankenwinkel möglichst
konstant zu halten, um konzentriertes Anlegen zu erzielen, da die Streuung
sonst merklich erhöht wurde.

P. E. Wiene: Wir haben eine kleine Verbesserung gefunden, wenn die untere
Kolbenstangenmutter mit einer Steigung 0,03 mm/1″ größer als das Stangen-
gewinde ausgeführt wurde; dabei wurde die Kraftverteilung günstiger. Der Gewinn ist aber zu klein im Verhältnis zu den praktischen Schwierigkeiten bei einer
solchen Ausführung.

D. G. Sopwith: Any small deviations from the correct form seems to be advant-
ageous.

In cooperation with the Author tests have been carried out at the MERL and
his results as to fatigue limit reproduced for 64 mm bolt diameter. On the other
hand the results for smaller diameter were not nearly so good.

P. E. Wiene: Angle deviation in one direction gives higher bending stress on the
screw thread and lower on the nut thread and vice versa.[1]

---

[1] Editors' note: cf. paper by Sopwith, Chapter 3.

# Variability in fatigue testing:
## Sources and effect on notch sensitivity

By

### F. A. McClintock

The information obtained from fatigue tests is obscured by the variability of the results. A knowledge of the sources of the variability is helpful in minimizing this difficulty. Once the variability has been reduced to that due to local variations alone, estimates can be made of how much of the size, shape, and notch sensitivity effects are due to statistical causes.

The observed life of a specimen is a function of variables affecting preparation, such as differences between ingots, the position of the bar in the ingot, the position of the specimen in the bar, the heat treatment, the machining history, and the surface finish; and is a function of variables affecting testing, such as the measurement of dimensions, the load, the temperature of the specimen, the speed, and the eccentricity of the specimen. Assume that the values of the $i$th variable $v_i$ vary from one specimen to another according to a statistical distribution with standard deviation $\sigma_i$. Then if the variables are independent, for small variations the standard deviation of the cycles to failure is given by

$$\sigma_{\log N} = \sqrt{\sum_i \left(\frac{\partial \log N}{\partial \log v_i}\right)^2 \left(\frac{\sigma_i}{v_i}\right)^2} \tag{1}$$

The values of the partial derivatives for several of the variables are listed in tab. 1.

Table 1. *Effect of variables on life*

| Variable | Material | $\dfrac{\partial \log N}{\partial \log v_i}$ | Reference |
|---|---|---|---|
| Stress | Steels | $-6$ to $-20$ (19/22) | [1] |
| | Aluminum alloys | $-7$ to $-14$ (14/16) | [2] |
| Temperature (for small | Steels | $-3$ to $-10$ (11/14) | [1] |
| variations | Aluminum alloys | $-5$ to $-10$ | [2] |
| near atmos.) | 75S - T6 Al. | $+4 \pm 2.5$ (95%) | Tests |
| | ,, | $+2.5 \pm 4$ (95%) | Tests |
| Speed | 1035 St. | $0.6 \pm 0.5$ (95%) | [3] |

Table 1. *(Continuation)*

| Variable | Material | $\dfrac{\partial \log N}{\partial \log v_i}$ | Reference |
|---|---|---|---|
| Speed | Armco | 0.7 ± 0.3 (95%) | [3] |
|  | 3130 St. | 0.6 ± 1.0 (95%) | [3] |
|  |  | $\partial \log N / \partial v_i$ |  |
| e/w (w = stat. | 4340 St. | 0 to − 1.5 | Theory and [4] |
| defl. under | 76S-T61 Al. | − 3 to − 5 | Theory and [5] |
| load ampl.) | 75S-T6 Al. | + 5 to − 3 (95%) | Tests |

The derivatives with respect to stress were obtained from a wide range of carbon and alloy steels of various heat treatments above the endurance limit. The numbers in parentheses give the fraction of the cases falling within the given range. In the case of aluminum, derivatives were obtained for 5 alloys at lives of from $10^5$ to $10^8$ cycles.

The temperature derivatives, based on absolute temperatures, were estimates from the effect on endurance limit multiplied by a stress derivative of 10. The size of this estimated temperature derivative is very disturbing, since specimen temperatures can vary during fatigue tests by several per cent. The data on 75 S-T 6 aluminum alloy were obtained in connection with tests reported below. The first results were obtained from 25 tests in which there were accidental variations in temperature, and the second from a series of 9 tests at two temperatures 50°C apart. In each case 95% confidence limits for the slope of the regression line were estimated by the appropriate statistical methods. These data indicate an increase in life at higher temperatures, in contradiction to the expected results. There was also some indication that for this material there was a corresponding increase of life at lower speeds; perhaps both effects are due to further age hardening of the material. Clearly there is need for more information on the effect of small variations in temperature.

The speed effect data reported for the steels may be confounded with a temperature effect, although the 1035 and 3130 steels were run below their yield point and yield strength at 0.1% offset, respectively.

The effect of an eccentricity in a rotating beam specimen is to produce vertical and horizontal vibrations. The horizontal vibrations only affect the shape of the stress cycle, whereas the vertical vibrations add to the major stresses. If the bearings and load are rigidly enough connected to be considered as a single degree of freedom system, then the amplitude of vibration $\delta$ is related to the eccentricity $e$, the speed of rotation $\omega$ and the natural frequency of vibration $\omega_n$ by the relation

$$\delta/e = 1 / (\omega_n{}^2 / \omega^2 - 1)$$

In most cases the speed of rotation is well above the critical speed. Then $\delta = -e$, and the specimen is simply straightened out. The moment required to straighten out the specimen superimposes a mean stress on the fluctuating stress. FINDLEY's data for 4340 steel [4] and 76S-T61 aluminum alloy [5] were used to find the derivative, in this case with respect to the variable, i. e. $\partial \log N/\partial(e/w)$. Tests were run on specimens having a ratio of eccentricity to deflection under load of 0.1, and compared with tests where eccentricities were one-tenth as large. Although the test results were practically identical, too few specimens were run to give assurance that the derivative was greater than $-3$.

## 1. Scatter due to local variations only

In previous papers [6], [7], it was shown that a criterion for the elimination of all the above sources of variation, so only local sources remain, could be obtained by comparing the standard deviation of life with the standard deviation of position of failure in specimens in which the stress varies from one cross section to another. In that analysis, it was assumed that fatigue failure was entirely a surface phenomenon. But if the variability in fatigue properties is due to a distribution of defects such as inclusions whose effect varies with their depth, then there will be an effect of stress gradient on the life. As a first approximation, one may assume that the effective stress on a cross-section falls off linearly with the distance from the surface. While the gradient of the effective stress would be expected to increase with an increase in the actual stress gradient, the two are not identical, for even when the actual stress gradient is zero as in the unnotched tension-compression test, failures rarely begin at any great distance below the surface. Thus the stress $S$ at a point $y$ beneath the surface, on a cross-section at a distance $z$ from the section of maximum stress $S_m$ will be approximated by

$$S = S_m (1 - az^2 - gy) \tag{2}$$

The quantities $a$ and $g$ are determined by the shape of the specimen and the method of loading. Following the previous analysis, let $-K$ be the slope of the $S$-$\log N$ curve, $C$ be the perimeter or width of a specimen, $p_2$ be a constant proportional to the density of elements with given strength, $\omega - S_m$ be the lower limit to $K \log N$, and $k+3/2$ be roughly the number of standard deviations from the lower limit to the mean of the distribution. Then the following results are obtained for the parameters of the marginal distributions of life and position of failure:

$$\overline{K \log N} = \omega - S_m + \left[ \frac{\sqrt{S_m a}\, S_m g}{p_2\, C \sqrt{\pi}} \cdot \frac{\Gamma(k+5/2)}{\Gamma(k+1)} \right]^{\frac{1}{k+3/2}} \Gamma\left(1 + \frac{1}{k+3/2}\right) \tag{3}$$

$$K\sigma \log N =$$

$$= \left[ \frac{\sqrt{S_{ma}}\, S_{mg}}{p_2\, C\, \sqrt{\pi}} \cdot \frac{\Gamma\,(k+5/2)}{\Gamma\,(k+1)} \right]^{\frac{1}{k+3/2}} \sqrt{\Gamma\left(1 + \frac{2}{k+3/2}\right) - \Gamma^2\left(1 + \frac{1}{k+3/2}\right)} \quad (4)$$

$$\frac{K\sigma_{\log N}}{S_{ma}\,\sigma_z{}^2} = (2k+3)\ \sqrt{\Gamma\left(1 + \frac{2}{k+3/2}\right) - \Gamma^2\left(1 + \frac{1}{k+3/2}\right)} \Bigg/ \Gamma\left(1 + \frac{1}{k+3/2}\right)$$

$$(5)$$

$$= 2.3 \pm 12\ \%\ \text{for}\ 0 < k < \infty \quad (5a)$$

$$\overline{y}/\sigma_z{}^2 = 2\,a/g \quad (6)$$

(5a) affords a check on whether or not there are present any extraneous variables affecting the scatter in life other than local variations within the various specimens. For if such extraneous variables are present, the scatter in life will be greater than that given by (5a) and measurements of $\sigma_z{}^2$, the scatter in the position of failure.

## 2. Experimental verification of the relation between scatter in life and in position of failure

Professor P. G. Fluck kindly made available his specimens [3] for measurement of the position of failure, with the results given in tab. 2. Since only twelve specimens were tested at each stress level, the results are not precise. None the less, the criterion is seen to check in each case, except for some of the preparations involving hand-polishing, and one involving superfinishing. In these cases there appears to be some extraneous variable affecting the life of specimens.

Table 2. *Relation between scatter in life and scatter in position of failure* (95% confidence limits are given, using method of [7] for first set)

| Material | Finish | Stress, psi | $K\sigma_{\log N}/2.3\, S_m\,a\,\sigma_z{}^2$ | $\dfrac{K\sigma_{\log N}}{S_m}$ |
|---|---|---|---|---|
| 1035 St. | Lathe formed | 38,000 | 0.24—1.6 | 0.015—0.036 |
| | | 36,000 | 0.28—1.85 | 0.011—0.029 |
| | Ground | 28,000 | 0.48—3.16 | 0.017—0.040 |
| | Ground polished | 38,000 | 0.55—3.6 | 0.027—0.065 |
| | Superfinished | 38,000 | 0.52—3.4 | 0.023—0.054 |
| | Partly hand-polished | 36,000 | 0.26—1.69 | 0.013—0.032 |
| 3130 St. | Lathe formed | 95,000 | 0.25—1.66 | 0.030—0.070 |
| | | 88,000 | 0.27—1.83 | 0.031—0.074 |
| | Partly hand-polished | 95,000 | 0.42—2.79 | 0.025—0.061 |
| | Hand-polished | 95,000 | 1.32—8.8 | 0.026—0.062 |
| | | 88,000 | 1.43—9.7 | 0.069—0.167 |

Table 2. *(Continuation)*

| Material | Finish | Stress, psi | $K\sigma_{\log N}/2.3\,S_m\,a\,\sigma_z{}^2$ | $\dfrac{K\sigma_{\log N}}{S_m}$ |
|---|---|---|---|---|
| | Ground | 95,000 | 0.44—2.91 | 0.022—0.052 |
| | | 88,000 | 0.45—3.0 | 0.035—0.083 |
| | Ground and | | | |
| | polished | 95,000 | 0.89—5.9 | 0.031—0.074 |
| | Superfinished | 95,000 | 1.26—8.5 | 0.049—0.119 |
| 1075 St. | | | | |
| Pearlitic | Polished | 38,800 | 0.96—4.0 | 0.017—0.032 |
| Shperoidized | Polished | 47,500 | 0.67—2.8 | 0.013—0.021 |
| 75 S-T6 Al. | Lathe turned | | | 0.0086— |
| | (power feed) | 46,000 | 0.34—1.29 | 0.015 |
| ZK60-T5Mg. | Lathe turned | | | |
| | (power feed) | 31,000 | 0.54—2.02 | 0.028—0.051 |

The data on the position of failure for the 1075 steel [7] were supplied in a private communication. Differences in heat-treatment between the various batches may account for the relatively high variation in life, and also thermal gradients may have been present in the pearlitic steel, which was tested above its yield point.

The 25 specimens for each of the non-ferrous alloys were cut from a single bar, or push, and finished in two cuts of 0.0035 and 0.0015 in. depth with a carbide tool having a 15° side rake, 0° front rake, 15° clearance, and a 0.02 in. nose radius, cutting dry at 1,500 r/min with a feed of 0.0017/rev. Final dimensions were 0.328 D with a $9^7/_8$ in. longitudinal radius of curvature. The order of specimens in the bar, the order of machining, and the order of testing were randomized in blocks of 5 according to a randomly selected latin square pattern.

For the 75S-T6 aluminum alloy, as previously mentioned, an effect of temperature was found, and this introduced a significant dependence on the order of testing. The variations between machining and bar-order groups were even less than expected from the residual and hence not significant.

The ZK60-T5 magnesium extrusions showed an increase in life from nose to butt of the push, but not enough to contribute significantly to the analysis of variance. Effects of testing and machining order were not significant.

## 3. Notch sensitivity effects

Inherent local variations in the strength of a material will cause a size effect, for a larger volume of metal will be more likely to contain a weak spot. This expected size effect can be estimated from (3), (4), (5), and (5a) for specimens of two different shapes, such as a smooth specimen $s$ and a notched specimen $n$ both subjected to the same maximum local stress. This size effect may be put in terms of the fatigue strengths for a given life exactly when the $S$-$\log N$ curve is linear, or apporximately when the variability is small [6]. Then defining $K_f = \bar{S}_s/(\bar{S}_n)_{\text{nom}}$ and $K_t = S_{\text{loc}}/S_{\text{nom}}$ and assuming there are only statistical effects on the fatigue strength so that $K_t = (\bar{S}_n)_{\text{loc}}/(S_n)_{\text{nom}}$, there results

$$\frac{K_t}{K_f} - 1 = \frac{\sigma_{S_s}}{\bar{S}_s} \left[ \left( \sqrt{\frac{a_n}{a_s}} \frac{g_n}{g_s} \frac{C_s}{C_n} \right)^{\frac{1}{k+3/2}} - 1 \right] \frac{2k+3}{2.3} \tag{7}$$

The right hand side of the equation, following a suggestion of Orowan, will be called the notch *insensitivity* term. A priori, one would expect $a_n$ and $g_n$ to be approximately $1/\varrho^2$ and $1/\varrho$, respectively, where $\varrho$ is the radius of curvature of the notch root. For the case of an elliptical hole with semi-major axis $b$ in a flat plate subjected to uniaxial tension, the gradients may be found from Inglis' solution [9]:

$$
\begin{array}{ccc}
 & a & g \\
b/\varrho = 1 & 4/3\,\varrho^2 & 7/3\,\varrho \\
b/\varrho \to \infty & 1/2\,b^{1/2}\varrho^{3/2} & 10/3\,\varrho
\end{array}
$$

Thus the *a priori* assumption will cause a slight overestimate of the statistical effect. For the smooth specimen of the same minimum radius $r$ and with a longitudinal radius of curvature of $R$, $a_s$ is of the order of $1/rR$ ref. [7] and $g_s$ is of the order of $1/r$.

For the smooth, U-, and V-notched rotating bending specimens of the identical material reported here [10] and assuming $\sigma_{S_s}/\bar{S}_s = K\sigma_{\log N}/S_m$, the following values are found for the notch insensitivity term $(K_t/K_f - 1)$:

| | Calculated | | Observed |
|---|---|---|---|
| | $k = 3/2$ | $k = \infty$ | |
| U-notch, $K_t = 1.56$ | 0.06—0.10 | 0.03—0.05 | 0.10—0.22 |
| V-notch, $K_t = 3.05$ | 0.24—0.43 | 0.06—0.10 | 0.37—0.57 |

The limits for the observed values were estimated by eye from the $S$-$N$ curves of [10] at $10^5$, $10^6$, and $10^7$ cycles. $K_f$ was essentially constant over this range and the theoretical local stresses were below the elastic limit.

It appears unlikely that the statistical effects are sufficient to account for all the notch insensitivity. Further studies of size and notch effects should include a determination of the statistical quantities so that the remaining sources of notch insensitivity can be more accurately isolated.

## 4. Conclusions

1. Rough limits are obtained for the effect of various testing variables on fatigue life.

2. Experimental data support the theoretical relation between scatter in position of failure and scatter in life due to local variations in strength:

$$K \sigma_{\log N}/2.3 \, S_m \, a \, \sigma^2{}_z = 1$$

3. From a statistical analysis taking into account the stress gradient normal to the surface, an estimate of notch insensitivity is obtained. Data from 75S-T6 aluminum alloy indicate that it is unlikely that notch insensitivity is due to statistical effects alone.

The author wishes to thank the late R. L. HARDY and F. M. WHITE for carrying out experimental work, W. WEIBULL for pointing out that the mathematical statistics could be expressed in closed form, and R. E. PETERSON for his interest.

This research was supported by the United States Air Force, through the Office of Scientific Research of the Air Research Development Command.

### Bibliography

[1] CAZAUD, R.: Fatigue of Metals, New York 1953.
[2] TEMPLIN, R. L.: Proc. ASTM, 54, 641 (1954).
[3] FLUCK, P. G.: Proc. ASTM, 51, 584—592 (1951).
[4] FINDLEY, W. N., F. C. MERGEN and A. H. ROSENBERG: Proc. ASTM, 53, 768 (1953).
[5] FINDLEY, W. N.: J. appl. Mech., 20, 365 (1953).
[6] McCLINTOCK, F. A.: J. appl. Mech., 22, 421—426 (1955).
[7] McCLINTOCK, F. A.: J. appl. Mech., 22, 427—431 (1955).
[8] DIETER, G. F., and R. F. MEHL: NACA TN 3019 (1953).
[9] INGLIS, C. E.: Trans. Instn. nav. Archit., Lond., 55 (I), 218 (1913).
[10] MACGREGOR, C. W., and N. GROSSMAN: NACA TN 2812 (1952).

# Über den Mechanismus der Zerstörung bei der zyklischen Belastung von Metallen

Von

## I. A. Oding

Mit 4 Abbildungen

Bei Erörterung von Prozessen, die in den Metallen bei zyklischer Belastung sich vollziehen und aus Verfestigung und Entfestigung [1] bestehen, muß man feststellen, daß immer noch die am wenigsten erforschten Prozesse jene sind, die das Material zur Entfestigung führen.

Der Versuch, die Metallzerstörung durch die bei der zyklischen Belastung eines Prüfstabs entstehenden Spannungen dritter Art zu erklären, der vorerst von W. I. Iweronowa [2] unternommen und von Terminasow [3] entwickelt wurde, ist nun durch die Arbeit von Glikmann und Techt [4] widerlegt, die gezeigt haben, daß eine bedeutende Entwicklung der restlichen Spannungen dritter Art noch nicht als Anzeichen der Metallermüdung dienen kann.

Dieser Artikel ist ein Versuch, den Prozeß der Mikrorißbildung in den Metallen bei zyklischer Belastung zu erklären unter Ausnutzung moderner Vorstellungen der Versetzungstheorie.

Die Versetzungen können bei ihrer Bewegung auf Hindernisse stoßen und aus der Gleitfläche hervortreten, was zu einer massenweisen Herausbildung von vakanten Stellen im Kristallgitter (Löcher) führt [5]. Die Anhäufung dieser Löcher zu selbständigen Kolonien oder die Ansammlung der Löcher an den günstig liegenden Mikroporen oder Mikrorissen wurde in den Arbeiten von Greenwood [6], Crussard [7], Oding und Iwanowa [8] als die Hauptsache behandelt, die die Dauerstandsfestigkeit des Metalls bei seinem Dienst unter Spannungen in hohen Temperaturen herabsetzt.

Unter Benutzung dieser Vorstellungen auch für den Fall einer zyklischen Belastung muß man in erster Linie konstatieren, daß hierbei die Bedingungen für die Bewegung von Versetzungen und für die Sammlung von Löchern sich nicht nur aus einem Zyklus in den andern, sondern auch in der Spanne eines Zyklus verändern. Wenn man der Einfachheit halber einen symmetrischen Zyklus erörtert, so muß man annehmen, daß der Versetzungslauf im ersten Zyklusviertel, d. h. bei der Belastung, zu solchen Veränderungen der Unvollkommenheit des

Kristallgitters führt, die einer Rückkehr der Versetzungen zu ihren Quellen im Rahmen des zweiten Zyklusviertels, d. h. bei der Entlastung des Prüfstabs, hinderlich sind. Eine Fixation der Versetzungen nach ihrem Lauf bei Belastung ist, wie LEIBFRIED und HAASEN [9] darauf hinweisen, durchaus möglich und wird durch eine Reihe von Ursachen hervorgerufen.

Deshalb ist im zweiten Zyklusviertel, bei der Entlastung, die Rückkehr der Versetzungen zu ihren Ausgangspositionen nicht sehr massenhaft.

Das dritte Zyklusviertel verläuft mit einer neuen Belastung, die aber ein entgegengesetztes Vorzeichen im Vergleich zur Belastung des ersten Zyklusviertels hat. Bekanntlich hat das dritte Zyklusviertel kleineren Widerstand gegen die plastische Verformung (Bauschinger-Effekt), was wahrscheinlich durch die teilweise Rückkehr derjenigen Versetzungen, die sich binnen des ersten Zyklusviertels verlagert haben und nicht die Möglichkeit hatten, in ihre Ausgangsstellung binnen des zweiten Zyklusviertels zurückzukehren, bedingt ist.

Das vierte Zyklusviertel widerspiegelt die Entlastung des Prüfstabs und unterscheidet sich prinzipiell durch nichts vom zweiten Zyklusviertel.

Die darauffolgenden Zyklen sind dem ersten Zyklus analog, und unterscheiden sich von ihm nur durch die Anzahl der in jedem Zyklusviertel teilnehmenden Versetzungen. Wird der Verankerungsprozeß der Versetzungen verstärkt, folglich, die Zahl der zu ihren Ausgangspositionen zurückkehrenden Versetzungen vermindert, so wird auch der Bauschinger-Effekt kleiner und führt zur Senkung der Hysteresis-Schleifenkurve, d. h. zur Verminderung der zyklischen Zähigkeit. Der Verankerungsprozeß begünstigt eine mechanische Alterung, die nach der Auslegung von COTTRELL [10] ein „Wolken"-gebilde, bestehend aus in dem Versetzungsfeld aufgelösten Atomen, ist.

Bei den effektiv verlaufenden Prozessen der Verankerung von Versetzungen muß keine Ermüdungszerstörung vor sich gehen, denn die Anzahl der an jedem darauffolgenden Zyklus teilnehmenden Versetzungen wird immer geringer, folglich wird auch die Herausbildung von Löchern herabgesetzt.

Sind die Spannungen, die durch Einwirkung von außenstehenden Kräften entstehen, so beschaffen, daß die Verankerung der Versetzungen wenig effektiv ist, so wird die Anzahl der an jedem darauffolgenden Zyklus teilnehmenden Versetzungen immer größer und die Hysteresis-Schleifenkurve wird sich ausweiten, die Zahl der Löcher sich vergrößern, bis eine Bildung von Mikrorissen auftritt.

Man kann annehmen, daß die Zahl der entstehenden Löcher proportionell der Anzahl wirkender Versetzungen ist.

Allein der Löcherbildungsprozeß bestimmt noch nicht im voraus die Effektivität der Prüfstabzerstörung. Man muß noch anderen Erscheinungen Rechnung tragen: 1. der Sammlung von Löchern in Kolonien und 2. ihrem Niederschlag auf der Oberfläche der Mikroporen und Mikrorisse. Die Bildung der Keimform eines Mikrorisses und dessen Entwicklung sind im Grunde genommen das wichtigste im Prozeß der Metallzerstörung. Betrachten wir nun, welche Bedingungen einer Sammlung und einem Niederschlag der Löcher günstig sind.

Die Versetzungsbewegung wird durch Schubspannungen hervorgerufen. Folglich wird die intensivste Entstehung von Löchern in den Flächen der maximalen Schubspannungen vor sich gehen (S-Fläche). Wenn in diesen Flächen normale Druck- oder Zugspannungen fehlen, so kann die Anhäufung von Löchern in Kolonien nur auf Kosten der Vereinigung der einzelnen Löcher bei ihrer Begegnung geschehen.

Im Ergebnis einer solchen Sammlung oder, wie J. I. FRENKEL [11] verwies, einer „Koagulation von Löchern" ist das Entstehen innerhalb des Kristalls von kleinen inneren Hohlräumen, zum Beispiel von Mikroporen, möglich. Man kann in diesem Falle kaum eine Herausbildung von an Mikrorissen erinnernden langgezogenen Kolonien der Löcher erwarten. Der Koagulationsprozeß von Löchern kann nur zu einer bedeutenden „Porosität" des Metalls in den den S-Flächen naheliegenden Volumen führen. Folglich kann in dem Fall, da in diesen Flächen Normalspannungen fehlen, die zu beobachtende „Auflockerung" des Kristallgitters als ein Prozeß der Verstärkung der Metallporosität auf Kosten der Anhäufung einzelner Löcher oder von Löchergruppen in mikroskopische Poren betrachtet werden. Zugleich mit der lokalen Verstärkung der Metallporosität wird auch eine entsprechende lokale Herabsetzung der Metallfestigkeit bis zu dem Augenblick vor sich gehen, wo die durch von außen wirkende Kräfte entstehende Spannung sich als genügend erweist, um das Metall in dem zu untersuchenden lokalen Ort zu zerstören.

Anders wird die Zerstörung bei der Einwirkung von Normalspannungen verlaufen. In der Tat, man muß aus thermodynamischen Gründen in diesem Falle erwarten, daß der Löcherstrom aus den stark elastisch-gezogenen Regionen in minder stark elastisch-gezogene Regionen und aus letzteren in elastisch-zusammengepreßte und von diesen wiederum in stark elastisch-zusammengepreßte Regionen umgeleitet werden wird.

Als Beispiel wollen wir die unweit der Mikropore gelegenen Kraftfelder untersuchen (Abb. 1). Die Zugspannung $\sigma$ ruft eine Konzentration der Spannung am Rande des Risses (alle drei Spannungen $\sigma_1$, $\sigma_2$ und $\sigma_3$ haben das Vorzeichen des Zuges) und der unter Druck stehenden Region $c$ hervor. Die in der Region $a$ sich herausbildenden Löcher werden sich ansammeln: 1. in der Nähe der Region $c$, was zur Abrundung der Risse führen wird, und 2. an der Grenze zwischen $a$ und $b$, was zur

Entwicklung der Pore in einer zur Spannungswirkung $\sigma$ senkrecht tehenden Richtung führen wird, d. h. zur Degeneration der Pore in einen Riß [8]. Dieser Fall der Metallzerstörung durch die Entwicklung des Mikrorisses unterscheidet sich prin- zipiell von dem oben untersuchten Fall einer Zerstörung wegen der Herausbildung lokaler Porosität. In diesem Fall hat der Terminus „Auflockerung" des Kristall-· gitters schon eine andere Bedeutung: die Degeneration der Mikroporen in Mikrorisse und die Weiterentwicklung der letzteren.

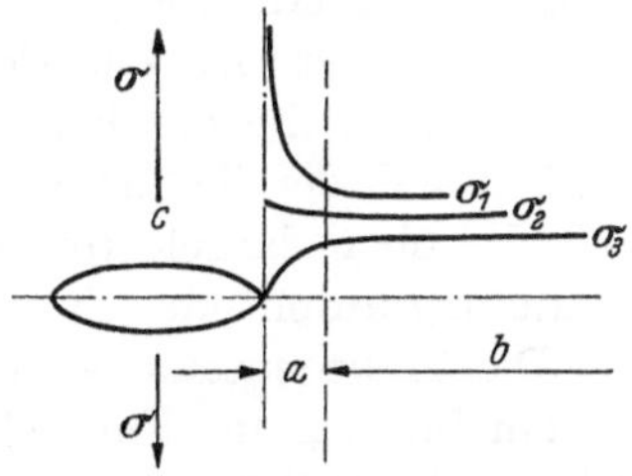

Als einleuchtender Beweis der dua- listischen Natur der Metallzerstörung

Abb. 1.

können die Experimente zur Erprobung der Metallermüdung bei Torsion mit Wechselvorzeichen dienen. Es ist bekannt, daß hierbei in den einen Fällen der Ermüdungsriß sich in den S-Flächen, in den anderen Fällen in den Flächen von maximalen Normalspannungen (N-Flächen) bildet. Wenn bei den aufgesetzten Experimentbedingungen der Ermüdungsriß in den S-Flächen entsteht, so bedeutet das, daß der Koagulationsprozeß der Löcher seiner Effektivität nach über den Prozeß des Niederschlags von Löchern prävaliert. Und umgekehrt: bildet sich der Ermüdungsriß in den N-Flächen, so bedeutet dies, daß die zyklische Festigkeit in diesen Flächen geringer ist, oder, mit anderen Worten gesagt, daß der Prozeß des Niederschlags von Löchern über den Prozeß der Koagulation von Löchern prävaliert.

Die prävalierende Bedeutung in der Effektivität des Koagulations- prozesses der Löcher muß die Größe der Zyklusamplitude haben, denn sie vertritt die Zahl der wirkenden Versetzungsquellen und die Effekti- vität der Bildung von Löchern. In dem Prozeß des Niederschlags von Löchern spielt die Hauptrolle die Stärke der maximalen Normalspannun- gen.

Es wäre falsch zu meinen, daß alle sich herausbildenden Löcher in der Koagulation und im Niederschlag aufgehen. In diesem Fall wäre die Ermüdungsgrenze im Grunde genommen die Elastizitätsgrenze, das heißt eine solche Spannung, bei der sich noch keine Löcher heraus- bilden. Es ist aber bekannt, daß bei der Ermüdungsgrenze oder bei Spannungen, die etwas niedriger als die Ermüdungsgrenze liegen, ein jeder Zyklus durch plastische Deformation begleitet wird. Deshalb muß man annehmen, daß die Hauptmasse der sich herausbildenden Löcher bei der Ermüdungsgrenze gleichenden Spannungen sich „ent- ladet" durch Begegnungen mit versetzten Atomen, welche auch bei der Bewegung von Versetzungen etwa in derselben Anzahl wie die Löcher entstehen. Die Prozesse des Niederschlags und der Koagulation von

Löchern beginnen in Erscheinung zu treten nur bei die Ermüdungs-grenze überschreitenden Spannungen.

Man kann folgende bekannte Gesetzmäßigkeiten in der Entwick-lung der Ermüdungsrisse feststellen: bei starken zyklischen Überlastun-gen entwickelt sich der Ermüdungsriß zumeist in den S-Flächen; bei Spannungen, die die Ermüdungsgrenze nur wenig überschreiten, ent-wickelt sich der Riß zumeist in den N-Flächen. Diese Tatsache stimmt mit der oben dargelegten Theorie überein, denn im ersten Fall ist die Spannungsamplitude relativ groß, und im zweiten Fall klein.

Die in bedeutendem Maße heterogene Struktur des Metalls führt oft zur Bildung und Entwicklung des Ermüdungsrisses in den N-Flächen. Ein diesbezügliches Beispiel ist Gußeisen. Das Bestehen von Graphit-einschlüssen in dem Gußeisen kann betrachtet werden als eine vor-bereitete Mikroporosität, d. h. in dem Gußeisen sind für den Prozeß des Löcherniederschlags bereits günstige Bedingungen geschaffen. Jedoch kann sich in einem solchen Material der Ermüdungsriß manchmal bilden und sogar in den S-Flächen entwickeln in dem Fall, wenn man zum Beispiel die Gußeisenprüfstäbe mit einem scharfen querliegenden Kerb versieht. Es kommt nicht selten vor, daß in diesem Falle die Ermüdungs-grenze, ausgedrückt in nominellen Spannungen, obwohl ein Spannungs-konzentrator besteht, sich gleichgroß oder sogar etwas höher als die Ermüdungsgrenze eines glatten Prüfstabs erweist. Im Gußeisen, manch-mal aber auch in anderen Metallen mit ausgeprägter heterogener Mikro-struktur, kann man bei nicht sehr scharfen Anschnitten einen gemischten Charakter des Ermüdungsrisses beobachten: ein Teil des Ermüdungs-risses liegt in der S-Fläche, der andere Teil liegt in der N-Fläche. Dies ist auch eine Bestätigung dessen, daß die Ermüdungszerstörung durch zwei verschiedene Prozesse hervorgerufen wird.

Möchten wir nun noch eine gutbekannte Tatsache behandeln. Eine Reihe von Materialien, die bei symmetrischer Torsion in der S-Fläche zerstört wird, beginnt sich zu zerstören in der N-Fläche bei asymme-trischen Zyklen, insbesondere wenn die Zyklus-Asymmetrie sehr groß ist.

Auf die Rolle der mittleren Spannungen in dem asymmetrischen Zyklus wurde in der Arbeit von Oding [12] verwiesen, der den Leitsatz vorbrachte, daß bei Grenzspannungen die vom Metall aufgenommene Energie von der Asymmetrie des Zyklus nicht abhängt. Unter Annahme, daß die Breite der Hysteresis-Schleifenkurve der maximalen Zyklus-spannung proportional ist, wurde folgende Abhängigkeit zwischen der Ermüdungsgrenze beim symmetrischen Zyklus $\sigma_w$ und den Grenz-spannungen (der Spannungsamplitude $\sigma_a = \frac{1}{2} (\sigma_{max} - \sigma_{min})$ und der mittleren Zyklusspannung $\sigma_0 = \frac{1}{2} (\sigma_{max} + \sigma_{min})$ des asymmetrischen Zyklus geliefert:

$$\sigma_w{}^2 = \sigma_a{}^2 + \sigma_a \sigma_0$$

Bei den Zug-Druck- und Zugprüfungen (mit Biegung) entspricht diese Gleichung ziemlich gut den experimentellen Angaben. Sieht man die Abb. 2, wo auf den Koordinatenachsen die Amplituden der Spannungen

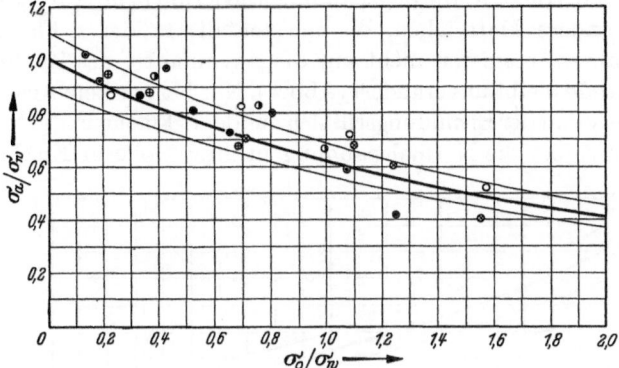

Abb. 2. Ermüdungsdaten bei asymmetrischen Zug-Druck und Zug-Biegung.

● Bronze
◐ Stahl mit 0,13 % C  } HAIGH [13]
⊗ Stahl mit 3,5 % Ni
⊕ Stahl mit 0,53 % C ($\sigma_B$ = 43 kg/mm²) } MOORE und JASPER [14]
⊗ Stahl mit 0,53 % C ($\sigma_B$ = 64 kg/mm²)
○ Stahl EJ-16 UZHIK [15]

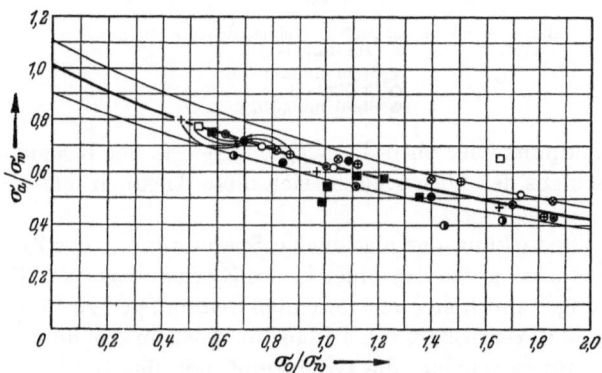

Abb. 3. Ermüdungsdaten bei asymmetrischer Wechseltorsion.
ZIMMERLY [16].

● $\sigma_w$ = 37,4 kg/mm²          ⊗ $\sigma_w$ = 33,9 kg/mm²
◐ $\sigma_w$ = 39,9 kg/mm²          ■ $\sigma_w$ = 37,4 kg/mm²
⊗ $\sigma_w$ = 33,9 kg/mm²          □ $\sigma_w$ = 14,0 kg/mm²
⊕ $\sigma_w$ = 29,0 kg/mm²          + $\sigma_w$ = 34,9 kg/mm²
○ $\sigma_w$ = 34,4 kg/mm²

und der mittleren Spannung des Zyklus vermerkt sind, die sich auf die Ermüdungsgrenze im symmetrischen Zyklus beziehen, so weiß man, daß die experimentellen Punkte der oben gebrachten Gleichung ziemlich gut entsprechen.

Bei der Prüfung auf Wechseltorsion entspricht ein Teil der Ergebnisse ebenfalls gut dieser Gleichung, wie man es leicht an den Daten der Abb. 3 ersieht. Das sind Materialien, die am meisten in den N-Flächen zerstört werden. Hier tritt die Zugspannung wiederum in ihrer Rolle hervor.

Jedoch andere Materialien, die meistenfalls in der S-Fläche Zerstörung erfahren, reagieren nicht auf die Asymmetrie des Zyklus; ihre Grenzamplitude bleibt unverändert (Abb. 4). Nur bei starkem Ausmaß der Asymmetrie, wenn der Ermüdungsriß sich aus der S-Fläche in die N-Fläche verlagert, tritt hier die Normalspannung in ihrer Rolle in Erscheinung.

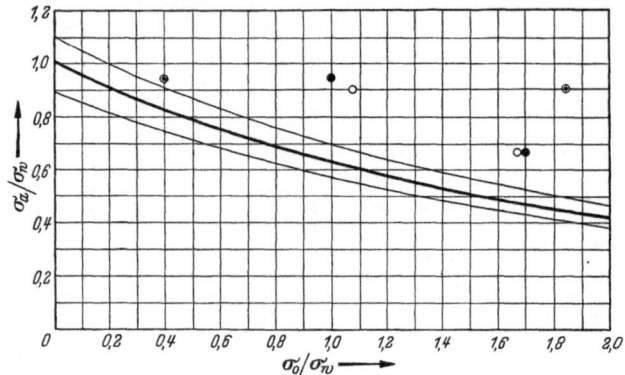

Abb. 4. Ermüdungsdaten bei asymmetrischer Wechseltorsion.
HANKINS [17].
⊕ Stahl mit 0,13% C
○ Cr-V Stahl
● Stahl mit 0,6% C

Vom Standpunkt der oben dargelegten Theorie der Koagulation und des Niederschlags der Löcher lassen sich diese Angaben folgendermaßen erklären.

Mit der Verstärkung der maximalen Spannung $\tau_{max}$ des Zyklus, d. h. mit der Verstärkung der Asymmetrie des Zyklus, beginnen die Quellen der Versetzungen mit höher aktivierenden Spannungen zu funktionieren. Dieser Umstand vergrößert die Intensität der Herausbildung von Löchern, was, wie es scheint, die Grenzamplitude des Zyklus $\tau_\alpha$ auch in dem Falle verringern müßte, wenn eine vorauseilende Zerstörung in den S-Flächen mittels der Koagulation von Löchern vorbereitet wird. Indem $\tau_{max}$ größer wird, nähert sie sich der Streckgrenze $\tau_s$ und viele asymmetrische Zyklen vollziehen sich bei $\tau_{max} > \tau_s$. In diesem Falle treten unweigerlich Prozesse in Aktion, die das Metall verfestigen, und schwächen die Wirkung der Versetzungen aus den Quellen mit höheren aktivierenden Spannungen. Ist die Effektivität der Verfestigung groß, so kann diese Kompensation sich auch auf bedeutende Teile der Asymmetrie ausdehnen.

Der Prozeß des Niederschlags der Löcher hängt von der Größe der

Normalspannungen ab. Bei der Zug-Druck-Spannung gleichen bekanntlich die maximalen Normalspannungen der doppelten Größe der maximalen Schubspannungen. Bei der Torsion jedoch gleichen sich zahlenmäßig $\tau_{max} = \sigma_{max}$. Folglich wird in diesem Fall die Effektivität der Normalspannungen vermindert. Ihre Rolle verstärkt sich mit der Erhöhung der Zyklusasymmetrie, denn hierbei wird sich die Größe $\sigma_{max}$, die für die Intensität des Prozesses des Löcherniederschlags verantwortlich ist, vergrößern, und $\tau_{\alpha}$ die für die Effektivität des Koagulationsprozesses verantwortlich ist, wird konstant bleiben oder sogar geringer. Dies muß unausbleiblich dazu führen, daß bei einer gewissen Größe der Zyklusasymmetrie der Prozeß des Löcherniederschlags die Effektivität der Koagulation der Löcher überschreiten wird. Der Ermüdungsriß wird sich herauszubilden beginnen in der N-Fläche und die weitere Erhöhung der Zyklusasymmetrie wird zur Verminderung der Größe der Grenzamplitude des Zyklus führen.

Aus diesen Beispielen ist zu ersehen, daß man zur Erklärung des Mechanismus der Ermüdungszerstörung von Metallen zur Theorie der vakanten Stellen greifen soll, denn dies kann sich äußerst nützlich erweisen.

### Literaturverzeichnis

[1] ODING, I. A.: Ustalost metalov Leningrad, 70 (1940).
[2] JDANOW, G. S. und J. S. UMANSKY: Rentgenografia metalov II, Moskau 1938, 212.
[3] TERMINASOW, J. S.: Zhur. Techn. Fiziki 18, Nr. 4 (1948).
[4] GLIKMAN, L. A. und W. P. TECHT: Nekotorie voprosi ustalostnoi prochnosti stali, Moskau 1955.
[5] SEITZ, F.: Advances in Physics 1, 43 (1952).
[6] GREENWOOD, I. N.: J. Iron St. Inst. 171, 380 (1952).
[7] CRUSSARD, C. and I. FRIDEL: Proc. Symp. Creep and Fracture, NPL, (1954.)
[8] ODING, I. A. und W. S. IWANOWA: Dokladi Akad. Nauk USSR 103, Nr. 1 (1955).
[9] LEIBFRIED, I. und P. HAASEN: Z. Physik 137 (1954).
[10] COTTRELL, A.: Rep. Conf. Strength of Solids, 30. London 1948,
[11] FRENKEL, J. I.: Wwedenie w teoriu metallov, Moskau 1950.
[12] ODING, I. A.: Zavodskaja Laboratoria, Nr. 4 (1937).
[13] HAIGH, B. P.: J. Inst. Metals 18, 55 (1937).
[14] MOORE, H. F. und T. M. JASPER: Univ. Illinois, Engr Exp. Station Bull. Nr. 136 (1923).
[15] UZHIK, G. W.: Vestnik Maschinostroenija, Nr. 4 (1949).
[16] ZIMMERLY, F. P.: Permissible Stress Range for Small Helical Spring, Univ. Mich. Dep. Engrng Res., Engrng Res. Bull. Nr. 26 (1934).
[17] HANKINS: Dep. Sc. Industr. Res., Engrng Res. Rep., Nr. 9.

### Diskussion

A. M. FREUDENTHAL: Tests with soap bubbles forming a Bragg "raft" exposed to cyclic force, give a relationship similar to the Wöhler curve for force vs. cycles necessary to form a cavity by aggregation of vacancies. This seems to confirm Author's theory.

# Torsion and tension relations for slip and fatigue

By

**R. E. Peterson**

With 7 figures

## 1. Introduction

A plot of ratios of torsion and bending fatigue limits for ductile materials is shown [1] in fig. 1, and it is seen that the results are in better agreement with the Mises criterion [2] than with the maximum shear theory [8]. It is generally recognized that fatigue failure in ductile materials starts by formation of slip bands [3], and it will therefore be of interest to consider differences in the formation of slip bands in torsion and tension. Published results [4], [5] on slip of all grains in a randomly oriented aggregate of cubic crystals in torsion and in tension showed close agreement with the Mises criterion. Since, however, slip of all grains is not a realistic requirement for fatigue, it was thought worthwhile to analyze the slip problem as a function of percentage of number of grains having slipped in terms of total number of grains.

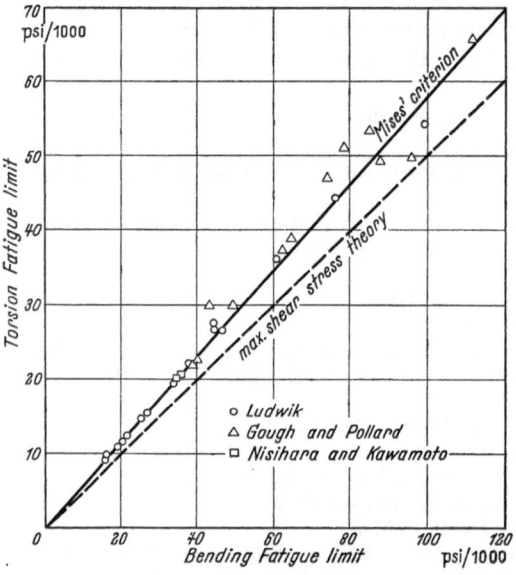

Fig. 1. Comparison of torsion and bending fatigue limits for ductile materials.

From the standpoint of design the difference between the above two theories may be said to be of some importance, but, it is not usually a major factor (maximum numerical difference is about 15%). It is therefore hoped that, in addition to the design aspect, the analysis presented herein will contribute some ideas which will be useful in further discussions concerning the mechanism of crack development under different states of stress.

## 2. Slip and yield criteria

First, we will recall some well-known facts about slip behavior [3]. In a crystal there are certain planes of maximum atomic density and in these planes there are certain directions of maximum linear atomic density. For example, in aluminum, which has a face-centered cubic structure, there are four such planes (octahedral planes) and in each plane three directions (face diagonals), or 12 maximum atomic density combinations. For any particular orientation with respect to applied stress, it is possible to compute the shear stress components corresponding to the 12 maximum atomic density combinations; these components are called resolved shear stresses. It has been shown that *slip occurs when the maximum resolved shear stress reaches a critical value*, independent of stress normal to the slip plane [3], [6].

Resolved shear stress values in terms of orientation with respect to applied tension and torsion stresses have been provided in the form of stereographic charts (fig. 2 is typical) for the face-centered cubic lattice (Al, Cu) by SACHS [4] and by COX and SOPWITH [5] and for the body-centered cubic lattice (Fe$_\alpha$, W, Cr, Mo) by COX and SOPWITH [5].

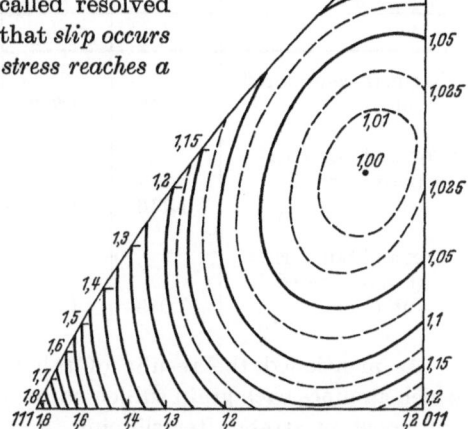

Fig. 2. Effect of orientation on ratio of maximum shear stress to maximum resolved shear stress for a face-centered cubic crystal subjected to tension (Sachs [4]).

Referring to fig. 2, the resolved shear stress distribution may be regarded as either that obtained by moving the stress direction (tension) through all possible positions with regard to the lattice of a single crystal, or it may be regarded as the distribution of resolved shear stress in the various grains of a randomly oriented aggregate with each grain subjected to the same applied tensile stress. On the basis of the latter viewpoint, assuming each grain subjected to equal applied stress up to slipping and constant stress after slipping, the above-mentioned authors computed the nominal tensile stress, $\sigma_N = \dfrac{P}{A}$, needed for slip in all grains of a tension specimen and the nominal shear stress, $\tau_N = T/K$ ($K$=sect. modulus in torsion), needed for slip in all grains of a thin tubular torsion specimen, both computations being made on the basis of slip of the first or most favorably oriented grain $\sigma_s$ and $\tau_s$, respectively (tab. 1). Stresses

$\sigma_S$ and $\tau_S$ may also be regarded as stresses required for slip if all grains had the orientation most favorable for slip.

The third column, $\tau_N/\sigma_N$ for slipping in all grains, is obtained by dividing $\tau_N/\tau_S$ by $2\sigma_N/\sigma_S$, since $\sigma_S = 2\tau_S$. The last three columns represent the same ratios as in the first three columns, but for conditions of first slip [4]. The Mises criterion gives $1/\sqrt{3}$ or 0.577 for the yielding of torsion and tension specimens [2] and the above-mentioned authors [4], [5] noted the close agreement with the values in the third column of tab. 1.

*Table 1*

| | Slip in all grains | | | First slip | | |
|---|---|---|---|---|---|---|
| | $\sigma_N/\sigma_S$ | $\tau_N/\tau_S$ | $\tau_N/\sigma_N$ | $\sigma_N/\sigma_S$ | $\tau_N/\tau_S$ | $\tau_N/\sigma_N$ |
| SACHS (face-centered cubic) . . . . . | 1.119 | 1.293 | 0.578 | (1) | (1) | (0.5) |
| Cox and SOPWITH (face-centered cubic) . . . . . | 1.116 | 1.281 | 0.574 Avg. 0.576 | 1 | 1 | 0.5 |
| Cox and SOPWITH (body-centered cubic) . . . . . | 1.068 | 1.232 | 0.577 | 1 | 1 | 0.5 |

As mentioned the results of tab. 1 are obtained from an analysis which assumes each grain subjected to equal applied stress up to slipping and constant stress after slipping. As pointed out by TAYLOR [7], this assumption is in error since the grains are not free to move independently. TAYLOR assumed that the deformation of each grain is the same, and found that five slip systems must be utilized to achieve this condition for tensile straining. BISHOP and HILL [8] pursued this further and found a torsion/tension ratio of 0.540 for slip of all grains of a face-centered cubic aggregate. There is reason to believe that uniform deformation is also not strictly correct. HERSHEY [9] has taken additional factors into account and has obtained numerical values from which can be calculated a corresponding value of 0.559. The problem is a very difficult one and it may be that a completely satisfactory exact solution will not be available for some time to come. However, it is interesting to note that the above values (including tab. 1) are all rather close, ranging from 0.540 to 0.578, the most recent value being about 0.56 (which happens to be about midway between the above values).

The values are all definitely above the maximum shear theory ratio (torsion/tension ratio 0.500), and tend to come closer to the Mises ratio (torsion/tension ratio $1/\sqrt{3} = 0.577$).

The Mises criterion was originally proposed as an applicable continuous mathematical expression [10] and the agreement of certain yield
tests with the Mises criterion has been interpreted as being due to
reaching critical values of shear energy [11] or octahedral shear stress
[12]. However, the observed behavior must be the statistical result of
the interaction of randomly oriented grains in which slip is due to
resolved shear stress and these relationships are so complex that agreement with the Mises criterion must be regarded as fortuitous [13]. These
remarks are not meant to detract from the usefulness of the Mises criterion in mechanics of materials and design, but are intended to emphasize that the detailed mechanism of slip in an aggregate is a different and
more complicated problem.

As mentioned in the introduction, the published analyses of slip
relations deal with slip of all grains. In the following section a similar
analysis will be made as a function of percentage of grains having slipped
in terms of total number of grains.

## 3. Conditions for slip as function of percentage of total number of grains

The stereographic charts (fig. 2 is an example) of SACHS [4] and of
Cox and SOPWITH [5] were utilized for this work.

Referring to fig. 2, we denote the area enclosed by 1.01 as $a_1$, the
area between 1.01 and 1.025 as $a_2$, etc. We denote by $r$ the ratio of

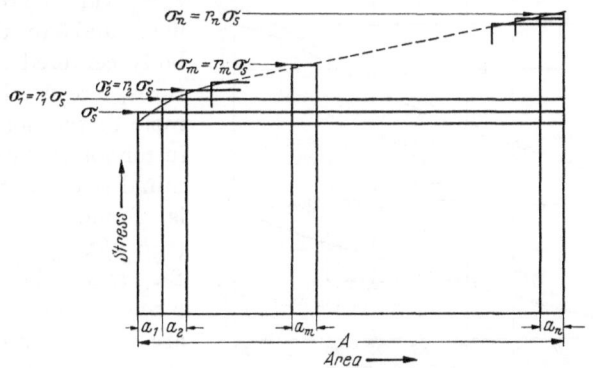

Fig. 3. Stress-area relation.

average stress $(\sigma_1, \sigma_2 \ldots)$ needed to cause slip in a given area $(a_1, a_2 \ldots)$
over the stress $\sigma_s$ corresponding to easiest slip (lattice plane and direction are oriented in such way that resolved stress and shear component
of applied loading are the same). Thus $r_1 = \dfrac{1 + 1.01}{2} = 1.005$, $r_2 = \dfrac{1.01 + 1.025}{2}$
$= 1.0175$, etc. Referring to fig. 3, the load to cause initial slip at point

1.00 is $P_s = \sigma_s A$. To cause slip over area $a_1$ the load must be increased to where an average stress of $\sigma_1 = r_1 \sigma_s$ exists over area $a_1$, $P_1 = r_1 \sigma_s A$. This approximation is sufficiently good since the number of areas is large.

To cause slip in area $a_2$ requires bringing area $(A - a_1)$ to the stress level $\sigma_2$, since area $a_1$ cannot be stressed higher than $\sigma_1$.

$$P_2 = r_1 a_1 \sigma_S + r_2 \sigma_S (A - a_1)$$

Extended to the $m$th element this becomes

$$P_m = \sum_{1}^{m-1} r a \sigma_S + r_m \sigma_S \left( A - \sum_{1}^{m-1} a \right)$$

The nominal stress, load/area, is

$$\sigma_N = \frac{P_m}{A}$$

Dividing by $\sigma_S$ we obtain

$$\frac{\sigma_N}{\sigma_S} = \frac{P_m}{\sigma_S A} = \frac{\sum_{1}^{m-1} r a + r_m \left( A - \sum_{1}^{m-1} a \right)}{A}$$

The above stress ratio is, of course, also the ratio of the load corresponding to the $m$th condition over the load at first slip, $P_m/P_s$.

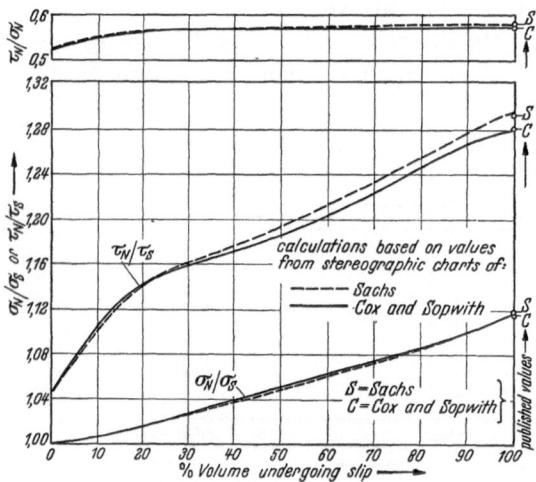

Fig. 4. Torsion and tension slip relations for aggregate of randomly oriented face centered cubic crystals.

The same procedure is followed for torsion.

The computed $\sigma_N/\sigma_S$ and $\tau_N/\tau_S$ values are shown in figs. 4 and 5 for the face and body centered cubic structures, respectively. The ratio of the nominal stress in torsion ($\tau_N$) over the nominal stress in tension ($\sigma_N$) is found by computing $(\tau_N/\tau_S)/(2\,\sigma_N/\sigma_S)$, since $\sigma_S = 2\,\tau_S$, and is shown in figs. 4, 5 and 6.[1] On figs. 4 and 5 are shown for comparison the values computed by SACHS [4] and by COX and SOPWITH [5]; these values are shown along the right hand edge since they are the only values (slip of all grains) which were computed in the quoted referen-

---

[1] In fig. 6 the curve for the face-centered cubic aggregate represents an average for the curves based on the SACHS and on the COX and SOPWITH stereographic charts.

ces. It will be seen that the agreement is good for each set of comparable values.

A rather interesting incidental feature of figs. 4 and 5 is the position of the $\tau_N/\tau_S$ curves at zero per cent volume (region of easiest slip).

On fig. 6 the positions of the Mises criterion and the maximum shear theory are also shown. It will be seen that a value midway between these criteria is reached when 5% of the volume has slipped in a face-centered cubic aggregate and 17% for a body-centered cubic aggregate. For larger percentages of the volume, the ratio increases so that at 50% it is 0.565 and beyond this increases slowly toward approximately the Mises value. The value of 0.500 (maximum shear theory) is obtained only for first slip, i. e., in a grain oriented for easiest slip.

The reason for the higher torsion values of figs. 4 and 5 lies in the restricted slip possibilities in torsion as compared to tension [5]. Referring to fig. 7, all planes tangent to an axially aligned 45° cone are planes of maximum shear stress for each element, whereas for each element of a torsion specimen only axial and radial planes are maximum shear planes.

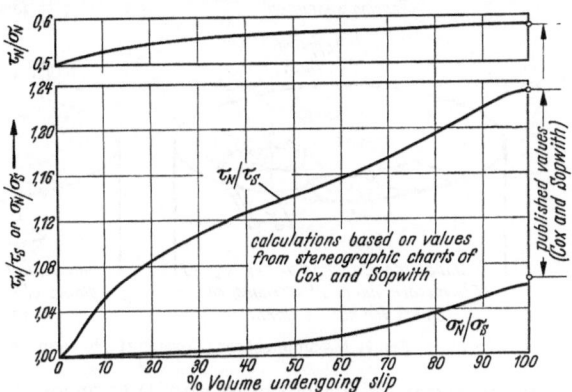

Fig. 5. Torsion and tension slip relations for aggregate of randomly oriented body centered cubic crystals.

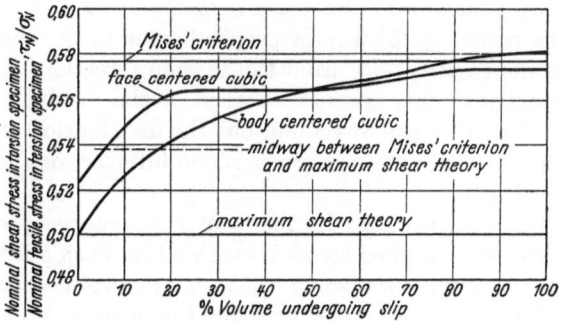

Fig. 6. Torsion/tension slip ratio for aggregates of randomly oriented crystals.

The region of orientation of easiest slip in the single crystal of fig. 2 is area $a_1$ enclosed by the dashed line 1.01. If we now consider an aggregate of randomly oriented crystals (test specimen), and utilize the assumptions of [4] and [5], it turns out that the ratio of the number of grains oriented for correspondingly easiest slip $n_1$ as compared to the total number of grains $N$ is $a_1/A$. For illustration, let us assume that $n_1$ is 10: if we distribute these around the periphery of the tension specimen of fig. 7 all 10 grains would have the same resolved shear stress; in the torsion specimen (fig. 7) if we align one grain for easiest slip and distribute the others (which have the same orientation in space) around the periphery, then it is clear that these other grains will not[1] be in a position of easiest slip. Consequently for each orientation area, $a_1 a_2 \ldots$, additional torque

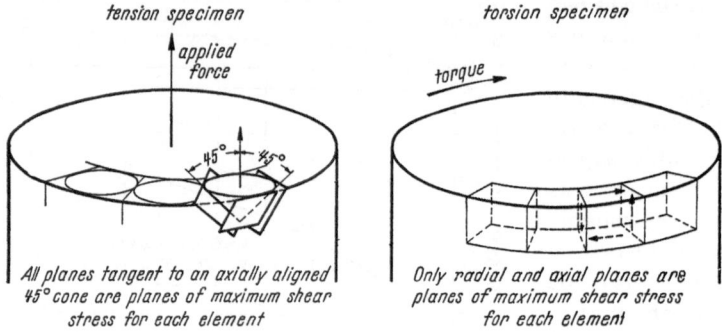

Fig. 7. Maximum shear planes in tension and torsion specimens.

will be required for slipping and this accounts for the higher torsion curves of figs. 4 and 5.

In this connection it is interesting to note that in a rectangular tension member, the maximum shear planes intersect the surface in the region $\pm 45°$ from a perpendicular to the tension direction but not in the region $\pm 45°$ from the tension direction. Slip lines do not behave exactly in this manner because of the resolved shear stress effect, as explained in the foregoing, but the distribution is roughly in accordance with maximum shear stress plane intersections for relatively low stress levels [4].

A criticism can be made of the analysis presented herein in that a constant applied stress is assumed for each grain before slip. However, as noted in the foregoing, the numerical values obtained from the various solutions do not differ greatly. But a more important consideration is that the relatively higher nominal torsion stress is due basically to the restricted slip possibilities in torsion as compared to tension, and this general conclusion is not altered by the above-mentioned initial assumption.

## 4. Discussion of results

The extent of slipping, in terms of number of grains, required to cause formation of a crack of sufficient length for propagation under cyclic stress is not definitely known. For a reasonably fine-grained material it may be necessary that slip and eventually separation under

---

[1] Except for the diametrically opposite grain.

cyclic stressing occur in several adjacent grains. Microscopical inspection indicates slipping in a considerable number of grains, but it must be admitted that specific examples of this kind are not conclusive and it seems that no systematic investigation has been made with the purpose of obtaining such data.

Returning to the initial paragraph of the paper, and fig. 1, ratios of torsion to bending fatigue limits $(\tau_f/\sigma_f)$ are usually found to be higher than 0.5. Or if based on shear stress $(\tau = \frac{\sigma_f}{2}$ in bending specimen), one obtains higher limit values in torsion than in tension. A number of factors can enter into such a comparison. We will assume that the obvious requirements are met, such as same diameter, contour radius, finish, etc. If torsion and bending are compared we also have the same stress gradient (linear) in both cases. One can therefore eliminate questions concerning statistical interpretation of different volumes of material being stressed. The remaining main differences appear to be the following:

   a) Anisotropy (relation of stress direction to rolling direction of bar),
   b) Normal stress component on shear plane,
   c) Slip distribution (as discussed in this paper).

With regard to a), the stress direction in the bending test is more favourably oriented with regard to rolling direction than the torsion test. Therefore, anisotropy cannot account for the observed result, i. e., relatively lower bending fatigue limit, based on shear. Since the plane of maximum normal stress does not coincide with the rolling direction in either case, the effect may be small.

With regard to b), if we consider an element subjected to tension, the maximum shear stress $\tau = \frac{\sigma}{2}$ occurs on a 45° plane and normal to this plane a component $\frac{\sigma}{2}$ is acting. In a torsion test there is no normal stress on the maximum shear planes. As mentioned in the foregoing, slip is independent of normal stress, but it is possible that under cyclic conditions normal stress could influence the development of micro-cracks in slip bands. If the normal stress component acting on a slip surface is a factor in fatigue, one would expect the bending test to have a relatively lower limiting value (based on shear stress) than the torsion test. The observed results are in the same direction.

With regard to c), the analysis in this paper shows that the slip distribution effect is also in the same direction as the observed results, even for conditions of slip in a fraction of the total number of grains (figs 4, 5 and 6). It is possible that both b) and c) contribute to the relatively higher torsion value, but factor c) could well contribute the major portion.

In conclusion, it is believed that slip relations must be considered as a basic factor in fatigue under different states of stress. If slipping in a considerable percentage of the total (for example, 25% or greater) number of grains at peak stress turns out to be a necessary condition for fatigue, then the major portion of the difference between torsion and bending fatigue strengths (based on shear stress) can be accounted for on the basis of the slip relation analysis presented herein. Conversely, if repeated slip in one grain (most favourably oriented for slip) is sufficient for fatigue then the relatively higher torsion values cannot be accounted for by slip relations. There is some evidence that in a relatively fine grained material considerable slip is needed for fatigue failure, but very little information on microstructural behaviour of aggregates under cyclic stress is available. The results of the present analysis and the discussion thereof point up the need for a detailed study of slip in terms of number of grains involved as an important factor in obtaining a better understanding of fatigue, particularly with reference to various states of stress.

Assistance was provided by Messrs. P. R. TOOLIN and J. R. WETHERBY in obtaining the corrected area values from the stereographic charts.

## Bibliography

[1] PETERSON, R. E.: Stress Concentration Design Factors, New York 1953, 7.
[2] TIMOSHENKO, S.: Strength of Materials, New York 1941, 473 (See also [12]).
[3] GOUGH, H. J.: Proc. ASTM, **33**, Part 2, 2 (1933).
   BARRETT, C. S.: Structure of Metals, New York 1952.
[4] SACHS, G.: Z. VDI, **72**, 734 (1928).
[5] COX, H. L. and D. G. SOPWITH: Proc. phys. Soc. Lond., **49**, 134 (1937).
[6] SCHMID, E.: Proc. 1st intern. Congr. appl. Mech., Delft 1924, 342.
[7] TAYLOR, G. I.: Timoshenko 60th Anniversary Volume, New York 1938, 218.
[8] BISHOP, J. F. W. and R. HILL: Phil. Mag., **42**, 1298 (1951).
[9] HERSHEY, A. V.: Trans. ASME, **76**, 241 (1954).
[10] von MISES, R.: Nachr. Ges. Wiss. Göttingen, 582 (1913).
[11] HENCKY, H.: Proc. 1st intern. Congr. appl. Mech., Delft 1924, 312.
[12] EICHINGER, A.: Proc. 2nd intern. Congr. appl. Mech., Zürich 1926, 325.
   NADAI, A.: J. appl. Phys., 8, 203 (1937).
[13] BEECHING, R.: Proc. Instn. mech. Engrs., **159**, 113 (1948).
   PRAGER, W. and P. G. HODGE: Theory of Perfectly Plastic Solids, New York 1951, 27.
[14] HEDGEPETH, J. M.: NACA TN 2777, 1952.

## Discussion

I. A. ODING: Das Problem der zwei- und dreiachsigen Wechselspannungen ist sehr kompliziert. Man muß hier nicht nur von den symmetrischen Zyklen ausgehen, sondern auch die asymmetrischen Zyklen im Auge halten.

Im Jahre 1937 habe ich diese Aufgabe analysiert. Kurz kommt man zu solchen Erfahrungen.

Soll sich die zyklische Torsionsspannung von $\tau_1$ bis $\tau_2$ und die Normalspannung von $\sigma_1$ bis $\sigma_2$ ändern, so ist bekanntlich die maximale und minimale Schubspannung

$$\left.\begin{aligned} \tau_{\max} = \frac{\sigma_1}{2}\sin 2\alpha + \tau_1 \cos 2\alpha \\[2mm] \tau_{\min} = \frac{\sigma_2}{2}\sin 2\alpha + \tau_2 \cos 2\alpha \end{aligned}\right\} \tag{1}$$

Diese wechselnden Spannungen fordern einen asymmetrischen Zyklus mit der mittleren Spannung und Spannungsamplitude

$$\left.\begin{aligned} \tau_m = \frac{\tau_{\max} + \tau_{\min}}{2} \\[2mm] \tau_a = \frac{\tau_{\max} - \tau_{\min}}{2} \end{aligned}\right\} \tag{2}$$

Früher wurde es gezeigt, daß eine asymmetrische Spannungsamplitude $\tau_x$ mit $\tau_a$ und $\tau_m$ durch

$$\tau_x^2 = \tau_a^2 + \tau_a \tau_m \tag{3}$$

verbunden ist. Oder mit (1) und (2)

$$\tau_x^2 = A\sin^2 2\alpha + B\cos^2 2\alpha + C\sin 2\alpha \ \cos 2\alpha \tag{4}$$

wo

$$A = \frac{\sigma_1^2 - \sigma_1\sigma_2}{8}; \quad B = \frac{\tau_1^2 - \tau_1\tau_2}{2}; \quad C = \frac{2\sigma_1\tau_1 - \tau_1\sigma_2 - \tau_2\sigma_1}{4}$$

Für die Grenzspannungen haben wir $\tau_x = \tau_w$

$$\frac{\mathrm{d}\tau_x}{\mathrm{d}\alpha} = 0 \quad \text{und} \quad \frac{B - A}{C} = \operatorname{ctg} 4\,\alpha,$$

wo $\tau_w$ die Ermüdungsgrenze bei symmetrischer Torsionsspannung ist.
Dann wird

$$\tau_w^2 = \frac{1}{2}\left(A + B + \sqrt{(B-A)^2 + C^2}\,\right)$$

Aus dieser Gleichung kann man die Grenzspannungen für beliebige asymmetrischen Zyklen für praktische Zwecke bestimmen. Man muß nur noch dafür sorgen, daß die maximale Schubspannung nicht die Streckgrenze überschreite:

$$\tau_s \geq 1/2\sqrt{\sigma_1 + 4\tau_1^2}$$

D. G. Sopwith remarked that, according to British experience the fatigue limit for combined normal and shear stresses will be found as in the figure, curve 1 for pure materials and curve 2 for materials with inclusions.

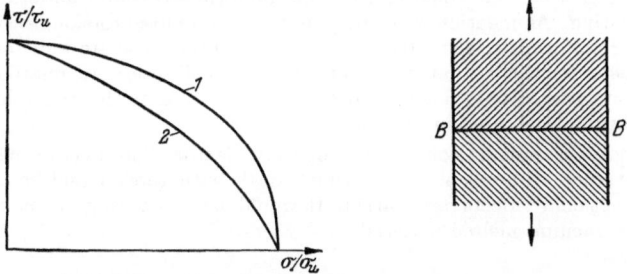

F. Wever: If single crystals with different orientation meet along a grain boundary $B\,B'$ (see fig.), X-rays reveal that the local transmission of stress across $B\,B'$

turns out to be something between what would be the result of the two assumptions: continuous normal stress and continuous strain. This result speaks against the uniform stress distribution as assumed by Author.

R. B. Heywood: An alternative theory giving the comparative fatigue behaviour of materials in bending or torsion is possible by postulating that strength is determined by the stress concentration around flaws within the material. Now Cox[1] has shown that for flaws of a cylindrical shape, the ratio of strengths in torsion to bending (or tension) is 0.75, whereas in practice a more realistic value would have been much less than this, about 0.6. A further difficulty that has been pointed out by Cox is that under combined bending and torsion the failure curve does not cut the torsional axis orthogonally, as has been found by experiments on ductile materials.

It can be shown that these difficulties associated with cylindrical flaws are overcome if one postulates that three-dimensional or ellipsoidal flaws are present within the material, and that failure depends on the stresses at the boundary of such flaws. At least two principal stresses at the boundary have values other than zero, and the strength in relation to the various combined stress criteria of failure has to be considered together with the shape and elastic properties of the flaw. An unpublished analysis of the simple case of a spherical cavity shows that ratios of torsion to bending strength are as follows

| Criterion of Failure | Ratio $\dfrac{\text{Torsion strength}}{\text{Bending strength}}$ |
|---|---|
| Maximum tension | 0.75 |
| Mises-Hencky | 0.6 |
| Maximum shear | 0.5 |

Thus both the shear and Mises-Hencky criteria give realistic values for the ratio of strengths. Moreover for both these criteria the failure curves under combined bending and torsion cut the torsional axis orthogonally, and this also is in agreement with observation as to the fatigue behaviour of ductile materials.

This alternative theory does not imply a rejection of the theory discussed by Peterson that failure occurs at slip planes in crystals; there is a possibility that a flaw (of undefined size) acts as a source of initiation for slip to occur in crystals, so ultimately causing failure.

R. E. Peterson: Wever's finding that the local transmission of stress is somewhere between what one would expect from uniform stress and uniform strain is quite interesting. As mentioned in the paper, the computed torsion/tension ratios are 0.576 for uniform stress and 0.540 for uniform strain; both are well above 0.500 and the reason for this is that in torsion the slip possibilities are relatively limited. This conclusion would not be expected to be altered by the above-mentioned choice of assumptions used in calculations.

Heywood's comments concern an important factor. The effect of macro-flaws has been studied in a recent paper[2] which deals with torsion and bending tests wherein directional effects are varied. It would be interesting to make similar tests with a vacuum melted material.

---

[1] Cox, H. L.: Aeronaut. Res. Counc., Rep. Mem. No. 2704, 1953.

[2] Findley, W. N. and P. N. Mathur: Proc. ASTM, 55, Part 2 (1955).

# Einige Besonderheiten der Kontaktermüdung

Von

## A. I. Petrussewitsch

Mit 5 Abbildungen

Der Spannungszustand beim Kontakt weist einige Besonderheiten auf. Die am meisten beanspruchten Teilchen aneinandergepreßter Oberflächenschichten werden der Wirkung allseitiger Druckspannungen ausgesetzt. Bei dem zu behandelnden Kontakt zweier Zylinder mit Parallelachsen unterscheidet sich die minimale Hauptdruckspannung bei einem Poissonschen Koeffizienten $m = 0,3$ von den zwei anderen Spannungen nur um 40 Prozent. Zugleich können bei Reibungskräften an den Kontaktoberflächen bedeutende Zugspannungen entstehen. Die Kontaktspannungs-Gradienten können sehr große Werte erreichen. Die Veränderungsgeschwindigkeit der Kontaktspannungen kann zeitmäßig viel größer sein als bei gewöhnlichen Ermüdungs- und Schlagexperimenten.

Sehr interessant und in der Praxis gewöhnlicher Ermüdungsexperimente nicht anzutreffen ist die folgende Besonderheit des Spannungszustandes bei Kontakt: die maximale Kontaktschubspannung ist in etwas tieferen Schichten des Materials größer als an der Kontaktoberfläche.

Wie theoretische Forschungen, die von N. M. BELJAJEW im Jahre 1924 veröffentlicht wurden [1], besagen, ist die maximale Schubspannung, die in jedem der zwei unter normaler Druckbelastung befindlichen Zylinder mit Parallelachsen in Punkten, die um $0,786\,b_1$ von der Oberfläche entfernt sind, gleich $0,3\,\sigma_c$, wo $b_1$ die Halbbreite des Kontaktstreifens und $\sigma_c$ die größte Druckspannung der Kontaktoberfläche ist, die nach der Hertzformel berechnet wird. Die Schubspannung ist an den Punkten der Kontaktoberfläche anderthalbmal kleiner als die maximale Schubspannung.

M. M. SAWERIN [2] ermittelte, daß beim Rollen von Zylindern die Schubspannung in einer Tiefe von $0,7\,b_1$ sich von $-0,065\,\sigma_c$ bis $0,3\,\sigma_c$ verändert, während in einer Tiefe von $0,5\,b_1$ die Schubspannung an den Horizontalflächen (Abb. 1) und an den entsprechenden Vertikalflächen sich innerhalb der Grenzen von $\pm\,0,25\,\sigma_c$ verändert, d. h. eine Doppelamplitude von $0,5\sigma_c$ besitzt.Bei einem Reibungskoeffizienten von 0,2 ist die Schubspannungsdoppelamplitude in einer Tiefe von $0,5\,b_1$ gleich

$0,51\,\sigma_c$ und in einer Tiefe von $0,2\,b_1$ gleich $0,44\,\sigma_c$. Offenbar ist die Spannungsdoppelamplitude von $0,5\,\sigma_c$ für die Ermüdung gefährlicher als die Spannungsdoppelamplitude von etwa $0,37\,\sigma_c$. Dies unterstrich bereits S. Way [3], der die von N. M. Beljajew entwickelten Formeln benutzte.

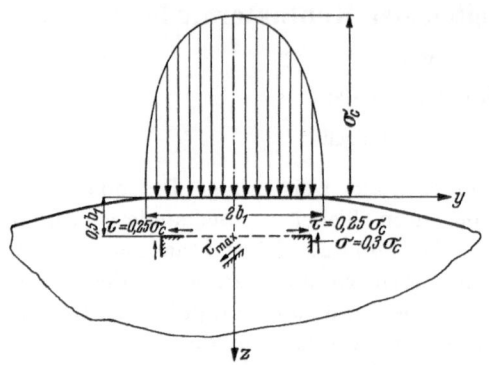

Bei einem Reibungskoeffizienten von $0,1$ ist die Schubspannungsdoppelamplitude in einer Tiefe von $0,5\,b_1$ zweieinhalbmal größer als an der Oberfläche [2]. Ungeachtet dessen aber sind die anfänglichen Ermüdungsrisse, die vor der Grübchenbildung (Pitting) auftreten, in der Regel in dünnen $10-25\,\mu$ starken Oberschichten entstanden.

Abb. 1. Die Tiefenlage der Schubspannungen mit maximaler Amplitude.

Um dies zu erklären, kann man annehmen, daß die Druckverteilung auf der Kontaktoberfläche bei Bestehen einer hydrodynamischen Schmierschicht sich stark von der halbelliptischen Verteilung unterscheidet, für die die oben angeführten Kontaktschubspannungen berechnet sind. Also sind die Kontaktschubspannungen in der Tiefe bedeutend

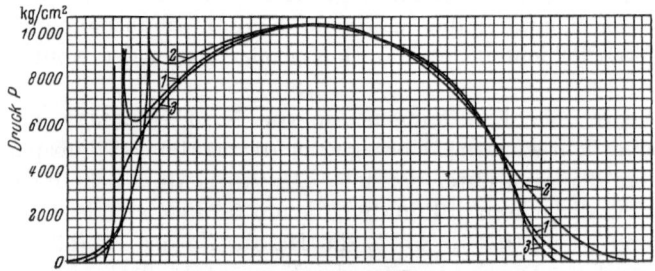

Abb. 2. Druckkurven $p$ bei einer Stärke der Schmierschicht von $1\,\mu$ (Kurve 1), $5\,\mu$ (Kurve 2) und $0,083\,\mu$ (Kurve 3) bei einem Krümmungsradius von 5 cm, und einem Elastizitätsmodul der sich in Kontakt befindlichen Zylinder von $2\,150\,000$ kg/cm². Die Abhängigkeit der Ölzähigkeit $\eta$ von dem Druck ist

$$\eta = \eta_0\,e^{p/500}.$$

kleiner als bei Fehlen einer Schmierschicht. Jedoch zeigen die Druckverteilungskurven in der Schmierschicht (Abb. 2), die für die in reinem Rollen befindlichen Zylinder unter Beachtung ihrer Deformation und der Abhängigkeit der Schmiermittelzähigkeit vom Drucke [4] ermittelt wurden, daß diese Hypothese abgelehnt werden muß. Wie wir aus Abb. 2

ersehen, unterscheiden sich nämlich diese Kurven nicht *so* stark von einer Halbellipse, um die Schubspannung in der Tiefe bedeutend zu verändern. Dies wird auch durch entsprechende Berechnungen bestätigt.

Man kann auch annehmen, daß die hohen Schubspannungen an den Kontaktoberflächen zur Oberflächenermüdung beitragen. Diese Spannungen sind durch die beim Kontakt entstehenden Reibungskräfte hervorgerufen und sind infolge des Bestehens einer hydrodynamischen Schmierschicht nicht nach dem Halbellipsengesetz, sondern nach einem anderen Gesetz verteilt. Obwohl der Spannungszustand in der Kontaktzone bei der Bildung einer hydrodynamischen Schmierschicht noch ungenügend erforscht ist, kann dennoch auf folgendes hingewiesen werden. Bei dem reinen Rollen ist die Ermüdungswirkung der Reibungskräfte nicht groß. Die Druckverteilungskurven in der Schmierschicht (Abb. 2) zeigen, daß der Wirkungsbereich mehr oder weniger bedeutend hydrodynamisch bedingter Schubspannungen an der Kontaktoberfläche auf sehr kleine Bereiche, die an dem Auslauf der Oberfläche in der Kontaktzone liegen, beschränkt sind.

Bei gleitendem Rollen leisten die vorrückenden Oberflächen einen viel größeren Widerstand der Kontaktermüdung als dieselben Oberflächen während eines reinen Rollens. Deshalb muß in diesem Falle die Wirkung der Reibungskräfte noch geringer sein als beim reinen Rollen. Und dennoch beginnt die Ermüdungszerstörung auch in diesem Falle ebenfalls von der Oberfläche. Da die Reibungskräfte vorrückender Oberflächen in einem irgendwie bedeutendem Ausmaß den Spannungszustand nicht ungünstig verändern können, können wir behaupten, daß in diesem Falle die Wirkung der Reibungskräfte in der hydrodynamischen Schmierschicht nicht die Hauptursache des Beginns der Ermüdung an der Oberfläche darstellt.

T. NISHIHARA und T. KOBAYASHI [5] vertreten den Standpunkt, daß die Ursache der Kontaktermüdung die hohe Druckspannung an den Kontaktoberflächen ist, die, sich nach dem pulsierenden Zyklus verändernd, hinsichtlich ihrer Ermüdung den pulsierenden Druckspannungen equivalent ist, die an zylindrischen Probestäben in den Pulsator-Prüfmaschinen erzeugt werden. Dieser Standpunkt kann nicht als genügend begründet betrachtet werden, wenn man im Auge behält, daß zum Unterschied von gewöhnlichen Experimenten an Pulsatoren, das Elementarvolumen des Materials an den auf der Mittellinie des Kontaktstreifens liegenden Punkten der Wirkung nicht einer, sondern dreier Haupt-Druckspannungen ausgesetzt wird: $\sigma_z = \sigma_c$, $\sigma_y = \sigma_c$ und (wenn der Poissonsche Koeffizient $m = 0,3$ ist) $\sigma_x = 0,6\,\sigma_c$. Von der Druckspannung $\sigma_c$ subtrahieren wir nun die gleichmäßige allseitige Druckspannung, die bekanntlich die Materialermüdung nur schwach beeinflußt. Der übrigbleibende Spannungswert $0,4\,\sigma_c$ ist gleichbedeutend

einer genauso starken einachsigen Druckspannung. Letzterer unterscheidet sich nach ihrem Ermüdungseffekt nur wenig von einer Schubspannung mit etwa halb so großer Doppelamplitude, d. h. mit einer
Doppelamplitude von 0,2 $\sigma_0$, wie dies Erfahrungen mit weichen Stählen
in Pulsatoren unter pulsierendem Druck oder aber in Ermüdungs-
maschinen vom Schenck-Typus bei Wechseldrehung besagen.

Wenn nur die Druckspannungen für die Kontaktermüdung ent-
scheidend wären, so könnte man schwerlich die starke Wirkung der
Schmiermittelzähigkeit auf die kontaktmäßige Ermüdungsfestigkeit
erklären, die im Zusammenhang mit der Veränderung des Reibungskoeffizienten an den Kontaktstellen steht wie das in einer Reihe von
Experimentalforschungen in der UdSSR festgestellt wurde. So z. B.
erwiesen die Experimente von G. K. Trubin an Zahnrädern mit geraden
Zähnen [6], daß die Veränderung des mittleren Reibungskoeffizienten
an den Zähnen von 0,029 auf 0,053, hervorgerufen durch die Tempe-
raturveränderungen des Zylinderöls von 45 auf 82° C, zur Verringerung
der Kontaktfestigkeit um 22 Prozent führte.

Die von N. F. Kusmin [7] unternommenen Experimente zeigten,
daß die Grübchenbildung an den Oberflächen der stählernen Zylinder-
prüflinge, die durch exzentrische Zahnräder miteinander so verbunden
sind, daß die Gleitgeschwindigkeit von einem bestimmten Wert bis zum
selben Wert mit entgegengesetztem Vorzeichen sich verändert, bei der
Anwendung verschiedener Schmieröle auf der nachschleppenden Oberfläche bei derselben Gleitgeschwindigkeit eintritt an der Stelle, wo der
Reibungskoeffizient sein Maximum erreicht.

Das Kriterium der Kontaktermüdung gemäß maximaler Druckspannung ergibt keinen Unterschied zwischen den vorrückenden und
nachschleppenden Kontaktoberflächen. Indessen aber ist die von der
Kontaktermüdung erlaubte Belastung bei den vorrückenden Oberflächen um mehrere Male größer als bei den nachschleppenden.

Also kann die Hypothese von der entscheidenden Rolle der maximalen Druckspannungen keine Antwort auf die Frage nach der Ursache
der größeren Neigung zur Kontaktermüdung bei den Oberschichten des
Materials liefern.

Schließlich kann man die Hypothese aufstellen, daß die Ursache der
Kontaktermüdungsprozesse von der Oberfläche an den immensen zu-
sätzlichen Spannungen, die durch den Kontakt der höchsten Punkte
der Flächenunebenheiten hervorgerufen sind, liegt. In der Tat kann
an der Kontaktoberfläche eine große Konzentrierung von Spannungen
an den Flächenunebenheiten insbesondere beim Kontakt von harten
und zugleich ungenügend glatten Oberflächen vorkommen. Jedoch
zeigen die Experimente des Referenten [8] sowie die von dem Referenten
zusammen mit J. A. Mischarin daß eine erhöhte Glätte der Ober-

flächen, die eine gewisse optimale Glätte übertrifft, bereits keine Wirkung auf die Entstehung der Kontaktermüdung ausübt.

Abb. 3 zeigt Wöhlerkurven der Kontaktermüdung von stählernen Rollen mit einem Durchmesser von 24 mm. Der Werkstoff war ein 0,45prozentiger Kohlenstoffstahl der auf 285—302 Brinell vergütet war. Jede Rolle befand sich im Kontakt mit zwei Walzen mit Durchmessern von 123—126 mm, aus demselben Stahl hergestellt, der jedoch auf 300 bis 320 Brinell vergütet war. Die Wöhlerkurven 1—5 fielen beinahe in eine Linie zusammen, obwohl die mittlere quadratische Höhe der Profilkurve der Oberfläche der Walzen (im Folgenden schlechthin als

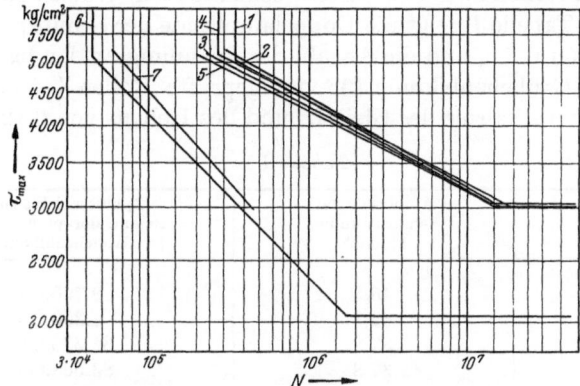

Abb. 3. Kontaktermüdung für 0,45prozentigen Kohlenstoffstahl ($H_B = 300$) bei verschiedenen Bearbeitungsmethoden der Oberflächen der Prüflinge:
*1* geläppte Rolle und polierte Walzen.
*2* geläppte Rolle und geschliffene Walzen.
*3* gedrehte Rolle und geschliffene Walzen.
*4* geläppte Rolle und gedrehte Walzen.
*5* gedrehte Rolle und gedrehte Walzen.
*6* geläppte Rolle und gefräste Walzen.
*7* gedrehte Rolle und gefräste Walzen.

Rauhigkeit bezeichnet), von denen in der Hauptsache die Kontaktfestigkeit der Rollen abhing, in der Achsenrichtung verändert wurde von 0,2 bis 7,6 $\mu$ und in der Tangentialrichtung von 0,1 bis 0,8 $\mu$. Die Linien 6 und 7 entsprechen der Achsenrauhigkeit der Walzen zwischen 1 und 2,3 $\mu$ und der Tangentialrauhigkeit von 4,3 bis 8,2 $\mu$.

Diese Experimente gestatten die Schlußfolgerung, daß auch die Hypothese von der entscheidenden Rolle der Kontaktspannungen an den Höhepunkten der Flächenunebenheiten mit den experimentellen Tatsachen unverträglich ist.

Folglich kann als festgestellt betrachtet werden, daß die Schubspannungen an der Oberfläche für die Ermüdung gefährlicher sind als die Tiefenspannungen derselben Größe. Mehr noch, es sind Ergebnisse vorhanden, die davon zeugen, daß das Material ohne Ermüdungs-

zerstörung sehr hohe Tiefen-Schubspannungen aushalten kann, wenn
an der Kontaktoberfläche Bedingungen geschaffen werden, die eine
Bildung von durch Ermüdung entstandenen Oberflächenrissen erschweren.

Wie bereits gesagt, entsteht bei einer gegen Walzen von gleicher
Oberflächenhärte gleitenden Rolle die Zerstörung immer an der nachschleppenden Oberfläche, d. h. an der Oberfläche derjenigen Zylinder,
die sich mit kleinerer Umfangsgeschwindigkeit dreht. Um die Kontaktermüdungsfestigkeit zylindrischer Rollen aus 0,45 prozentigem vergü-
tetem Kohlenstoffzahl zu bestimmen, die sich mit einer größeren Umfangsgeschwindigkeit drehen als die benachbarten Rollen, wurden diese
zylindrischen Rollen zwischen harten (zementierten) Walzen zusammen-
gepreßt. Die Tabelle 1 zeigt die Doppelamplitude der Schubspannung in
einer Tiefe von 0,5 $b_1$ und die Anzahl der Spannungszyklen bis zur fort-
schreitenden Grübchenbildung für vier geprüfte Rollen bei einem Ge-
schwindigkeitsverhältnis des Gleitens und des Rollens von 0,12.

*Tabelle 1*

| Brinell Härte | Amplitude der Schubspannung kg/mm² | Zykluszahl bis zum Beginn der progressiven Grübchenbildung |
|---|---|---|
| 285 | 46,3 | 8.790.000 |
| 228 | 42,3 | 4.300.000 |
| 222 | 37,8 | 34.530.000 |
| 213 | 37,8 | 83.568.000 |

Für den in der Tab. 1 aufgeführten Kohlenstoffstahl der betreffenden
Härte wird die Drehwechselermüdungsgrenze etwa bei 20 kg/mm² liegen.
Somit haben die Tiefen-Wechsel-Schubspannungen, die in der Tab. 1
aufgeführt sind, die Drehwechselfestigkeit 1,9—2,3 mal überholt und
dennoch hatte die Ermüdungszerstörung gewöhnlichen Charakter d. h.
sie begann in der dünnen Oberschicht.

H. D. Mansion [9] machte Experimente an Zahnrädern mit stufen-
weise erhöhter Belastung. Die Belastung wurde jede Stunde mit 41,2
kg/cm vergrößert. Die Zähne der Zahnräder waren aus Ni-Cr-Mo-Stahl,
gehärtet bis zur Vickers-Härte $H_v = 517—536$. Die Grübchenbildung
begann an der Oberfläche bei einer Belastung von 520—560 kg/cm. Zugleich aber hatten zyanierte Zahnräder aus demselben Stahl mit einer
0,15 mm starken Zyanschicht bei einer Kernhärte $H_v = 533$ und bei
einer Oberflächenhärte $H_v = 663$ keine Grübchenbildung aufgewiesen,
sogar bei einer Belastung von 1.190 kg/cm, obwohl die maximalen
Schubspannungen im letzteren Falle in einer Tiefe von 0,26 mm lagen.
In einer Tiefe von 0,165 mm, d. h. auch unterhalb der zyanierten Schicht
betrug dabei die Schubspannungsdoppelamplitude noch immer 57
kg/mm².

Eine von dem Referenten geprüfte Rolle aus Kugellagerstahl, der bis $H_v = 730-760$ gehärtet war, wies beim Walzen ohne zwangläufiges Gleiten keine Grübchenbildung nach 235 Millionen Zyklen bei einer Schubspannungsdoppelamplitude (in einer Tiefe von 0,5 $b_1$) von 82 kg/mm² auf.

All das besagt, daß der Stahl, ohne zerstört zu werden, sehr große wechselartige Tiefen-Schubspannungen aushalten kann.

S. WAY [3] erklärt dies mit der Fähigkeit des Materials, eine hohe Wechselspannung zugleich mit einer allseitigen Druckspannung auszuhalten. Jedoch hat der Referent errechnet, daß auf einer Fläche (einer Vertikalfläche) mit der maximalen Schubspannungsdoppelamplitude von 0,25 $\sigma_c$ (in einer Tiefe von 0,5 $b_1$) die Druckspannung gleichzeitig nur 0,3 $\sigma_c$ beträgt (Abb. 1). Kann nun eine Druckspannung von derselben Größenordnung wie die Schubspannung den Widerstand des Stahls im Vergleich zu der Wechseldrehbeanspruchung ohne Normalspannung mehr als zweimal vergrößern? Aus der Analyse der experimentellen Resultate an Proben bei wechselnder Druckspannung muß diese Frage verneinend beantwortet werden.

Die oben aufgeführte Analyse gestattet es, als erwiesen zu betrachten, daß die Tiefen-Schubspannungen auf die Ermüdungsfestigkeit des Materials weniger einwirken als die betreffenden Oberflächenspannungen. Vielleicht ist dieser Effekt mit einer „Selbstheilung" der Mikrorisse verbunden, wenn zu ihren Oberflächen andere Stoffe keinen Zutritt haben (gemeint sind Sauerstoff aus der Luft, Wasserdämpfe u. ä.). Es ist verständlich, daß die Entwicklungsprozesse der Ermüdungsschädigungen in die Tiefe des Materials nach der Bildung oberflächlicher Ermüdungsrisse davon abhängen, wie groß die Tiefen-Schubspannungen sind.

Kann aber behauptet werden, daß die Tiefen-Schubspannungen überhaupt nicht imstande sind allein Ermüdungszerstörungen hervorzurufen? Augenblicklich ist es noch schwer, diese Frage zu beantworten, da die manchmal anzutreffenden Fälle einer Entstehung von Ermüdungszerstörungen in der Tiefe des Materials und der Abschichtung bei Kontaktspannungen von diesem Standpunkt aus in vollem Ausmaß noch nicht untersucht worden sind. Es ist möglich, daß diese Erscheinung auf einen Eigenspannungszustand im Zug des Materials zurückzuführen ist, wie das z. B. der Fall ist bei der Entstehung von Ermüdungszerstörungen unter der nitrierten Schicht bei zylindrischen Dauerbiegeproben.

In den Forschungen V. A. KISLIKS, N. R. MIRSAS und N. P. STSCHAPOWS [10] wurde festgestellt, daß die unter der Oberfläche eintreffenden Ermüdungsbrüche in Eisenbahnradreifen in der Regel eine Folge von Silikat-Schlacken-Einschlüssen sind.

Es ist festgestellt, daß die Kontaktermüdungsfestigkeit bei der Vergrößerung der zementierten Schichtstärke bis zu einer gewissen optimalen

Stärke anwächst. Dasselbe betrifft die nitrierte und zyanierte Schicht. Offenbar steht es im Zusammenhang mit der Veränderung der Eigenspannungen in den Oberflächen-Schichten sowie mit der leichten Durchdrückung der festen Schicht in die weichere Innenschicht bei Überbelastungen und bei der Entstehung bedeutender plastischer Deformationen unter der festen Schicht. Deshalb bieten die angeführten Tatsachen keinen Zweifel an der früher gemachten Schlußfolgerung, daß die Tiefen-Schubspannungen weniger zur Ermüdung beitragen als die der Oberfläche. Mithin gestatten dieselben nicht zu behaupten — bis diesbezügliche spezielle Forschungen angestellt worden sind — daß die Tiefen-Schubspannungen überhaupt nicht dazu beitragen, Ermüdungszerstörungen hervorzurufen.

Man muß den Vorbehalt machen, daß die Schlußfolgerung von der kleineren Gefahr der Tiefen-Spannungen sich nicht auf die Biege-, Zug- oder Druckspannung bezieht, da die maximalen normalen Kontaktspannungen an der Oberfläche selbst entstehen und daß deshalb die Erforschung der Kontakt-Ermüdungsprozesse keine Daten ergeben kann für den Vergleich der Effektivität der Normalspannungen an der Oberfläche und in den Tiefen. Aber aus vielen Beobachtungen kann man folgern, daß die dünne Oberflächen-Schicht eine sehr große Rolle bei der Materialermüdung spielt auch bei den Zug- und Biegebruchspannungen.

In dieser Hinsicht sind zum Beispiel bezeichnend die kürzlich veröffentlichten Experimente von G. W. Karpenko [11], bei denen festgestellt wurde, daß neben der Korrosionsermüdung eine Ermüdung existiert, die Karpenko Adsorptionsermüdung nannte. Diese Ermüdungsart entwickelt sich in Prüfmedien, die auf das Metall nicht einwirken, aber an ihren Oberflächen aktive Stoffe ansammeln, die die Deformation adsorptionell erleichtern und die Ermüdungsfestigkeit herabsetzen. Die Ermüdungskurve ist bei der Adsorptionsermüdung ihrem Charakter nach vollkommen analog der Ermüdungskurve, die man in dem nichtaktiven Prüfmedium erhält. Es besteht nur der Unterschied, daß die Ermüdungsgrenze um 10—20% niedriger liegt. Mineralische Öle mit einem Zusatz oberflächen-aktiven Stoffes wie z. B. die Oleinsäure wirken auf eine sehr dünne Oberflächenschicht der Prüflinge ein. Aber auch dies genügt, um eine wesentliche Herabsetzung der Ermüdungsgrenze des Metalls hervorzurufen.

Andererseits führte bekanntlich die Ermüdungsprüfung in einem Vakuum bei einer verhältnismäßig kleinen Verdünnung (bis $10^{-3}$ mm Quecksilbersäule) zu einer wesentlichen Erhöhung der Ermüdungsfestigkeit [12], [13]. Dabei war also in der Umgebung des Prüflings der Sauerstoffgehalt äußerst gering, geschweige denn der Gehalt des im Metall gelösten Sauerstoffs.

E. Siebel und G. Stähli [14] haben bei überbeanspruchten Wechsel-
biegeproben mit glatten Probestäben 50 und 150 μ starke Schichten
abgeschliffen. Nach den verschiedenen Lastwechselzahlen führten sie
sodann die Probestäbe bis zum Bruch und bestimmten, inwiefern sich
nach dieser Zwischen-
bearbeitung die summa-
rische Lastwechselzahl
bis zum Bruch verän-
dert. Es erwies sich, daß
die Zerstörungsschäden
durch eine bedeutend
stärkere Verfestigungs-
wirkung des Materials
überholt werden. Bei
einer rechtzeitigen Ent-
fernung von sogar nur
10—20 μ starken Metall-
schichten gelang es,
die Ermüdungsbeschädi-
gungen vollkommen zu
heben.

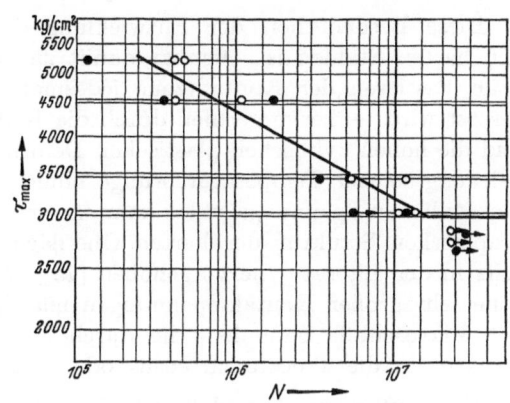

Abb. 4. Kontaktermüdung für 0,45prozentigen Kohlenstoffstahl ($H_B \approx 300$):
o geläppte Rolle und geschliffene Walzen.
• gedrehte Rolle und· geschliffene Walzen.

Die manchmal vor-
kommenden Fälle der
Entstehung von Ermü-
dungsrissen unter den
zementierten oder ni-
trierten Schichten kann
erklärt werden durch die
Wirkung hoher Eigen-
zugspannungen unter der
harten Schicht oder
durch den Bestand nicht
metallischer Einschlüsse
und Weichstellen in dem
Metall.

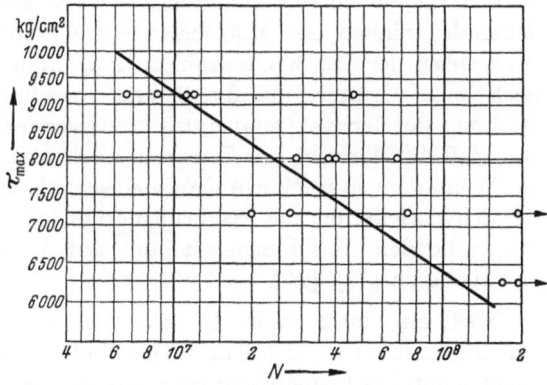

Abb. 5.
Kontaktermüdung für zementierten Chromnickelstahl.

Die zweite Besonderheit der Kontaktermüdung, auf die hier die
Aufmerksamkeit gelenkt werden muß, ist die Verschiedenheit der Er-
müdungskurven der weichen Stähle und der Stähle mittlerer Festig-
keit einerseits, sowie der Stähle mit harten Oberflächenschichten ander-
seits. Bei den ersteren wird die Ermüdungsgrenze gewöhnlich bei der
Lastwechselzahl von 1—20 Millionen erreicht (Abb. 4), bei den harten
Stählen ist beim gleitenden Rollen die Lastwechselzahl, die der wahren
Ermüdungsgrenze entsprechen, noch nicht festgestellt worden. Unsere

Experimente mit zementierten Prüflingen aus Chrom-Nickel-Stahl erwiesen, daß beim Rollen mit einem 8 bis 10%-igem Gleiten der ab-
sinkende Zweig der Ermüdungskurve nicht in die Horizontale übergeht,
wenn die Zahl der Überrollungen unter 200 Millionen liegt (Abb. 5).

Diese Besonderheit der Entwicklung der Ermüdungsprozesse bei
den harten Stählen ist offenbar damit zu erklären, daß das Material
beim Passieren der Kontaktzone jedesmal erhöhter Temperatur ausgesetzt wird — hervorgerufen durch die Reibung in der Kontaktzone
und die hohen zyklischen plastischen Deformationen. Die summarische
Wirkung solcher Temperatursprünge binnen Dutzender und Hunderter
von Millionen Spannungszyklen kann zu einer Veränderung der metallographischen Struktur der harten Oberflächenschicht führen. Wie bereits in der Literatur hervorgehoben [15], [16], wird in der Wirkungs-
zone sehr großer Kontaktspannungen manchmal eine erhöhte Ätzung
der Mikroschliffe gefunden, die durch den Übergang der Martensit-
struktur in die Troostomartensit- oder Troostitstruktur erklärt wird.

Man muß vermerken, daß es bei der Prüfung von Proben mit Kontaktspannungen, bei denen die Lastwechselzahl Dutzende und Hun-
derte von Millionen ausmacht, nicht gelingt, wesentliche strukturelle
Veränderungen im Metall festzustellen. Es gelingt auch nicht, ein be-
deutendes Sinken der Mikrohärte der Oberfläche abhängig von dem
Anwachsen der Lastwechselzahl zu konstatieren. All das bietet jedoch
noch keine Gründe, um die bereits vorgebrachte Annahme von der
Wirkung der Kontakttemperaturen zu verwerfen. Es ist an sich möglich, daß die Wirkung der Temperaturerhöhung am Kontakt ganz lokal
ist. Wenn dem so ist, hätte man vielleicht dadurch auch eine Erklärung
der Schwierigkeiten, die Erfahrungen mit langsam laufenden, reibenden
und rollenden Maschinenelementen auf hohe Geschwindigkeiten zu
extrapolieren [17], [18].

Noch eine interessante Besonderheit der Kontaktermüdung bietet
das in bestimmter Hinsicht ungewöhnliche Verhalten des Materials,
wenn Kontaktschwingungsversuche niedriger Belastungsamplitude und
hoher Lastwechselzahl mit vereinzelten kurzdauernden Überbelastungen
kombiniert werden. Wie die Experimente von S. P. Pawlow [19] zur
Erforschung der Kontaktermüdung von Zahnrädern aus 0,45%igem
Kohlenstoffstahl, der bis $H_B = 170-197$ vergütet war, erwiesen, ver-
mindern bedeutende Überbelastungen keineswegs die Zykluszahl bis zu
einer progressiven Grübchenbildung, sondern erhöhen diese Zykluszahl.
In der Tab. 2 ist die Zykluszahl bis zur progressiven Grübchenbildung
bei einer Wechselbelastung unter verschiedenen Regimen aufgeführt.
Der Vergleich der Zykluszahlen, nach denen eine progressive Ermüdungszerstörung der Oberflächenschichten unter konstanter und wechselnder

Belastung eintritt, bezeugt einen günstigen Einfluß aller Überbelastungen, außer der in den letzten Zeilen von Tab. 2 genannten.

*Tabelle 2*

| Spannung nach Hertz ($\sigma_c$) und die Zykluszahl ($N_c$) in der Periode des Belastungszyklus | | | | Mittlere Zykluszahl vor Beginn der progressiven Grübchenbildung |
|---|---|---|---|---|
| bei kleinerer Belastung | | bei größerer Belastung | | |
| $\sigma_c$ | $N_c$ | $\sigma_c$ | $N_c$ | |
| 85 | 100.000 | 95 | 20.000 | 5.128.000 |
| | | 105 | 20.000 | 2.680.000 |
| | | 115 | 20.000 | 1.035.000 |
| 85 | 116.000 | 105 | 4.000 | 3.500.000 |
| | 110.000 | | 10.000 | 2.465.000 |
| | 100.000 | | 20.000 | 2.680.000 |
| | 80.000 | | 40.000 | 1.092.000 |
| | 60.000 | | 60.000 | 553.300 |

Man kann zur Erklärung dieser Besonderheit der Kontaktermüdung die Hypothese aufstellen, daß bei einem Wechselregime der Arbeit der Zahnräder der Einlaufprozeß der Zähne eine längere Zeitspanne einnimmt, als bei einer konstanten Belastung, und daß die Oberflächenschichten sich schneller verschleißen, als daß sich die Ermüdungsprozesse bis zur Bildung von Ermüdungsrissen entwickeln können.

Dies bezeugt wiederum die wichtige Rolle, die die dünnsten Oberflächenschichten in der Entwicklung der Ermüdungsprozesse des Materials spielen.

Leider ist es mangels zuverläßlicher experimenteller Daten nicht möglich, noch eine wichtige Besonderheit der Kontaktermüdung zu analysieren, nämlich daß die Ermüdungsgrenzen bei Vergrößerung der Probestücke bedeutend weniger Veränderungen erfahren, als bei gewöhnlichen Ermüdungsexperimenten.

Zum Schluß sei bemerkt, daß es beim Fehlen des Schmiermittels zu keiner Grübchenbildung kommt. Es erübrigt sich hier, auf die Gründe dieser Erscheinung einzugehen, da es zum Thema des Referats nicht gehört. Wir möchten nur auf die Experimente von J. M. Schwezowa und I. W. Kragelski an Probestücken aus Chlorsilber [20] hinweisen, die ergaben, daß der Kontakt der Oberflächen sich an einzelnen Höhepunkten der Flächenunebenheiten konzentriert, was in einer Reihe anderer Forschungen indirekt und auch theoretisch festgestellt wurde [21]. Die Entwicklung der Ermüdungsprozesse in denjenigen Teilchen, die sich in der unmittelbaren Nähe der tatsächlichen Kontaktflächen befinden, gehört mit zu den Hauptgründen des Metallverschleißes. Die Gesetzmäßigkeiten dieser Art der Kontaktermüdung sind jedoch bisher nur sehr wenig erforscht worden.

Somit sind auf Grund der Analyse von Prozessen der Kontakt-ermüdung einige Gesetzmäßigkeiten festgestellt worden, deren Kennt-nis bei der Inangriffnahme des gesamten Ermüdungsproblems von Nutzen sein kann.

### Literaturverzeichnis

[1] BELJAJEW, N. M.: Örtliche Spannungen bei der Zusammenpressung ela-stischer Körper, Sammelband, Ingenieurbauten und Baumechanik, Lenin-grad 1924.

[2] SAWERIN, M. M.: Die Kontaktfestigkeit des Materials, Moskau 1946.

[3] WAY, S.: Mach. Design, 11, (1939).

[4] PETRUSSEWITSCH, A. I.: Wichtigste Schlüsse aus der Kontakthydrodyna-mischen Schmierungstheorie. Izvestija Akademija nauk SSSR. Otd. techn. nauk. Nr. 2, 209 (1951).

[5] NISHIHARA, T. und T. KOBAYASHI: Trans. Soc. mech. Engrs., Japan, Nr. 3 (1937).

[6] TRUBIN, G. K.: Die Kontaktermüdung der geradzähnigen Zahnräder, Moskau 1952.

[7] KUSMIN, N. F.: Über den Reibungskoeffizient im Schwerbelastungskontakt, Vestnik mašinostroenija, 34, Nr. 5, 18—26 (1954).

[8] PETRUSSEWITSCH, A. I.: Zahnrad- und Schneckengetriebe, Nachschlagebuch Maschinenbau, Moskau 1948.

[9] MANSION, H. D.: Automobile Engr. 32, (1942).

[10] KISLIK, W. A., N. R. MIRSA und N. P. STSCHAPOW: Die Erforschung des Radreifenstahls, Moskau 1938.

[11] KARPENKO, G. W.: Die Wirkung der oberflächenaktiven Stoffe auf die Stahl-ermüdung, Doklady Akademija nauk SSSR, 73 (1950).

[12] GOUGH, H. J. und D. G. SOPWITH: Engineering, 162, 197 (1946).

[13] GOUGH, H. J. und D. G. SOPWITH: J. Inst. Metals, 72, 415—421 (1946).

[14] SIEBEL, E. und G. STÄHLI: Arch. Eisenhüttenw., 15, 519—527 (1942).

[15] JONES, A. B.: Steel, 119, Nr. 14, 68—70 (1946).

[16] BARWELL, F. T.: Properties of Metallic Surfaces, Institute of Metals Mono-graph Nr. 13, 101—122 und 330—364 (1952).

[17] NIEMANN, G.: Z. VDI. 87, 521—523 (1943).

[18] BUCKINGHAM, E. und G. I. TALBOURDET in J. T. BURWELL Jr.: Mechanical Wear, Amer. Soc. Metals, Cambridge 1950.

[19] PAWLOW, S. P.: Die Dauerarbeitsfestigkeit der Zahnräder bei einer Wechsel-belastung, Vestnik mašinostroenija, 33, Nr. 3 (1953).

[20] SCHWEZOWA, J. M. und I. W. KRAGELSKI: Von der geometrischen Charakte-ristik der Oberflächen der Maschinenelemente, Vestnik mašinostroenija, 33, Nr. 3 (1953).

[21] PETRUSSEWITSCH, A. I.: Die Oberflächengüte und die Festigkeit bei Kontakt-spannungen, Moskau 1946.

### Diskussion

F. K. G. ODQVIST: Ein ähnliches Thema wie das des Verfassers wurde von uns vor 20 Jahren in Angriff genommen, wobei Kugeln durch pulsierenden Druck ermüdet wurden. Es entstanden dabei Grübchen („Pittings") die aus Ermüdungs-rissen in 45° zur Oberfläche gebildet waren. Es konnte aber dabei nicht festgestellt werden, ob die Risse an der Oberfläche selbst oder aber im Innern entstanden. Dies Ergebnis ist unpubliziert geblieben. Bei statischen Versuchen entstanden jedoch die ersten Fließfiguren unter der Oberfläche im Gebiet der höchsten Schubspannung, vgl. F. K. G. ODQVIST, Plasticitetsteori (schwedisch), Stockholm 1934, 65. Die Ergebnisse des Verfassers ergänzen hier wesentlich unsere Arbeiten und stellen einen wichtigen Fortschritt dar.

D. G. SOPWITH gave a short description of tests carried out at the MERL with pulsation load on rollers of different diameter. The region of maximum stress was explored by ultra sound and certain indications of cracks from below the surface noted. Subsequent cutting and polishing failed to reveal visible cracks.

R. E. PETERSON: It may be of interest to mention some results obtained by S. WAY with rotating rollers, normally loaded but without slip. It was not possible to produce the fatigue phenomenon commonly denoted by "pitting" without use of lubricant. The hydraulic wedge theory seams logical since the crack direction (about 15° to tangency) is such that the "mouth" of the crack enters the contact zone first. This direction changes from left to right with change of direction of rotation from clockwise to counterclockwise (lower roller). The "pitting limit" is a function of hardness of material, surface smoothness and viscosity of lubricant.

A. I. PETRUSSEWITSCH dankte den Diskussionsteilnehmern und stellte die gute Übereinstimmung ihrer Ergebnisse mit seinen eigenen fest.

# Some observations on the propagation of fatigue cracks

By

**C. E. Phillips**

With 10 figures

The current researches on crack propagation in Materials Division of MERL mainly arose from two short fatigue determinations which formed a very small part of a paper [1] by the author and a colleague.

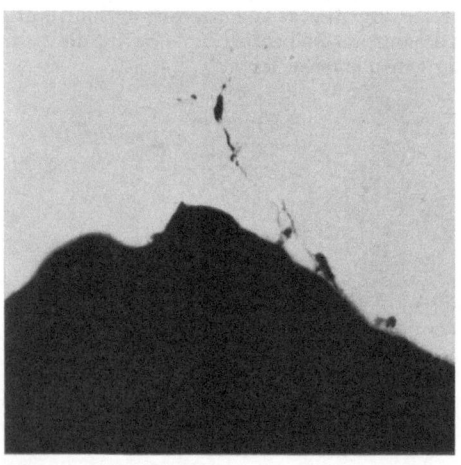

It was shown that mild steel bars of about 2 inches diameter, containing a circumferential V-notch 0.2 inch deep, had the same fatigue strength under reversed direct stress whether the root radius of the notch was 0.002 inch or 0.025 inch. Further considerations of this matter were described in another paper [2] in which it was shown that cracks occurred at the bottom of the sharp notches at a very early stage of the fatigue test. Fatigue cracks in mild steel notched specimens were formed at a stress of $\pm 2$ tsi after an endurance of 10,000 cycles; cracks of about the same length were present in similar specimens after 30 million cycles of the same stress level. Fig. 1 and 2 give photographs of typical cracks found after widely differing endurances. The existence of non-propagating cracks was thus clearly established.

Fig. 1. Crack in mild steel after $5 \cdot 10^4$ cycles. $\times 350$.

The behaviour of other materials under reversed direct stress (aluminium alloys in particular) is being studied by FROST [3]. He has already shown that cracks can easily be detected at the bottom of a circumferential curve of small root radius in a medium-strength aluminium alloy (L65) when tested at stresses below the notched fatigue limit of the material. The length that such cracks attained depended upon the value of the applied stress. Application of NEUBER's analysis to determine the theoretical stress distribution in the material at the bottom of the notch gave a surprising result; each crack propagated until its end reached the point in the original stress field due to the notch at which the theoretical stress was equal to the fatigue limit of the material. The crack would not propagate further unless the applied stress range was increased.

The conclusion that may be drawn from these results is that the stress gradient at the root of a crack is so very steep and acts over such a very short distance that its effect on the original stress field is negligible.

The maximum length of non-propagating crack found, however, was 0.006 inch, and it is to be expected that the original stress distribution in the vicinity of the notch has been materially altered by the growing crack. Moreover, at stresses just above those necessary to cause cracks 0.006 inch long, complete fracture of the specimen always occurred — in other words, the fatigue limit of the material had been exceeded. No complete explanation has been found to account for the fact that slight increase of stress range caused such a marked difference in crack behaviour.

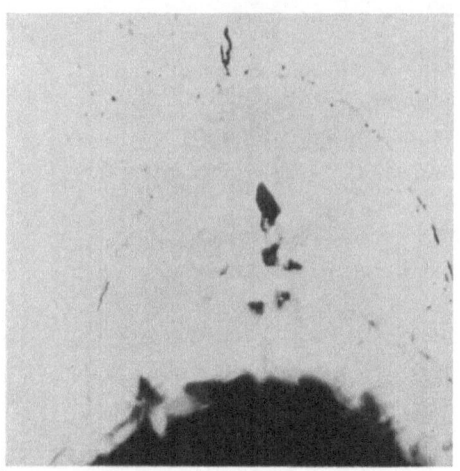

The shortest non-propagating cracks found were about 0.001 inch long. At stresses below those necessary

Fig. 2. Crack in mild steel after $100 \cdot 10^6$ cycles. × 350.

to cause such short cracks, no cracks at all were found. One salient feature of the short cracks is that they were invariably at an angle of about 45° to the axis of a specimen — all other cracks were transverse to the direction of loading. Examples of cracks referred to are given in fig. 3, 4 and 5. The smallest cracks appear to be propagating under the influence of shear stress rather than of tension stress.

The work by Cox and FIELD [4] on square section test-pieces of mild steel subjected to combined torsion and bending fatigue stresses, showed that for this material fatigue cracks were initiated under the influence of tension stress in preference to shear stress, when the ratio tension stress range to shear stress range exceeded 1.6. An extension of this work is now including similar tests on various light alloys, viz., DTD. 683,

DTD. 684 and RR 59. Fatigue cracks in these alloys all followed directions normal to that of the principal stress at any point, regardless of the ratio of principal tension stress to principal shear stress.

It is not reasonable, therefore, to attribute the direction of the smallest cracks found at the bottom of V-notches by FROST to any possible dominant effects of shear stress in crack propagation.

Similar tests are also in progress on square section test-pieces of nearly pure copper in an isotropic condition. Macroscopical examination indicates that cracks in this material behave similarly to those found in the mild steel reported on by COX and FIELD [4]. Microscopical examination of the cracks, on the other hand, indicates that there is a possibility

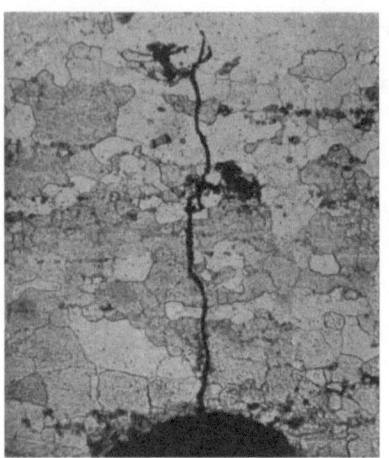

Fig. 3. Crack in aluminium alloy after 31 · 10⁶ cycles at ± 2.5 tsi. × 300.

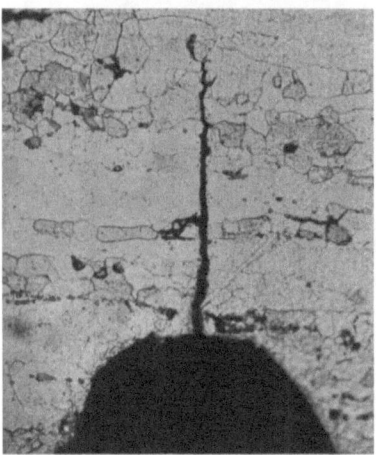

Fig. 4. Crack in aluminium alloy after 28 · 10⁶ cycles at ± 2 tsi. × 300.

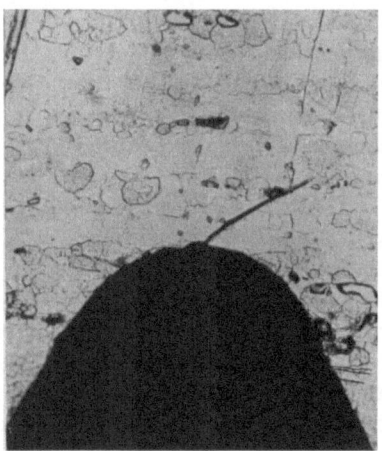

Fig. 5. Crack in aluminium alloy after 14 · 10⁶ cycles at ± 1.5 tsi. × 300.

that the cracks were, in fact, following alternately one or other of the two orthogonal systems of maximum shear stress directions. The macroscopic course of such a crack would, of course, depend upon the extent to which the two systems were alternatively followed. Such cracks are illustrated in fig. 6 and 7.

Careful examinations have now been made of cracks in specimens from all of the above branches of the work and no correlation has been found between direction of propagation of the crack and the characteristics of the individual grains of the material. In the case of non-propagating cracks in the V-notch specimens, the terminal point of a crack was randomly situated either within a grain or on a grain boundary.

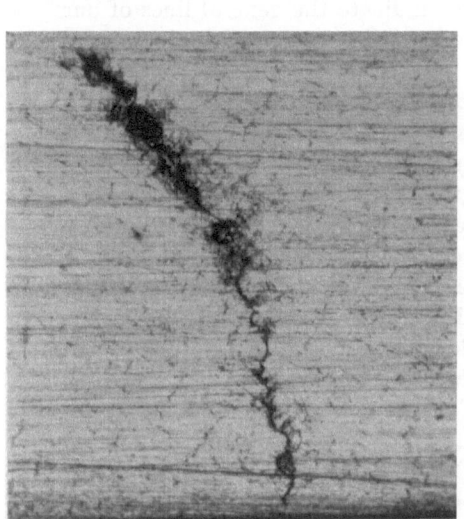
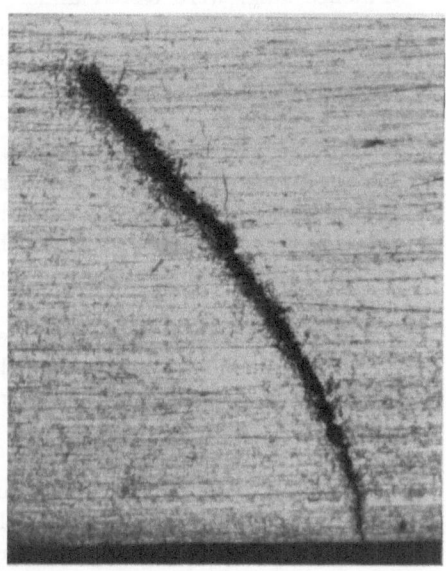

Fig. 6.                                    Fig. 7.

Fig. 6 and 7.   Cracks on faces of copper specimens of square section.
Applied stress system (combined bending and torsion) the same in both cases.
In both specimens, the general macroscopic direction of the crack tends to follow a curve which is at all points normal to the direction of the principal tensile stress.

The existence of non-propagating cracks in areas of high stress concentration naturally leads to the examination of the stress concentration arising from a crack per se. There is now ample evidence that a sharp notch can cause a crack to form at a certain stress level, but that continuous propagation of the crack at that stress need not occur; in other words, a notch may cause a crack to form but the crack itself does not necessarily cause a further crack to develop. This must lead to the reconsideration of the usual interpretation of a crack as being the extreme case of a sharp notch as far as the effect on fatigue resistance is concerned. In order to determine the strength reduction factor of a fatigue crack, experimentally, it was necessary to evolve a technique for cracking under fatigue stresses, unnotched specimens of the various materials being examined. It was eventually found possible to stop the test on any given 1 inch diameter specimen in a 4-point loading rotating beam fatigue machine at such a stage in the test that any fatigue crack or cracks formed had not penetrated the section to any appreciable distance. A supply of notched specimens was thus available for fatigue strength determinations, the notch in each case being a fine crack. The specimens, each of which had an effective portion 1 inch diameter and 3 inches long, were tested under conditions of rotating bending stress and direct stress. Some of the results so far are of sufficient interest for them to be mentioned here in order to indicate the general lines of our thoughts in this matter; a detailed paper will be prepared in due course for publication.

The technique for stopping a rotating beam machine in which a specimen was being tested at a stress above the fatigue limit, depended upon the change of deflection of the specimen as a crack or cracks were forming, or about to be formed. In the case of aluminium alloy and a nickel-chrome steel, the slightest increase of deflection after an endurance of a few thousand cycles had been exceeded, invariably indicated the presence of a crack. The rapidity with which removal of load and stopping of the machine was accomplished determined the size of the resulting fatigue crack. In the case of mild steel and copper at stresses just above the fatigue limit, progressive increase of deflection of a specimen occurred as the number of cycles of stress increased. Practice and experience were necessary to determine the precise stopping point of a test in order to ensure that unduly large cracks were not present, but for those softer materials the surprising degree of consistency in the number of cycles to initiate a crack of suitable length was of considerable assistance.

It is of interest to note that only one crack was formed in the aluminium alloy and the nickel-chrome steel specimens; the mild steel specimens were always found to contain several cracks of various lengths, whilst the copper specimens exhibited a very large number of cracks.

Specimens cracked in the manner described above were then retested, either under rotating bending stress or reversed direct stress, suitable modifications to the specimen ends being made, where necessary, in order to hold them in different types of testing machines. After fracture, the area of the initial crack was always plainly visible, so it was possible to re-assess the applied load and to determine the true range of stress applied to that section of a specimen at which failure did eventually occur.

The length on the surface of a specimen of each crack was duly noted; in the case of the direct stress tests, the crack or cracks on each specimen were visible throughout the testing period. Although careful observation was made, no progressive growth of any crack was observed. The initial fatigue cracks retained their original length until a very short time before final failure. In the case of the mild steel, where a number of cracks were present on the surface before the re-test took place, observations showed that after fracture only one crack extended

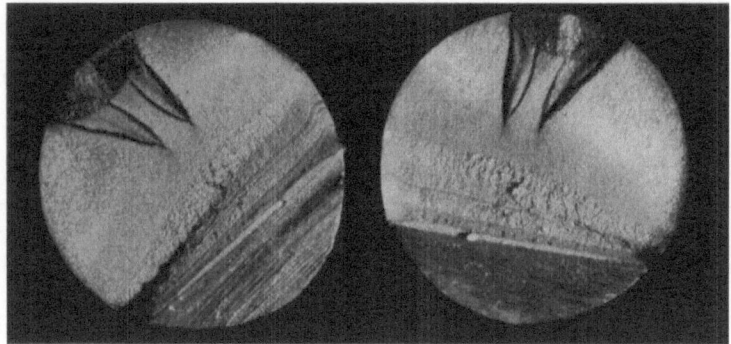

Fig. 8.  Nickel-chromium steel.

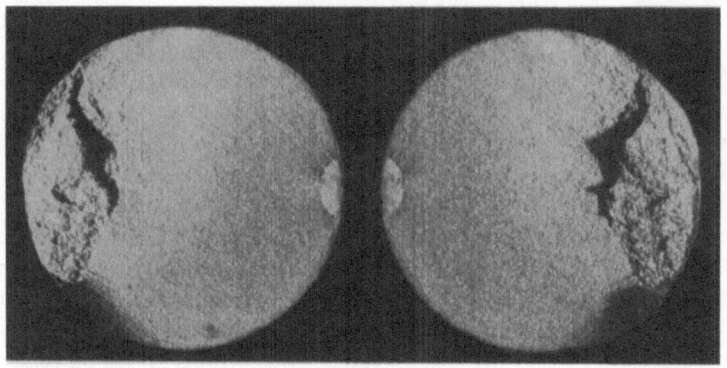

Fig. 9.  Mild steel.

in length and that was invariably the crack which eventually propagated completely across the section.

Another matter of interest in the case of the mild steel is that the final fracture did not always begin from the longest of the original fatigue cracks on the surface of a specimen. Again, metallurgical examination of the material around the ends of the non-propagated and propagated cracks revealed no significant differences which might account for the difference in behaviour. Photographs of some typical specimens after fracture are shown in fig. 8 and 9. It was invariably found that under rotating bending stress, fracture occurred by propagation of the initial crack from its two ends on the surface of the specimen. With the reversed direct stress specimens, the original crack spread all along its inner surface, and in many cases the original contours of the fracture surface were continued across the section. Visual appearance of all the fractures suggested the rapid growth from the original crack, and no evidence was found of any slow progressive damage.

Typical results of the fatigue tests on cracked specimens of mild steel are shown in fig. 10. The fatigue limit of cracked specimens appears to be well above that reported by FROST [3] for the case of notched specimens. The work so far completed on nickel-chrome steel and aluminium alloy appears to be giving similar results in so far as the fatigue limits are above those previously reported on the same material for notched specimens.

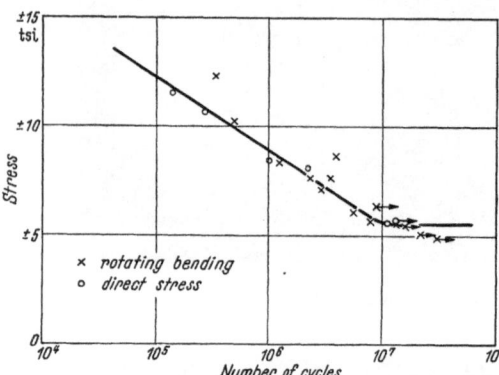

Fig. 10. *S-N* curve for cracked specimens of mild steel. Stress range is twice maximum calculated stress.

In estimating the stresses applied to a cracked specimen, due allowance was made for non-axiality of loading arising from the presence of the crack. In some cases the crack was so small that the allowance was negligible. The general conclusions to date suggest that the strength reduction effect of a crack is independent of the depth of crack over the range of crack areas investigated, and that the results from rotating bending and reversed direct stress tests are in agreement. It should also be mentioned that the initial cracking conditions, i.e., applied stress range and number of cycles, varied considerably from specimen to specimen, and it would appear from the smoothness of the curves obtained, that the strength reduction effect is also independent of the pre-cracking conditions.

Further work is in hand and some modifications to specific conclusions may be necessary as other information becomes available. It is hoped, eventually, to be able to correlate conditions of crack propagation under various stress systems.

It seems clear that the conditions necessary to cause a fatigue crack to form in a material, and then to develop, cannot be generalized for all materials; different materials may require different conditions. In most cases, however, it would appear that principal maximum tension stresses play a predominant part in crack initiation and propagation; moreover, it is an average stress acting over a small but finite quantity of material, which must be exceeded before failure begins.

It appears probable that under zero mean stress conditions, the strength reduction factor due to a fatigue crack is independent of its size, and of the size of the component containing it, and is less than that due do mechanically-formed sharp notches.

The work described has been carried out as part of the research programme of the Mechanical Engineering Research Board of the Department of Scientific and Industrial Research. The paper is published by permission of the Director of Mechanical Engineering Research.

### Bibliography

[1] PHILLIPS, C. E., and R. B. HEYWOOD: Proc. Instn mech. Engrs, 165, 113—124 (1951).
[2] FENNER, OWEN and C. E. PHILLIPS: Engineering, 171, 637 (1951).
[3] FROST, N. E.: Engineer, 200, 464—467, 501—503 (1955).
[4] COX, H. L., and J. E. FIELD: Aeronaut. Quart., 4, 1 (1952—54).

### Discussion

W. WEIBULL asked for the length of the cracks.

C. E. PHILLIPS: The fatigue cracks develop all round the test piece with separate intermittent cracks somewhat displaced in axial direction.

E. GASSNER: Could there be any influence from residual stresses due to manufacture.

C. E. PHILLIPS: Some of the test pieces were stress relieved after manufacture but gave same result as non-stressrelieved.

P. KUHN remarked that tests with two different steels according to the same specification had shown entirely different behaviour. In one cracks were stopped and in the other the cracks propagated to failure.

G. V. UZHIK said that the stop of cracks could be explained taking account of work hardening and diminished hysteresis.

R. E. PETERSON: In confirmation of PHILLIPS' findings with respect to non-propagating cracks, it may be of interest to mention HORGER's bending fatigue tests of railway axles. Failure started at the wheel fit. HORGER determined a "breaking-off limit" and a "crack limit", the latter being of the order of half of the former. Between the two limits the cracks do not progress to failure. As one might imagine, this raises an interesting question as to what action should be recommended, when small cracks are found during periodic inspection of railway axles.

C. E. PHILLIPS: I have already referred to HORGER's tests on large railway axles. HORGER was one of the first investigators to demonstrate the existence of large non-propagating fatigue cracks in areas of high stress concentration; it is of interest to note that the lowest values of stress quoted by HORGER as being necessary for the production of non-propagating fatigue cracks agrees with our own values.

I do not think UZHIK's explanation of work hardening and diminishing hysteresis for the cessation of propagation is a reasonable one, as a very small increase in applied stress could cause propagation of a crack completely across the section.

# Some investigations on cumulative damage

By

**F. J. Plantema**

With 5 figures

## 1. Introduction

Life estimates for aircraft structural components, which are subjected to repeated loads of varying amplitudes and frequencies, must be based on some cumulative damage hypothesis. Such a hypothesis enables the calculation of the endurance of the component under a more or less complicated load spectrum from the normal $S$-$N$ curve. Practical calculations have up till now been based on MINER's hypothesis [1]

$$\sum_i n_i/N_i = 1, \tag{1}$$

where $n_i$ and $N_i$ are the total number of applied load cycles at a mean stress $S_{mi}$ and a stress amplitude $S_{ai}$, and the endurance of the component at the same combination of stresses respectively.

If $\sum_i n_i/N_i = 1$ fatigue failure should occur according to this hypothesis.

As shown by SCHIJVE [2] MINER's hypothesis can be derived from two assumptions, viz. 1) that the state of fatigue damage is completely determined by one parameter and 2) that this parameter can be taken as $n_i/N_i$. It is not to be expected that the fatigue process is governed by such simple rules (see [2]) and it was therefore decided to verify the validity of (1) by means of some series of tests on simple specimens loaded according to elementary load spectra. Under these circumstances it may be possible to explain deviations from (1) or to establish rules or assumptions of more general validity with respect to these deviations.

The investigations reported in this paper were therefore not intended to yield results of immediate use in the design of aircraft structures for fatigue. However, within the limits set the experiments were adapted as far as possible to aircraft design problems. Thus, as material of the test specimens a standard clad 24 S-T aluminium alloy was chosen. One of the types of specimens was a typical simple riveted joint.

## 2. Test specimens, test equipment and types of test

Three types of test specimens were used, viz.

A. Unnotched 24 S-T alclad strips, the dimensions of which are given in fig. 1 a.

B. 24 S-T alclad strips, notched by two grooves with a semi-circular bottom. The dimensions are given in fig. 1 b.

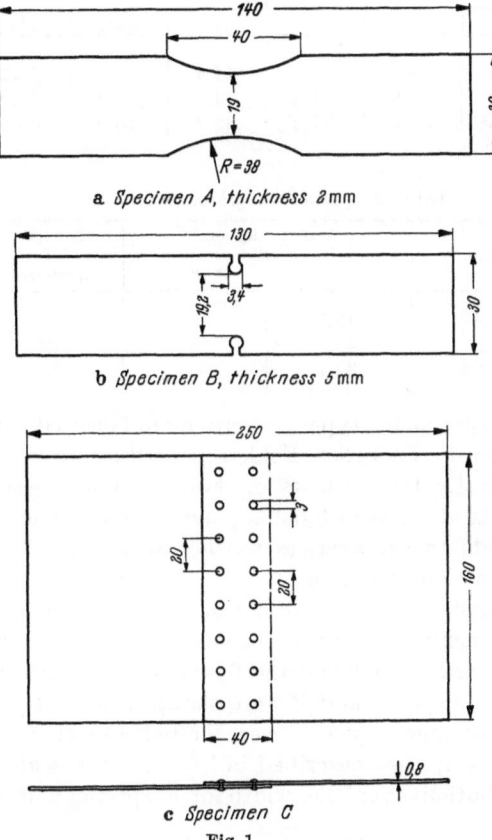

a *Specimen A, thickness 2* mm

b *Specimen B, thickness 5* mm

c *Specimen C*
Fig. 1.

C. Single-lap riveted joints of 24 S-T alclad sheets connected by two rows of eight 17 S-T snap rivets each. The dimensions are given in fig. 1 c.

All specimens of type A were manufactured from one sheet of 2 mm nominal thickness, some static properties of which are given in table 1. The type B specimens were all made from one sheet of 5 mm nominal thickness; table 1 also contains its static properties. The notched and unnotched specimens were milled to the accurate length and width. The unnotched specimens were then turned to the reduced section of fig. 1 a.

The notches shown in fig. 1b were made by drilling and reaming two holes and sawing out the slots to the holes. No special surface finishing was given. The results of some static tests on completed specimens are given in table 2.

Table 1. *Results of material tests*

| Material for specimens | $S_{0.2}$ kg/mm² | | | $S_u$ kg/mm² | | | Number of tests |
|---|---|---|---|---|---|---|---|
| | min. | max. | av. | min. | max. | av. | |
| A | 35.9 | 38.0 | 36.9 | 44.4 | 45.7 | 45.2 | 13 |
| B | 33.8 | 34.6 | 34.2 | 44.5 | 45.3 | 45.0 | 3 |
| C | 32.3[1] | 35.7[1] | 34.0[1] | 42.4 | 48.0 | 45.5 | 10 |

[1] $S_{0.1}$.

Table 2. *Static strength of specimens*

| Specimen | Mean $S_u$ kg/mm² | | Number of specimens |
|---|---|---|---|
| | virgin | fatigued | |
| A | 46.7 | — | 2 |
| B | 45.8 | 45.8 | 22   2 + 5 |
| C | 33.7 | — | 2 |

The riveted specimens type C were manufactured by the Royal Netherlands Aircraft Factories Fokker according to standard workshop practice. Static tensile tests on two specimens gave failure by shear of the rivets at loads of 3,630 kg and 3,640 kg. The mean of these values corresponds to an average tensile stress $S_u = 33.7$ kg/mm² in the critical net section of the sheet.

The fatigue tests were run on Amsler high-frequency Vibrophore resonance-type machines. For the specimens of types A, B and C the test frequencies were 4,200, 6,000 and 6,000 cycles per minute respectively. The specimens types A and B were clamped in the standard clamping heads; the specimens type C were bolted and clamped in special steel grips. These grips are described in [3], where it is also shown that the stress distribution over the width of a specimen is satisfactorily uniform.

Fatigue failure was defined as the degree of crack formation at which the fatigue machine switched off automatically. The switch-off mechanism was adjusted such that in all cases a sizable crack had grown and the adjustment was kept as constant as possible.

Normal fatigue tests were first carried out to determine the mean endurances at two stress levels, to be used for the cumulative damage tests. For the specimens A and B these tests were run in repeated tension (stress ratio $R = 0$) and for some specimens of type C the same type of test was chosen, except that the constant lower load limit was

100 kg instead of zero. The remainder of the riveted joints were tested at a mean stress, representing the 1 $g$ level, of 9 kg/mm², which corresponds to an ultimate load factor of 3.75.

The cumulative damage tests were of three simple types. In the first two types various cycle ratio's at the low and the high stress level respectively were first applied and then the test was continued to failure at the second stress level. These tests will be called L-H and H-L tests respectively in the following, and together they are called two-step tests. In the two-step tests the first stress, applied during $n_1$ cycles, is called pre-stress and the second stress is called test stress ($n_2$ cycles). The third type of tests will be called interval tests. In these tests cycle ratio's of 0.05 at both stress levels were applied alternately. As for the normal fatigue tests, the tests on specimens A and B and some specimens C were run at constant lower load limits of zero and 100 kg respectively, the remainder of the tests on the specimens C being carried out at a mean stress of 9 kg/mm².

## 3. Results of the normal fatigue tests

The two stress levels were chosen such that the mean endurances were of the order of 100,000 and 1 million respectively. From the test results the mean and the standard deviation of log $N$ were computed, as well as the antilogarithm $\overline{N}$ of the mean log $N$.

The latter was used in the determination of the cycle ratio's $n/N$ of the cumulative damage tests. A summary of the test results is given in table 3; the detailed results can be found in [2], [4], [5]. The standard deviations $\sigma$ given in table 3 have been computed from the mean of log $N$, i.e. log $\overline{N}$, and the standard deviation $\sigma_1$ of log $N$ as follows:

$$\left.\begin{array}{l}\log N_1 = \log \overline{N} + \sigma_1; \ \log N_2 = \log \overline{N} - \sigma_1, \\ \sigma = \frac{1}{2} \cdot (N_1 - N_2).\end{array}\right\} \tag{2}$$

In agreement with normal experience the standard deviation is relatively smaller at the higher stress levels.

Table 3. *Results of normal fatigue tests*

| Type of specimen | Stress level | $S_a$ kg/mm² | $S_m$ kg/mm² | $\overline{N}. 10^{-3}$ log. mean | $\sigma. 10^{-3}$ see eq. (2) | Number of specimens |
|---|---|---|---|---|---|---|
| A | H | 11.5 | 11.5 | 196 | 52 | 20 |
| A | L | 8.0 | 8.0 | 1290 | 496 | 18 |
| B | H | 5.25 | 5.25 | 185 | 30 | 20 |
| B | L | 3.25 | 3.25 | 1168 | 497 | 30 |
| C | H 1 | 5.16 | 5.96 | 185 | 41 | 9 |
| C | L 1 | 2.38 | 3.18 | 1920 | 490 | 9 |
| C | H 2 | 7.2 | 9.0 | 116 | 16 | 20 |
| C | L 2 | 3.2 | 9.0 | 1019 | 232 | 20 |

The unnotched specimens A have a theoretical stress concentration factor $k_t$ of about 1.15, ref. [6]. For the notched specimens B, [7] and [6] give values of $k_t$ of 2.55 and 2.85 respectively. The fatigue strength reduction factors $k_f$ for this specimen can be computed somewhat conservatively by multiplying the fatigue strength of specimens A by 1.15 and dividing by the fatigue strength of specimens B. Then at $N = 2 \cdot 10^5$ it is found that $k_f = 2.55$ and at $N = 1.3$ million $k_f = 2.89$. It is therefore probable that the value of $k_t$ from [6] is the more correct one.

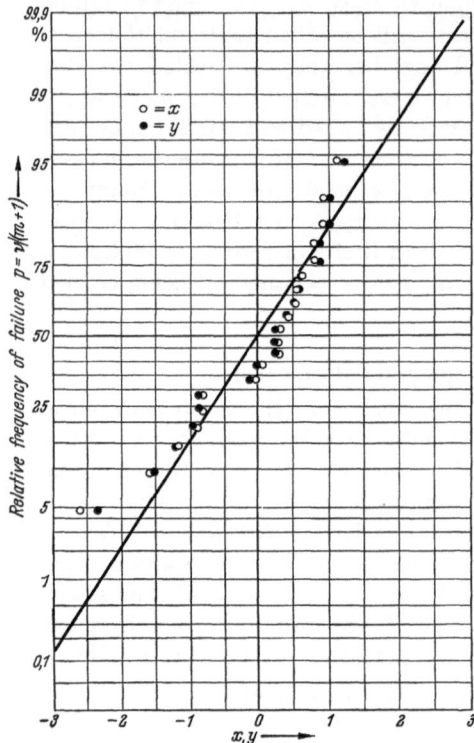

Fig. 2. Fatigue strength distribution for notched specimens B at $S_a = S_m = 5.25$ kg/mm².

It is interesting to investigate the distribution of the fatigue strength. To this end the test results for the notched as well as for the unnotched specimens were plotted on probability paper. Fig. 2 gives a plot for the notched specimens B at a stress amplitude and mean stress $S_a = S_m = 5.25$ kg/mm². The ordinate in this graph is the probability of failure.

$$P = \nu/(m + 1), \qquad (3)$$

where $\nu$ is the number of the specimen (when these are arranged in the order of increasing $N$) and $m$ is the total number of specimens (in this case $m = 20$).

The abscissa in this graph is the normalized value of log $N$ or of $N$, viz.

$$y = \frac{1}{\sigma_1}(\log N - \log \overline{N}), \text{ or } x = \frac{1}{\sigma_2}(N - N_m). \qquad (4)$$

In (4) $\sigma_1$ and $\sigma_2$ are the standard deviations and log $\overline{N}$ and $N_m$ are the mean values of log $N$ and $N$ respectively.

If the distribution were normal, the test results would plot on or randomly near the straight line drawn in the figure. It is seen that the distributions of $x$ and $y$, i.e. of $N$ and log $N$, are remarkably equal, but that they are definitely not normal. For the fatigue strength of the notched specimens at $S_a = S_m = 3.25$ kg/mm² the distribution proved to be not normal either and, moreover, it was quite different from that of fig. 2 (see [2]). It is clear that the standard deviations $\sigma_1$ and $\sigma_2$, which were computed in the normal way, do not have the same meaning as the standard deviation of a normal distribution. They do give, however, a good measure for the scatter of the test results.

For the unnotched specimens A, a normal distribution of $N$ as well as of log $N$ seemed to be an acceptable approximation. However, it was shown by SCHIJVE [2] that the fatigue test results were affected by inhomogeneity of the sheet from which the specimens were cut and, therefore, the agreement may be only accidental.

For the riveted joints C the distributions of $N$ and log $N$ were again nearly the same. The distributions of log $N$ for both stress levels are given in fig. 3. At the high stress amplitude the deviations from a normal distribution are more pronounced than at the low stress amplitude, but the distributions are similar in character.

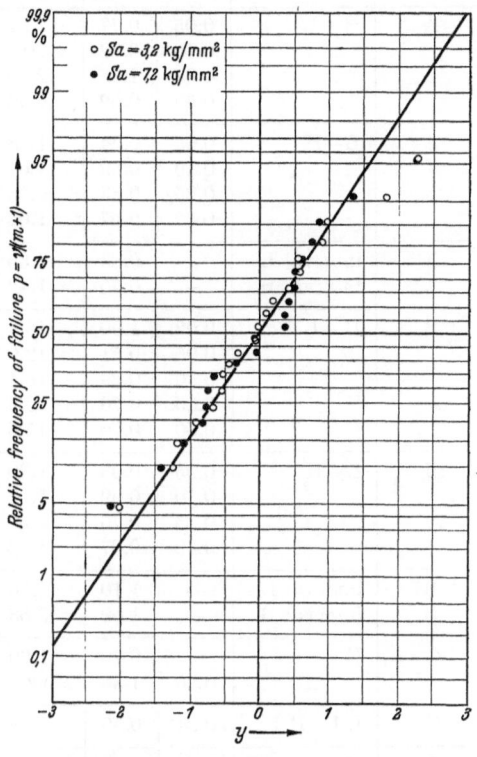

Fig. 3. Fatigue strength distribution for riveted joints C at $S_m = 9$ kg/mm² and $S_a = 7.2$ or $3.2$ kg/mm².

From the figures 2 and 3 it must be concluded that it is not possible to extrapolate the test results and thus determine a reliable value of the endurance for a low value of the probability of failure.

## 4. Results of the cumulative damage tests

The test results are summarized in table 4; the detailed results can be found in [2], [4], [5].

Considering the results given in table 4 it may be said that the scatter is reasonable and that the mean values of $\Sigma n/N$ in general show a consistent behaviour. The worst in these respects are the test series H-L for specimens B. The results are rather different for the various types of specimens and tests.

In general, a high pre-stress followed by a lower test stress (H-L test) gives $\Sigma n/N > 1$, so that the pre-stress has a strengthening effect. This

Table 4. *Results of cumulative damage tests*

| Type of specimen | Type of test[1] | $\dfrac{n_1}{N_1}$ | $\Sigma\, n/N$ | | | σ stand. dev. | Number of specimens |
|---|---|---|---|---|---|---|---|
| | | | min. | max. | mean. | | |
| A | H—L | 0.05 | 0.77 | 2.37 | 1.38 | 0.462 | 10 |
| | | 0.10 | 0.82 | > 20[2] | 1.37[2] | 0.355[2] | 9 |
| | | 0.25 | 1.05 | 2.70 | 1.65 | 0.622 | 9 |
| | | 0.50 | 0.59 | 6.33 | 2.36 | 1.592 | 11 |
| A | L—H | 0.05 | 0.54 | 1.28 | 0.84 | 0.214 | 10 |
| | | 0.10 | 0.59 | 1.07 | 0.75 | 0.158 | 10 |
| | | 0.25 | 0.63 | 0.95 | 0.75 | 0.090 | 10 |
| | | 0.50 | 0.57 | 1.02 | 0.85 | 0.141 | 9 |
| A | interval L | — | 0.83 | 1.35 | 1.05 | 0.165 | 10 |
| A | interval H | — | 0.76 | 1.42 | 1.01 | 0.199 | 10 |
| B | H—L | 0.02 | 1.00 | > 15.4 | > 6.50[3] | — | 7 |
| | | 0.05 | 0.51 | > 12.0 | 1.77[3] | — | 12 |
| | | 0.10 | 0.29 | > 18.1 | 5.10[3] | — | 10 |
| | | 0.25 | 0.70 | > 20.2 | 5.35[3] | — | 10 |
| | | 0.50 | 0.70 | > 15.5 | 1.67[3] | — | 10 |
| B | L—H | 0.05 | 0.93 | 1.30 | 1.10 | 0.099 | 10 |
| | | 0.10 | 0.99 | 1.52 | 1.27 | 0.183 | 10 |
| | | 0.25 | 0.76 | 1.59 | 1.21 | 0.216 | 10 |
| | | 0.50 | 0.67 | 1.62 | 1.15 | 0.254 | 10 |
| B | interval L | — | 1.10 | 2.80 | 1.81 | 0.426 | 10 |
| B | interval H | — | 1.00 | 2.53 | 1.77 | 0.466 | 10 |
| C | H 1—L 1 | $n_1 = 1$ | 0.70 | 1.60 | 1.15 | — | 2 |
| | | 0.26 | 1.30 | > 32[2] | 5.87[2] | 4.69[2] | 9 |
| C | L 1—H 1 | 0.24 | 0.59 | 1.18 | 0.86 | 0.239 | 9 |
| C | H 2—L 2 | $n_1 = 1$ | 0.56 | 1.88 | 1.12 | 0.346 | 10 |
| | | 0.01 | 0.67 | 1.40 | 0.98 | 0.221 | 10 |
| | | 0.05 | 0.79 | 1.97 | 1.15 | 0.315 | 10 |
| | | 0.25 | 0.74 | 1.28 | 1.00 | 0.151 | 10 |
| C | L 2—H 2 | 0.25 | 0.96 | 1.53 | 1.24 | 0.176 | 10 |
| | | 0.50 | 0.59 | 1.43 | 0.91 | 0.274 | 10 |
| C | interval H 2 | — | 0.81 | 1.86 | 1.31 | 0.292 | 10 |

[1] The notations L—H, H—L and "interval" are explained at the end of section 2. Interval L and interval H mean that the first interval of 5% was applied at the low and at the high stress level respectively. The stress levels are given in table 3.

[2] One test was stopped at high $n_2/N_2$ without the specimen having failed. The mean value and the standard deviation of $\Sigma\, n/N$ were computed by omitting this result and the lowest value of $\Sigma\, n/N$.

[3] One or more (up to 4) tests were stopped at values of $\Sigma\, n/N$ equal to or less than the value given in the column "max.". Instead of the mean the median of $\Sigma\, n/N$ is given for these tests.

effect is much more pronounced for the notched specimens B and the riveted joints C at constant minimum load than for the unnotched specimens A. In the latter case it is probably caused by general strain hardening, whereas for notched specimens a stress redistribution may have an additional beneficial effect. It is also to be expected that the strengthening at the low stress level will be more pronounced as this stress level is nearer the original endurance limit and this may have been the case for specimens B and C, as compared with specimens A. The application of one pre-stress cycle to specimen C gave no strengthening, so that evidently the effect of the plastic deformations and consequent stress redistribution is not yet large for this pre-stress. In such a case, it seems that reversals of the pre-stress are essential in order to cause strengthening. For the specimens A the strengthening is increasing up to $n_1/N_1 = 0.5$, whereas for the specimens B it has decreased considerably at this high pre-stress cycle ratio. Is is probable, and it has in fact been observed for one specimen, that small cracks had already originated at the end of the pre-stress period in some of the specimens B and these will undoubtedly considerably reduce the remaining life at the lower test stress (also see section 5).

There is a remarkable difference between the results of the H2-L2 tests at a constant mean stress on specimens C and the other H-L tests (at $R = 0$ or constant minimum load). The former tests confirm MINER's hypothesis quite well and this also applies to all other tests on specimens C at a constant mean stress. It is not easy to explain this difference and it is highly desirable to investigate the effect of the mean stress further.

For the L-H tests, where a low pre-stress is followed by a high test stress, the results for different specimens are again rather different. For specimens A the mean $\Sigma n/N$ is slightly below unity, as well as for specimens C in the L1-H1 tests. This result is difficult to explain. For specimens B $\Sigma n/N$ is roughly equal to $1 + n_1/N_1$, which would mean that the low pre-stress has been ineffective from the point of view of fatigue damage, except for $n_1/N_1 = 0.50$. In the latter case the pre-stress has lasted long enough to cause fatigue damage. It may be that the pre-stress for specimens B was nearer the fatigue limit than for specimens A. The L2-H2 tests for specimens C show a very good agreement with MINER's hypothesis and so do the interval tests at a constant mean stress.

The interval tests for specimens A also agree remarkably well with the hypothesis. This is not the case for specimens B. If, as suggested above, the low stress would be ineffective in this case, the result would be $\Sigma n/N = 2$. In fact, this sum is somewhat lower, viz. 1.8, approximately. This can be explained by observing that the low stress will definitely contribute to the fatigue damage after a crack has initiated. Of both the specimens A and B, about half failed at the higher and half at the lower stress level.

In [2] the results of the tests on specimens A and B are extensively discussed and compared with similar published information. It is suggested that in general, a high pre-stress may give considerable strengthening if the pre-stress does not last too long and if the fatigue process at the lower test stress is much less crude than at the pre-stress. In the case of a low pre-stress, under these same conditions $\Sigma n/N$ will approach $1 + n_1/N_1$, whereas otherwise it may be about unity. For tests with random load spectra it may be expected that in general Miner's hypothesis will be somewhat conservative.

## 5. Crack propagation

The interval tests on specimens A and B have given interesting results concerning the rate of crack propagation. If the crack lasts during several intervals and the specimen is fractured completely in fatigue or broken statically after the fatigue test, the fracture surface

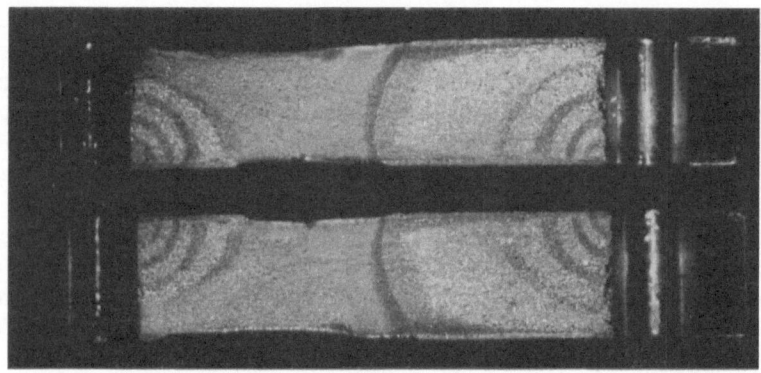

Fig. 4.

shows the well-known oyster shell markings. A clear example is given in fig. 4, which is typical for the specimens B, except that in most cases the crack formed only at one side.

For the unnotched specimens A no or at most one oyster shell markings were visible, which means that the remaining life after the initiation of the crack is less than or at most about 5% of the endurance for the stress level at which the specimen failed.

For the 20 notched specimens B the number of oyster shell markings ranged from 7 to 12. This scatter is much less than the scatter in $\Sigma n/N$. Considering that the average of $\Sigma n/N$ is about 1.8 (table 4), it follows that the average life remaining after the initiation of a crack is about 25% of the total life. Of course, this result is valid only for this type of specimen and this material.

The specimens were broken after the fatigue test, and the remaining static strength was determined. The relation between the crack size and the remaining static strength is given in fig. 5. It is seen that the static strength decreases rapidly as the crack grows.

In drawing the upper part of the curves, it was assumed that as long as no crack is visible the static strength is still equal to the original static strength. This assumption is based on some test results included in table 2 and on the general experience gained in other fatigue work.

The relation between the crack area and the remaining life was also determined and with the aid of these data the percentages of life consumed were indicated in fig. 5. It may be concluded that up to 95% of the total life the remaining static strength exceeds 80% of the origin-

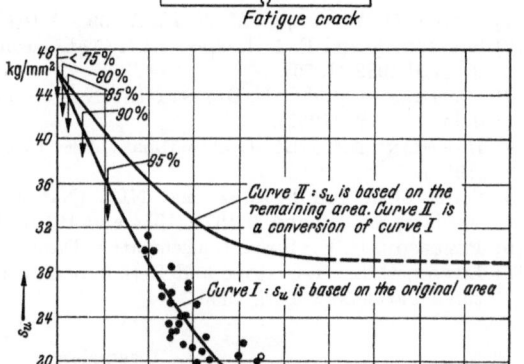

Fig. 5. Ultimate static strength and remaining life for notched specimens B after interval tests.

al static strength and that the crack is growing slowly. This is encouraging with regard to the possibility of detecting fatigue cracks in similar aircraft structural components before catastrophic failures are to be feared. Further research on other types of specimens and other materials is, however, highly desirable.

## 6. Conclusions

Fatigue tests on 24 S-T alloy specimens with only two stress levels, applied either successively or alternately, partly with constant lower load limit (in most cases zero) and partly at a constant mean stress, show that the deviations from MINER's cumulative damage hypothesis depend upon the type of specimen, the load sequence and the mean stress.

This research has been made possible through support and sponsorship by the Netherlands Aircraft Development Board and the Air Research and Development Command, United States Air Force, through its European Office under contract No AF 61 (514)—812.

## Bibliography

[1] MINER, M. A.: J. appl. Mech. 12, A 159—A 164 (1946).
[2] SCHIJVE, J. and F. A. JACOBS: NLL (Nat. aeronaut. Res. Inst.) Rep. (Amsterdam) M 1982 (1955).
[3] HARTMAN, A. and G. C. DUIJN: NLL (Nat. aeronaut. Res. Inst.) Rep. (Amsterdam) M 1857 (1952).
[4] HARTMAN, A.: NLL (Nat. aeronaut. Res. Inst.) Rep. (Amsterdam) M 1923 (1953).
[5] SCHIJVE, J. and F. A. JACOBS: NLL (Nat. aeronaut. Res. Inst.) Rep. (Amsterdam) M 1970 and M 1974 (1954 and 1955) (Restricted).
[6] PETERSON, R. E.: Stress Concentration Design Factors, New York 1953.
[7] LIPSON, C. L., G. C. NOLL and L. S. CLOCK: Stress and Strength of Manufactured Parts, New York 1950.

## Discussion

F. R. SHANLEY: We have found (at the RAND Corporation) that when test data are reduced to an *equivalent stress* basis the discrepancies between theory and test are greatly reduced. The Author's data would undoubtedly show even closer agreement with predicted values if this method of comparison were used.

From the philosophical point of view, the prediction of an "allowable" equivalent fatigue stress may be regarded as being about midway between the prediction of fatigue life (with the cumulative damage equation) and an ideal analysis based on reducing the probability of failure to a certain acceptable minimum (LUNDBERG method), in which both stress and life are treated on a probability basis.

A. S. PETRUSSEWITSCH asked about the significance of the bands in the fractured surface.

F. J. PLANTEMA: Each band of the fractured surface indeed corresponds to one interval of load cycles and the dark bands correspond to the intervals with the high stress amplitude.

It was remarkable that the scatter in the crack stage was much smaller than the scatter in the pre-crack stage.

J. SCHIJVE: The rate of the crack propagation was derived from the area of the bands. These area's were determined by means of an optical enlargement.

F. TURNER: Why have the bands different colour?

J. SCHIJVE: As far as I know the different colours on the failure surface are due to a kind of deformation and oxydation process.

E. GASSNER attributed different appearance of fracture to occurrence of shear and cleavage fracture respectively.

# A guide to statistical methods for use in fatigue testing

By

## J. T. Ransom[1]

In this talk I will describe a manual which is being prepared by a Task Force in the ASTM Committee E-9 on Fatigue. The purpose of this manual is to provide an outline of step-by-step procedures for using statistical methods in fatigue testing. The manual is intended for testing engineers without statistical training. We hope that the availability of such simplified outlines will permit everyone to make more use of these methods. This in turn will lead to the collection of information which in the future will permit more precise recommendations to be made. We welcome this opportunity to receive your suggestions on how this manual may be made most useful.

The manual will consist of three principal sections. In the first we clarify those basic statistical concepts which will be useful in fatigue testing. In the second section we present statistical procedures which have been used to study fatigue strength, that is, the maximum stress which can be tolerated for a given life. In the third section we outline procedures for analyzing fatigue life data, that is, data obtained at a given stress or groups of data obtained at several stresses. Let me now describe each of these sections in more detail.

In the introductory section we develop the concept of the population and the sample, using a fatigue problem as an example. We emphasize that the end product of the analysis of data from tests of a sample will be estimates of the characteristics of the population. This leads naturally to definitions of the confidence limits which can be placed upon the estimates. We indicate the reasons for the different treatments required for fatigue strength and fatigue life types of problems by illustrating the frequency distributions on the stress and life scales of the *S-N* curve. Finally in this section we stress the importance of good sampling techniques and randomization procedures.

The first method outlined for determining the fatigue strength is the *Probit method* because it illustrates clearly the principles involved in this type of problem. The total number of specimens in the sample is divided into several groups. All of the specimens in one group are

---

[1] Absent. Paper read by A. M. Freudenthal.

tested at the same stress but the stress for each group is different. This method gives points for the survivorship curve directly and statistical procedures are used to make the best fit of the curve to the data. We recommend that a minimum of ten specimens be tested at each of five different stress levels in order to estimate the mean fatigue limit within plus or minus a few per cent of the true value. We outline only the graphical analysis for the mean fatigue strength, the standard deviation and the standard deviation of the estimate of the mean. In choosing the five stress levels we recommend that they be included within an interval of plus or minus 1.5 standard deviations about the mean. In order to do this a few preliminary tests are recommended, and expected values of the standard deviation are given as ranging from 1,500 psi for normalized or hot-rolled steels to 5,000 psi for steels quenched and drawn to high hardness levels. The Probit procedure has the advantage of providing data for a rather complete analysis of the fatigue strength distribution. It has the disadvantage of requiring approximately 30% more specimens than some of the other methods. An illustrative example is given for each of the steps in the procedure.

The *Staircase* or *Up-and-Down method* is the second statistical procedure described for estimating the fatigue strength. In this method specimens are tested sequentially; that is, the stress at which the second specimen is tested is greater or less by a fixed increment than the stress for the first specimen, depending upon whether the first specimen ran out or failed, respectively, before reaching the prescribed number of cycles. The stress for the third specimen depends upon the results of the second specimen, and so forth. The incremental steps are recommended to be one standard deviation high. Equations are given to analyze the data for the mean, standard deviation, and various confidence limits. A minimum of 25 specimens is proposed. This procedure has the advantage of requiring many fewer specimens than, for example, the Probit method. However, the sequential nature is a disadvantage because of the long time required to complete a program.

Following the description of the Staircase procedure there are presented two modifications of the Staircase method which are designed to alleviate certain of the shortcomings of the basic method. One of these modifications provides for a more correct analysis for sample sizes as small as 10. It uses a variable step-size in order to get the test stress into the range of the true mean without wasting too many specimens. The other modification provides for using several simultaneous small Staircase groups in order to avoid the long time required to test the same number of specimens as a single group.

In the final section on methods for determining fatigue strength, increasing load methods are analyzed. In presenting these methods

·extreme caution is urged in applying them to materials which exhibit understressing or overstressing tendencies. However, inasmuch as the methods are used extensively for problems in which the specimens are very expensive or limited in number, their inclusion in this manual seems only logical. In the *Stepped increasing load method*, the fatigue strength of an individual specimen is obtained by starting the specimen at an initial stress level equal to about 70% of the estimated mean fatigue strength. The test is run for a fixed number of cycles, say 10 million for steel and 50 or 100 million for non-ferrous alloys. If failure does not occur, the stress is raised by an amount usually equal to less than one standard deviation of strength, and another 10 million cycles (or whatever number of cycles was used for the first test) are run. This is continued until failure occurs. The fatigue strength for this specimen is taken at the stress level half-way between the final breaking stress and the highest stress at which the specimen survived. The data are then analyzed graphically in a manner similar to the analysis for the Probit method. A minimum of ten specimens is recommended.

In the *Prot method* of increasing load, the stress is continuously increased from below the fatigue strength of the specimen until the ˙ specimen fractures. One obtains a distribution of failure stresses for several different rates of increasing the load. The data are analyzed graphically on the basis of extrapolating the failure stress back to zero rate of increasing load. We recommend a minimum of ten specimens be tested at each of three rates of increasing the load.

In the third main section of the manual we have described several procedures available for analyzing fatigue life types of problems. These are not yet completely written down and hence the following discussion is of our plans and not of our accomplishments. We plan first to reiterate a general discussion about the type of information to be gained from use of these techniques. In particular we point out that we will obtain estimates of mean life-to-failure and some measure of the distribution about the mean. We can then estimate extremes of life and can compare the means or extremes of different groups of specimens. We explain why procedures based upon the "normal" frequency distribution are used and the uncertainty in using these methods for estimating extreme life properties.

The analysis for the use of normal statistics is given in two sections, one is analytical and the other is graphical. The analytical procedures which are given can be found in any standard book on statistics. However, we have tried to reduce these to an outline of specific steps. Recommendations must still be worked out for the numbers of specimens which will be required in order to be able to predict a given life with a given confidence, or in order to be able to compare the mean lives of two groups of specimens, or to be able to compare the variability ot lives of two groups of specimens. Examples are given for each of these analytical steps. The graphical procedure for analysis is based upon a mortality ratio to obtain a plotting position for each specimen in a group. The data are then plotted on log-normal probability paper and a curve fitted by eye. Further mathematical analysis of the data then can be carried out as given in the Probit method.

Non-parametric methods are described for obtaining median fatigue life and confidence limits based on the range between longest and shortest life in the group. These methods have the advantage of being very simple, quick, and free of assumptions regarding the frequency distribution of life to failure. We plan to develop these methods into procedures which can be used for quality control work.

It is expected that this manual will become a special technical paper of the ASTM. By virtue of sponsorship by the ASTM, it will probably be widely used. Therefore, we are most anxious to make this manual absolutely correct, as complete as possible, and most useful to all practical engineers. You can help us in several ways. First, you can make recommendations about the details of the techniques that have been described; for example, how many specimens should be recommended for the different problems considered? Second, you can help us by indicating techniques which we have overlooked. Third, you can help us with suggestions which will improve the simplicity and clarity of the manual. We of the ASTM want to thank the Colloquium for the opportunity to enlist world-wide cooperation in this effort.

### Discussion

R. J. TAYLOR and G. P. KENNEDY asked whether the extreme value distribution (WEIBULL) would fit test data better than the log-normal distribution.

A. M. FREUDENTHAL: No difference is obtained at test series of usual numbers. The margins are more important to the designer than the averages.

W. WEIBULL: There seems to be some danger in presuming a priori that the distribution of fatigue life is log-normal, as may be concluded from fig. 4 of my paper. For a number of tests of, say, 10 almost any distribution function will do. For a number of 100, it is obvious that the distribution is not log-normal, but the decision between the remaining three functions requires several thousands of tests, in spite of the fact that the functions behave quite differently at low probabilities.

B. LUNDBERG: We are all concerned with the determination of the complete $P$-$S$-$N$ family of curves. With reference to fig., it is fairly easy to determine points on $P$-$S$-$N$ curves for the higher load levels, for instance of the magnitudes $S_1$ and $S_2$ in the figure. At lower load levels, $S_3$, difficulties arise because many or most of the test specimens do not fail due to the extremely large scatter in $N$ in the region of the endurance limit. It has occurred to me that the following test procedure might be worth while to employ in order to overcome this difficulty. $P$-$N$ testing is first conducted at one or a number of load levels ($S_1$ and $S_2$) above the endurance limit and thereby the corresponding part of the $P$-$S$-$N$ field can be at least approximately determined, for instance for $P = 50$, 10 and 1.0% probability of failure. With this it is possible to make an approximate extrapolation downwards of a $S$-$N$ curve for a low $P$ value, for instance $P = 1.0\%$. When this has been done, samples of specimens are tested at one or a few low load levels of constant amplitude, $S_3$, and the tests are run to a $N$ value, $N_3$, in the neighbourhood of the crossing with the extrapolated $S$-$N$ curve for $P = 1.0\%$. The continued testing is then conducted with a stepwise or con- tinuous increase in load level right across the scatterband as indicated by the oblique line. As a result one would be able to determine the scatter distri- bution along this line. The advantage with this method would be that all the specimens could be run to failure. The method has the advantage, as compared

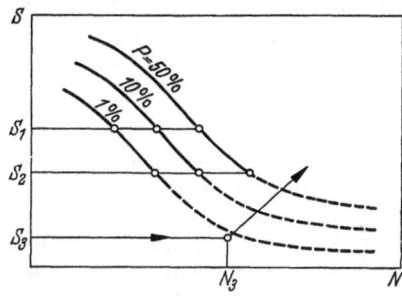

with the PROT method, that it is to the largest part a $S$-$N$ testing, the testing with increasing load being limited to the region of the endurance limit. Non- validity of the cumulative damage theory would cause small errors, as the "oblique" running is limited to a small range in load.

F. A. McCLINTOCK: In my opinion, much of the scatter in fatigue life reported in the literature is due to variations in specimen preparation and testing technique rather than inherent variations in the material itself. I therefore believe that a description of analysis of variance and latin square techniques, by which such extraneous variations can be sorted out, should be included in any manual on statistical techniques for fatigue testing.

Although the small sample statistical theory is not as well developed for extreme-value as for log-normal distributions, the problem of estimating tolerance limits (such that one can state with a certain confidence that less than some arbitrary fraction of the population will lie below the limits) has been solved for the extreme value distribution of the first kind in a NACA technical note by JULIUS LIEBLEIN. Furthermore, he has stated in a private communication that no mathematical difficulties are present in the corresponding theory for the ex- treme-value distribution of the third kind (with finite lower limit). Since tolerance limits are of practical interest, the use of these theories is strongly recommended to give an idea of the effect of the shape of the distribution function on the quan- tities being estimated.

K. SCHIJVE: You will allow me to give some general thoughts on the PROT accelerated-fatigue method.

Fig. 1 explains the principle of testing in this method, which will be well known $A$, $B$ and $C$ are different failure points of PROT-tests, which are replotted in fig. 2

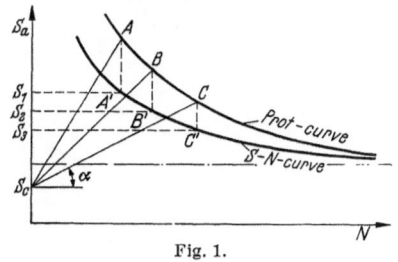

Fig. 1.

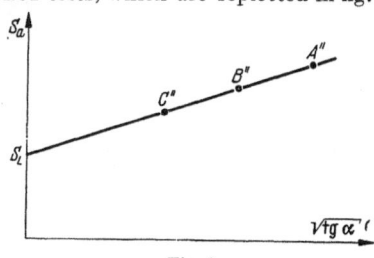

Fig. 2.

points $A''$, $B''$ and $C''$. In this figure $(\mathrm{tg}\alpha)^{1/2}$ is plotted on the horizontal axis [also $(\mathrm{tg}\,\alpha)^n$, $n \neq 1/2$ has been used]. It is claimed that $A''$, $B''$ and $C''$ could fit a straight line. By a linear extrapolation the endurance limit $S_L$ is obtained.

In fig. 1 also the normal $S$-$N$ curve has been given. Both curves of fig. 1 should have the same asymptotical $S_a$-value for $N \to \infty$.

If the straight line of fig. 2 is converted to the ordinate system of fig. 1 the relation of the PROT-curve becomes ($m$ = slope of line in fig. 2)

$$N = m^2 \frac{S_a - S_c}{(S_a - S_L)^2} \tag{1}$$

The extrapolation method of fig. 2 actually means an extrapolation in fig. 1 according to relation (1).

It may now be stated:

1) The PROT-method is essentially an extrapolation method using relation (1).

2) If an extrapolation method is thought to be acceptable for the determination of the endurance limit other extrapolation methods may be used equally well.

It then is advisable to use normal fatigue test results for instance tests at three stress levels $S_1$, $S_2$ and $S_3$ which require as much time as the three PROT-tests, see fig. 1. An extrapolation formula must be chosen, for instance such one as proposed by WEIBULL.

Comparing such a method with the PROT method, disadvantages of the latter are:

1) Fatigue test results $A$, $B$ and $C$ are difficult to interpret. This is not the case with $A'$, $B'$ and $C'$. In aircraft problems mostly a complete $S$-$N$ curve is required.

2) It remains questionable whether the PROT method gives the endurance limit.

3) A complication of the fatigue machine is necessary, which is easy to overcome in rotating beam tests, but not so easy in other types of fatigue machines.

These disadvantages are not inherent to an extrapolation method, using normal fatigue test results.

A. M. FREUDENTHAL: Yes, but it should be remembered that engineers prefer straight lines.

With reference to aeronautical engineering data collected at the NACA and in the United Kingdom it has been stated that for load distribution curves neither $N$ nor log $N$ was normally distributed.

# Die durch große Zug- und Druckermüdungsbelastungen hervorgebrachte mechanische Hysterese in Stählen

Von

## J. Salokangas

Mit 7 Abbildungen

## 1. Allgemeines über die Messung der Dämpfung

Es sind zahlreiche Messungen des Dämpfungsvermögens bei Stählen ausgeführt worden. Im allgemeinen wurden diese Messungen an Hand der Dämpfung der freien Torsionsschwingung vorgenommen. Desgleichen sind mehrere Apparate konstruiert worden, in denen die Dämpfung der Biege- oder Zug-Druckschwingungen gemessen worden ist. Größtenteils beziehen sich die Messungen auf geringe mechanische Spannungen. Die Firma Schenck hat eine Maschine konstruiert, mittels welcher aus erzwungenen Torsionsschwingungen die mechanische Hystereseschleife des Materials erhalten wird. In diesem Apparat erfolgt die Messung der Phasenverschiebung zwischen Spannung und Formveränderung dadurch, daß ein Lichtstrahl von einem im Takt der Spannungsänderungen schwingenden Spiegel und alsdann von einem zweiten Spiegel abgelenkt wird, der die Formveränderungen verfolgt, wonach der Lichtstrahl einen Schirm trifft. Hierdurch zeichnet er die mechanische Hystereseschleife des Probestabes auf. Dieser Apparat eignet sich nur zur Ausführung der Messung bei großen mechanischen Spannungen. Eine Biegeermüdungsmaschine ist von Lazan und Wu [1] konstruiert worden; bei derselben wird die Phasenverschiebung zwischen Spannung und Formveränderung in einem rotierenden Probestab aus der Horizontalabweichung seiner Durchbiegung bestimmt. Mit diesem Apparat läßt sich auch die durch Spannungen von nur verhältnismäßig großem Betrag hervorgebrachte Dämpfung messen.

## 2. Die bei der Messung benutzten Vorrichtungen

**a) Der Resonanzpulsator.** Das Prinzip der Ermüdungsmaschine baut auf der Resonanzerscheinung auf. Der Apparat in seiner Gesamtheit stellt ein schwingendes System mit einem Exzenter mit Motorantrieb als Resonator dar. Der Probestab wird im Apparat einer Zug-Druck-ermüdungsbelastung unterworfen. Die Kraftamplitude, die sich im Ap-

parat ergibt, ist von der Exzentrizität des Exzenters und von dessen
Winkelgeschwindigkeit abhängig. Eine gewisse Winkelgeschwindigkeit $\omega$
zeitigt ein Maximum der Kraftamplitude, und dies stellt somit den Re-
sonanzfall dar. Der Apparat wird jedoch nicht im Resonanzpunkt, sondern erheblich unterhalb desselben betrieben. Hierbei bewirken kleine
Änderungen der Winkelgeschwindigkeit bedeutend geringere Änderungen der Kraftamplitude als im Resonanzpunkt. Die Kraft wird mit
einem Dynamometer gemessen, das nach der Angabe am Probestab be-
festigter elektrischer Dehnungsmeßstreifen geeicht ist. Die Eichung ist
mit einer Genauigkeit besser als 1% ausgeführt worden. Die Kraft kann
in der Maschine auf höchstens $\pm$ 900 kg gesteigert werden. Die Schwingungszahl des Apparats, d. h. die Umdrehungszahl des Resonators ist
geeigneterweise innerhalb der Grenzen 50 bis 60 Hz zu regeln.

Der Konstruktion des Pulsators zufolge beschreibt der Balken, den
der rotierende Exzenter in Schwingungen versetzt, einen Kreisbogen,
womit also der Probestab eine leicht exzentrische Drückung erfährt.
Dies gibt Anlaß, in der Druckphase eine Knickung zu befürchten. Durch
Messungen und Berechnungen konnte festgestellt werden, daß in keinem
der Versuche eine Knickung des Probestabes hat eintreten können.

**b) Die Bestimmung der Hystereseschleife.** Wenn man eine Kraft auf
den Probestab einwirken läßt, entsteht in diesem sofort eine Spannung,
welcher die Formveränderung nach einer gewissen Zeit nachfolgt. Zwischen Spannung und Formveränderung besteht somit eine Phasenverschiebung. Die Messung der Phasenverschiebung im Pulsator erfolgt dadurch, daß das obere und untere Ende des Probestabes je eine Leitungs-
spule trägt, die sich im magnetischen Feld bewegen. Die eine der Spulen
bewegt sich im Takt der Formveränderung $x$ des Stabes, während die
zweite Spule die Bewegungen des Dynamometers, d. h. die Änderungen
der Kraft $F$ erfaßt. In den Spulen wird eine elektromotorische Kraft
induziert, die im Takt mit der Formveränderung $x$ bzw. mit der Kraft $F$
variiert. Wird die eine Spule mit den waagerechten und die andere mit
den senkrechten Ablenkungsplatten eines Kathodenstrahloszillographen
verbunden, so erscheint auf dem Bildschirm das Kraft-Dehnungsdiagramm. Falls im Probestab überhaupt keine plastischen Verformungen
eintreten, ist das Kraft-Dehnungsdiagramm eine gerade Linie. In einem
Probestab unter dynamischer Belastung finden aber stets plastische
Verformungen statt, und das Kraft-Dehnungsdiagramm ist dann keine
Gerade, sondern es hat die Gestalt der sog. Hystereseschleife, die im
Bereich der reversiblen Formveränderung eine Ellipse ist. Im plastischen
Bereich hat sie die in Abb. 1 gezeigte Gestalt. Der Flächeninhalt der
Hystereseschleife stellt die verlorene Energie dar, die hauptsächlich in
Wärme übergeht. Um einen dementsprechenden Betrag wird die Schwin-

gungsbewegung des Probestabes gedämpft, insofern nicht von außen neue Energie zugeführt wird. Die Dämpfung ist auf die durch die innere Reibung des Materials bewirkte Phasenverschiebung zurückzuführen.

Bei den Versuchen mit dem Pulsator ist die Hystereseschleife auf dem Bildschirm des Kathodenstrahloszillographen sichtbar und ihre Veränderung kann somit während des Ermüdungsversuchs fortlaufend bis zum Bruch des Probestabes verfolgt werden. Das oben beschriebene Verfahren zur Umwandlung der Kraft- und Formveränderungsvariationen in entsprechende elektrische Ströme ermöglicht das Erfassen von Belastungen erheblicher, die statische Streckgrenze überschreitender Größe. Wäre man statt dessen genötigt, die Schwingungen mittels elektrischer Dehnungsmeßstreifen aufzunehmen, so würde im allgemeinen schon vor dem Bruch

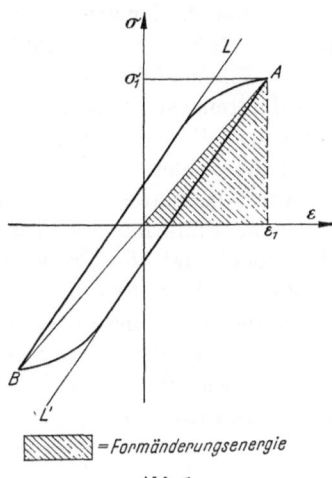

Abb. 1.

des Probestabes ein Zerreißen dieser Geber durch Ermüdung stattfinden, insbesondere bei so großen Belastungen wie die der ausgeführten Versuche.

c) **Über die Konstruktion des Resonanzpulsators sowie die von der Schwingungszahl abhängige Phasenverschiebung.** Die Messung der Phasenverschiebung der Dämpfung wurde mit einem Stoff von bekanntem Dämpfungsvermögen bei verschiedenen Schwingungszahlen des Pulsators vorgenommen. Bei diesen Messungen wurde ein Duraluminstab benutzt, mit der Dämpfung $\psi = 0,0005$ bei der in Frage stehenden Spannung, sowie ein harter Stahlstab, dessen Dämpfungskonstante der gleichen Größenordnung war. Bei den ausgeführten Messungen ergab sich als Hystereseschleife eine gerade Linie, womit also die Phasenverschiebung $\varphi$ sehr nahe gleich Null war.

## 3. Die Hystereseschleife

a) **Die Form der Hystereseschleife.** Wenn der Probestab unter einer periodisch veränderlichen Zug-Drucklast steht, hat die Spannungs-Formveränderungskurve die Gestalt der Abb. 1. Die Geraden $L$ und $L'$ sind parallel, und ihr Winkelkoeffizient kann approximativ dem statischen Elastizitätsmodul $E$ gleichgesetzt werden, insofern die Schwingungszahl nicht sehr hoch ist. Der Winkelkoeffizient der Geraden $AB$ stellt den mittleren Elastizitätsmodul des Materials dar, der auch als mittlerer dynamischer Elastizitätsmodul des Materials bezeichnet werden kann.

Wenn die Form der Hystereseschleife sowie der Winkelkoeffizient der Geraden $L$, der wie gesagt als statischer Elastizitätsmodul des Materials aufgefaßt werden kann, bekannt sind, läßt sich durch Planimetrieren der Flächeninhalt der Hystereseschleife bestimmen. Wählt man das Koordinatensystem derart, daß die relative Formveränderung als Abszisse und die Spannung als Ordinate erscheint, so gibt der Flächeninhalt der Schleife die Hystereseenergie je Volumeinheit an.

Wenn das Material nicht völlig elastisch ist, ist die Formveränderung auch eine Funktion des vorangegangenen Spannungszustands oder der „Vorgeschichte" des Probestabes. Besteht zu irgendeinem Zeitpunkt $t'$ im Probestab die Spannung $\sigma(t')$, während des kurzen Zeitintervalls $dt'$, so ist die durch diese Spannung zu einem späteren Zeitpunkt $t$ in der Formveränderung hervorgerufene elastische Nachwirkung, dem Intervall $dt'$ sowie einer Funktion der verstrichenen Zeit $(t - t')$ proportional, welche Boltzmann [2], [3] als Erinnerungsfunktion bezeichnet. Demgemäß wird die Formveränderung durch folgende Gleichung ausgedrückt:

$$x(t) = \frac{\sigma(t)}{E_\infty} + \frac{1}{E_\infty} \int_{-\infty}^{t} \Phi(t - t') \, \sigma(t') \, \mathrm{d}t' \tag{1}$$

wo $E_\infty$ der Grenzwert des Elastizitätsmoduls für $\omega \to \infty$ ist. Eine nähere Betrachtung zeigt, daß $\sigma(t')/E_\infty$ die Formveränderung zum Zeitpunkt $t'$ während des Zeitintervalls $dt'$ und $\Phi(t - t')$ die Kriechgeschwindigkeit je Einheit der Formveränderung vertritt. Die Erinnerungsfunktion $\Phi$ kann mit Hilfe der Maxwellschen [2] Relaxationszeit $\tau$ bestimmt werden. Man erhält so für die Erinnerungsfunktion den Wert

$$\Phi(t) = \frac{E_\infty - E}{E} \, \tau^{-1} e^{-t/\tau} \tag{2}$$

Nach ausgeführten Messungen treffen (1) und (2) recht gut zu (Gross, Zener), insofern nur die Spannung unterhalb einer gewissen Grenze liegt. Bei Stahl ist die Theorie bis zu einer Dehnungs-Amplitude von $10^{-5}$ stichhaltig, entsprechend einer Spannung von 0,2 kg/mm$^2$.

Außer vom Material und von der Spannung hängt die Dämpfung auch von der Art der Spannung (Zug, Druck, Torsion, Biegung) sowie von Gestalt und Größe des Probekörpers ab. Demnach ist es offenbar, daß das Material bei großen Spannungen sich besser der erfahrenen Behandlung „erinnert" als die Erinnerungsfunktion (2) voraussetzt. Es liegt auch auf der Hand, daß dann die Boltzmannsche Erinnerungsfunktion nicht mit Hilfe der Maxwellschen Relaxationszeit bestimmt werden kann. Bei großen Spannungen dürfte sich die die Spannungs- und Verformungsgeschichte des Materials wiedergebende Funktion besser dem wirklichen Sachverhalt angleichen lassen, indem man die experimentell gewonnenen Hysteresebilder sowie eine bessere Kenntnis der Nachwirkung im Material heranzieht, als sie die MAXWELLsche Theorie vermittelt.

**b) Experimentelle Untersuchungen.** Stahlsorte St 34.12 (C = 0,10%, Si = 0,50%, Mn = 0,68%, P = 0,011%, S = 0,019% und N = 0,011%) warmgewalzt.

Mit der vorhandenen Apparatur kann die Veränderung der Hystereseschleife während des Ermüdungsversuchs fortlaufend bis zum Bruch des Probestabes verfolgt werden. Auf diese Weise läßt sich die Hystereseenergie nur bei großen, die Ermüdungsfestigkeit übersteigenden Belastungen bestimmen. Es wurden Messungen zur Bestimmung der Hystereseenergie bei zwei Stahlsorten vorgenommen. Die Hystereseschleife auf dem Bildschirm des Kathodenstrahloszillographen wurde in bestimmten Zeitabständen im Verlauf des Ermüdungsversuchs photographiert; der Probestab stand dauernd unter der gleichen Zug-Druckermüdungsbelastung. Als Ermüdungsfestigkeit für die Stahlsorte St 34.12 nach der DIN-Norm ergab sich mit dem Resonanzpulsator $\pm 20$ kg/mm². Erst bei Spannungen über $\sigma = \pm 28$ kg/mm² erhält man eine deutlich wahrnehmbare und ausmeßbare Hystereseschleife. Gleichzeitig mit den Aufnahmen der Hystereseschleife wurde jeweils die Temperatur im Probestabe mit Hilfe eines an die Staboberfläche angeschweißten Thermoelements aufgezeichnet. Die Bilderreihe in Abb. 2 zeigt die Hystereseschleifen bei der Spannung $\sigma = \pm 32$ kg/mm². Abb. 3 gibt die gemessenen Werte der Hystereseenergie in Abhängigkeit von der Zahl der Belastungswechsel bei verschiedenen Spannungen wieder. Aus diesen Kurven ersieht man, daß die Hystereseenergie mit zunehmender Zahl der Belastungswiederholungen andauernd steigt. Bei kleineren Spannungen ist der Anstieg der Kurve langsamer als bei großen Spannungen. In Abb. 4 ist die Temperatur im Probestab während des Ermüdungsversuchs als Funktion der Zahl der Belastungswiederholungen eingetragen. Die Kurve für $\tau = \pm 32$ ist für $T > 100°$ etwas zu steil eingezeichnet und sollte etwa mit $T = 170°$ bei $n = 7 \cdot 10^3$ enden. Die Temperaturkurven zeigen einen ähnlichen Verlauf wie diejenigen der Hystereseenergie.

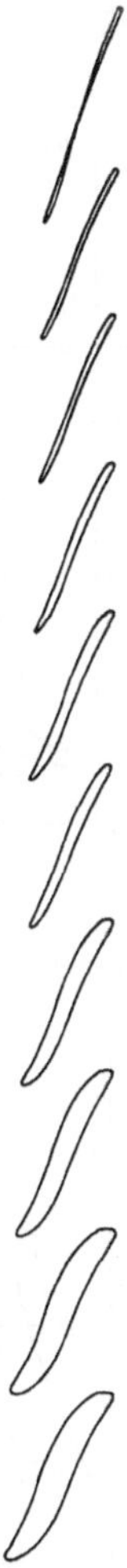

Abb. 2.

Stahlsorte St 50.11 (C = 0,22%, Si = 0,28%, Mn = 0,70%, P = 0,010%, S = 0,050% und N = 0,010%), normalisiert.

Die Ermüdungsfestigkeit des Stahls nach Angabe des Resonanzpulsators betrug $\pm 22$ kg/mm². Die Hystereseschleifen und die Stabtemperatur wurden in gleicher Weise wie im Vorangehenden ermittelt. Die Bilderreihe in Abb. 5 zeigt die Hystereseschleifen bei der Spannung $\sigma$ = $\pm43$ kg/mm², Abb. 6 die Hystereseenergie in Abhängigkeit von der Zahl der Belastungswiederholungen bei verschiedenen Spannungen so- wie Abb. 7 die entsprechenden Temperaturen. Aus den Hy- stereseenergiekurven geht her- vor, daß die Hystereseenergie nach einigen hundert oder einigen tausend Belastungs- wiederholungen zuerst ein Ma- ximum erreicht und dann auf einen konstanten Wert herab- geht, den sie bis zum Ende des Versuchs beibehält.

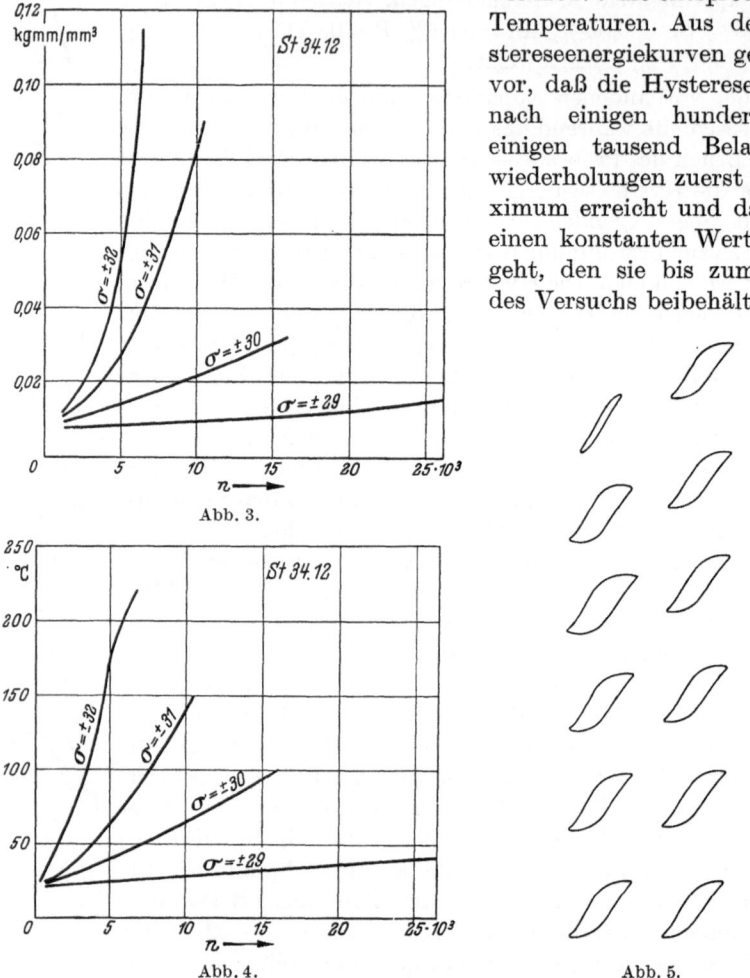

Abb. 3.

Abb. 4.

Abb. 5.

Zu einer nahezu gleichartigen Gestalt der Hystereseenergiekurven bei Belastungen oberhalb der Ermüdungsgrenze sind Lazan und Wu [1] ge- langt. Sie haben Messungen im Biegeversuch mit einem rotierenden Probestab ausgeführt. Als Versuchsmaterial hatten sie warmgewalzten Stahl SAE 1020 nach amerikanischer Norm, mit 0,20% Kohlenstoff. Die Temperatur des Probestabs war die ganze Zeit hindurch $27 \pm 12°$C.

## 4. Deutung der Form der Hystereseenergiekurven

Nach der nunmehr eingebürgerten Auffassung (Cottrell [4], Nabarro [5]) geht die plastische Verformung im Metall hauptsächlich gemäß der sog. Dislokationstheorie in der Weise vor sich, daß im Metallkristall ein Gleiten einer Gitterebene in bezug auf die benachbarte Gitterebene stattfindet. Das Gleiten erfolgt in Schritten, jeweils in einem Teil der Gleitebene, wobei dann in diesem Teil eine Gleitung um höchstens einen Atomabstand erfolgt ist, die als Dislokation oder Versetzung bezeichnet wird. Die Verformung kommt nun dadurch zustande, daß die Versetzung längs der Gleitebene fortschreitet. Ein ebensolches Gleiten findet auch beim Verdrehen statt. Nach der Dislokationstheorie hat man sich vorzustellen, daß die Versetzungen beim Gleiten benachbarte Versetzun-

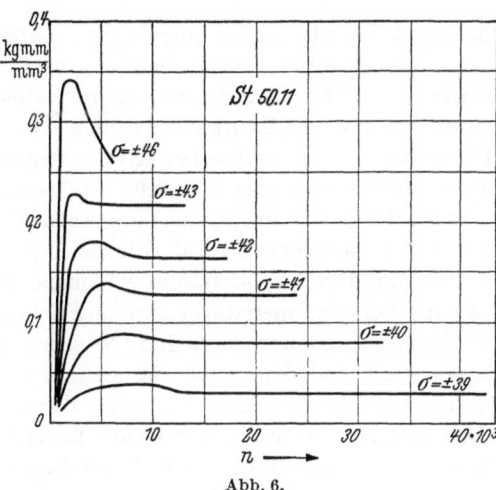

Abb. 6.

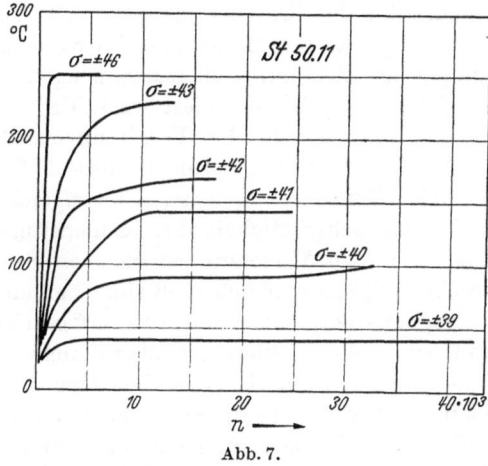

Abb. 7.

gen mitziehen, wobei sog. Versetzungslinien entstehen, deren Gestalt krummlinig ist. Es ist noch keine endgültige Klarheit darüber gewonnen worden, in welcher Weise die Versetzungen entstehen und sich in Bewegung setzen. Man hat festgestellt, daß sich die Zahl der Versetzungen durch Bearbeitung vermehrt, so daß stärker bearbeitetes Metall zahlreichere Versetzungen aufweist.

Bei der Entstehung einer Versetzung wird die Translationszelle des Atomgitters verzerrt und ihre Dimensionen ändern sich. Demzufolge ändern sich auch die Einlagerungsmöglichkeiten der interstitiellen Atome, der Kohlenstoff- und Stickstoffatome. Diese ordnen sich derart um, daß die nach der Verzerrung günstigsten Plätze ausgefüllt sind. Es ist natürlich, daß die interstitiell eingelagerten Atome die Bewegung der Versetzungen erschweren. Durch dieselben werden die Versetzungen gewissermaßen verankert. Um die Versetzung erneut in Bewegung zu setzen, ist dann eine größere Kraft erforderlich. Das Material verfestigt sich also. Die Schar der interstitiellen Atome nennt man eine Wolke. Beispielsweise erklärt man das deutliche Auftreten einer Streckgrenze im Zugversuch des Stahls in Zimmertemperatur dadurch, daß die Versetzungen durch die Kohlenstoff- und Stickstoffwolken verankert sind, wodurch der Formänderungswiderstand erhöht ist und abermals kleiner wird, sobald die Versetzungen durch eine hinreichend rasche Belastung von ihren Wolken losgerissen worden sind (Nabarro [5]). Die interstitiellen Atome, Kohlenstoff und Stickstoff, die sich in der $\alpha$-Eisen-Elementarzelle des ferritischen Stahls einlagern, rufen darin außer dem Volumenzuwachs auch eine erhebliche Deformation hervor. Für die Einlagerung dieser Atome in der normalen Elementarzelle des $\alpha$-Eisens beträgt im Ferrit der Halbmesser des größten Interstitiums etwa 0,36 Å, während der Atomradius des Kohlenstoffs etwa 0,77 Å ist.

Es liegt auf der Hand, daß die Kohlenstoffatome bei ihrer Einlagerung in der Elementarzelle zusammengedrückt werden und daß zugleich die Zelle elastisch deformiert wird. Von der Diffusion des Kohlenstoffs ist die Verankerung der Versetzungen abhängig. Überwiegt die Geschwindigkeit der Versetzungen diese Diffusionsgeschwindigkeit, so findet keine Verankerung statt. Mit steigender Temperatur wird auch die Diffusionsgeschwindigkeit des Kohlenstoffs stärker und vermag somit besser mit den Versetzungen gleichen Schritt zu halten. Wenn beide Geschwindigkeiten gleich groß sind, befindet sich der Stahl in der Blausprödigkeitstemperatur, die etwa 200° beträgt [4]. Bei Zimmertemperatur sind somit die Kohlenstoffwolken nicht imstande die Bewegung der Versetzungen, wohl aber das Einsetzen dieser Bewegung zu verhindern. Beim Anstieg der Temperatur auf etwa 200° C vermögen die Kohlenstoffwolken die Bewegung der Versetzungen zu bremsen, womit z. B. die im Zugversuch erhaltene Dehnung erheblich abnimmt, obwohl die Belastungsgeschwindigkeit die gleiche ist. In stark bearbeitetem Stahl [4] mit einer Versetzungsdichte von $10^{12}$ Versetzungen/cm² hat man wenigstens 0,01 % Kohlenstoff im Ferritgitter zur maximalen Verankerung der Versetzungen bei Zimmertemperatur als notwendig gefunden, d. h. es würden bei den Störungsstellen keine weiteren Wolken Platz finden.

Beide in den vorliegenden Versuchen benutzten Stähle enthalten mehr Kohlenstoff als die obenerwähnte Menge. Aus den Hystereseenergiekurven für den Stahl St 50.11 mit 0,22 % Kohlenstoff bei großen Belastungen, ersieht man, daß nach einigen Hundert oder einigen Tausend Belastungswechseln ein konstanter Wert erreicht wird, der nahezu bis zum Augenblick des Bruchs bestehenbleibt. Die Temperatur im

Stahl steigt hierbei rascher auf ihren endgültigen Wert, 40 bis 250° C je nach dem Betrag der Belastung. Wenigstens unter einigen Belastungen liegt die Temperatur im Stahl in der Gegend der Blausprödigkeitstemperatur, bei welcher die Kohlenstoffwolken dank ihrer Diffusion am besten imstande sind, den bei der angewandten Lastwechselzahl 55 Hz unter starker Bearbeitung stattfindenden Bewegungen mit den Versetzungen gleichen Schritt zu halten. Bei den anderen Temperaturen ist die Diffusion des Kohlenstoffs derart hoch, daß die Kohlenstoffwolken eine solche Verankerung der Versetzungen herbeizuführen vermögen, die es bewirkt, daß die Hystereseenergiekurve von einer gewissen Lastwechselzahl an einen konstanten Wert beibehält. Der konstante Endwert der Kurve erhält hiermit seine Erklärung. In den Hystereseenergiekurven für den Stahl St 34.12, mit 0,10% Kohlenstoff, bei großen Belastungen findet man einen dauernden Anstieg der Kurve. Die Temperatur im Stahl steigt ebenfalls und erreicht bei den angewandten Belastungen Werte zwischen 30 und 170° C. Die Temperatur bleibt in diesem Fall unterhalb der Blausprödigkeitstemperatur und die Verformung ist derart stark gewesen, daß die Kohlenstoffwolken nicht imstande waren, die Bewegungen der Versetzungen genügend zu bremsen, weshalb der Wert der inneren Reibung dauernd zunimmt.

### Literaturverzeichnis

[1] LAZAN, B. J. und T. WU: ASTM Preprint Nr. 22 (1951).
[2] ZENER, C: Metals Techn. (1946, Aug.).
[3] GROSS, B.: J. appl. Physics 18, 212—221 (1947).
[4] COTTRELL, A. H.: Progress in Metal Physics Nr. 4 (1953).
[5] NABARRO, F.: Report of a Conference on Strength of Solids, London 1948, 38—45.

### Diskussion

Nach einer Frage von Herrn ODING bestätigte der Verfasser, daß die Streuung in der Dämpfungsarbeit groß ist, und zwar innerhalb den Ergebnissen mit demselben Werkstoff und sogar innerhalb derselben Charge.

# Der Mechanismus des Dauerbruchs metallischer Werkstoffe

Von

## C. Schaub und W. Liedtke

Mit 2 Abbildungen

Im Herbst 1951 wurde unter Zusammenarbeit des Nationalkomitees für Mechanik und des Jernkontoret ein gemeinsamer Forschungsausschuß zum Studium des Mechanismus des Dauerbruches bei metallischen Werkstoffen gebildet. Den Anlaß hierzu bildete eine Eingabe des zuerst genannten Verfassers vom Frühjahr 1951, wonach es eine allgemein anerkannte Vorstellung von den Vorgängen bei der Ermüdung metallischer Werkstoffe noch nicht gab.

Als Ausgangspunkt für die kommende Arbeit wurde somit eine neue Arbeitshypothese angenommen, deren Inhalt in Kürze wie folgt zusammengefaßt werden kann.

„Bei Dauerbeanspruchung metallischer Werkstoffe findet wiederholte örtliche plastische Deformation (Gleitung) statt, die in der Grenzschicht gegen ein anderes umgebendes oder eingeschlossenes Medium liegt. Hierdurch wird eine örtlich wechselnde Aktivität des Werkstoffes in physikalisch-chemischer Hinsicht verursacht. In Gegenwart gewisser Metalloide (insbesondere Sauerstoff) im umgebenden Medium spielen sich infolge dieser Aktivität örtlich begrenzte reaktionskinetische Vorgänge ab, die bei fortlaufender Auflösung der metallischen Bindungen zu lokalen Anrissen und schließlich zum Dauerbruch führen."

Ein ausführliches Literaturstudium der bis dahin veröffentlichten Arbeiten, insbesondere über Fragen, die den Mechanismus des Dauerbruches behandeln, ist im Rahmen des Ausschusses von STRÖM [1] durchgeführt worden und soll hier durch seine Zusammenfassung wiedergegeben werden.

„Während der letzten 100 Jahre ist eine sehr umfassende Forschungsarbeit ausgeführt worden, um Klarheit über den Mechanismus des Dauerbruches metallischer Werkstoffe zu verschaffen.

Besonders mikroskopische und röntgenographische Untersuchungen von Wechselfestigkeitsproben haben ergeben, daß eine bedeutende plastische Deformation in den Bereichen auftritt, in denen sich später die Ermüdungsanrisse ausbilden. Benachbarte Bereiche hingegen können nahezu frei von jeglicher plastischen Deformation sein.

Hierin liegt einer der grundlegenden Unterschiede zum statischen Bruch, bei dem sich die Deformation gleich stark über größere Bereiche erstreckt. Röntgenographische Untersuchungen haben außerdem ergeben, daß die Oberflächenschicht metallischer Werkstücke eine niedrigere Streckgrenze aufweist als die Werkstücke in ihrer Gesamtheit. Dies sowohl wie korrodierende Einflüsse der umgebenden Atmosphäre bedingen, daß in den meisten Fällen die Anrisse in der Oberfläche der Wechselfestigkeitsproben beginnen trotz gleichförmiger Verteilung der Belastung über den ganzen Querschnitt.

Ausgehend von den experimentellen Ergebnissen sind mehrere Theorien gebildet worden, um den Mechanismus des Dauerbruches und die Form der Wöhlerkurve zu erklären. Von diesen Theorien sind besonders diejenigen von DEHLINGER und KOCHENDÖRFFER sowie diejenige von OROWAN behandelt worden."

Es lassen sich nun nach der Ansicht der Verfasser aus dieser Arbeit folgende Schlüsse ziehen:

1. Das Problem des Dauerbruches ist bisher (DEHLINGER, OROWAN u. a.) stets von der mechanischen Seite her angegriffen worden und kann nach unserer Ansicht auf diesem Wege wahrscheinlich nicht zu einer endgültigen Lösung führen.

2. Es ist bisher nichts bekannt geworden, was in Widerspruch zu unserer Arbeitshypothese steht.

Demgegenüber soll im folgenden die Aufmerksamkeit auf einige Forschungsergebnisse gelenkt werden, welche man nach unserer Ansicht als wesentliche Stützen der angegebenen Arbeitshypothese ansehen muß.

Bei Versuchen mit sauerstofffreiem, sogenanntem OFHC-Kupfer, sowohl polykristallinen als auch Einkristallproben in Zug- und Druck-Wechselbeanspruchung bei 1.000 Hz konnte THOMPSON [2] folgende Feststellungen machen:

Nach 5% der zu erwartenden Lebenslänge wurden Gleitlinien an der Oberfläche festgestellt. Durch elektrolytisches Polieren konnte die Mehrzahl dieser Gleitlinien beseitigt werden, und nur einige, die sogenannten „beständigen" Gleitlinien, waren dann noch sichtbar. Diese verschwanden erst nach einer Materialabtragung von 10 bis 20 μ Dicke. Abwechselnde Ermüdung bis zu 25% der zu erwartenden Lebenslänge mit darauffolgender elektrolytischer Materialabtragung konnte bis zu neunmal, d. h. also dem $2^1/_4$ fachen Wert der zu erwartenden Lebenslänge wiederholt werden, ohne daß die Probe Anzeichen einer stattgefundenen Schädigung aufwies. Eine einstündige Glühbehandlung im Vakuum bei 600° C hatte demgegenüber keinen Einfluß, weder auf die Wechselfestigkeit noch auf die beständigen Gleitlinien. Weiterhin konnte THOMPSON nachweisen, daß die Entstehung der sich zu Anrissen ausbildenden beständigen Gleitlinien verzögert wurde, wenn die Versuche in trockenem Stickstoff statt in Luft ausgeführt wurden. Die Erhöhung der Lebenslänge durch Abtragung der offensichtlich durch Wechsel- beanspruchung allein geschädigten Oberflächenschicht konnte durch Arbeiten von Lissner [3] an Stahl im Rahmen unseres Ausschusses bestätigt werden.

Die Versuche von Thompson zeigen weiterhin deutlich, welchen Wert man der Anwesenheit von Sauerstoff für die Ausbildung der be- ständigen Gleitlinien beimessen muß. Dies ist übrigens im Prinzip schon aus Arbeiten von Gough und Sopwith [4] bekannt, da sie nachweisen konnten, daß unter Anwendung eines Vakuums von $10^{-3}$ mm Hg eine Erhöhung der Dauerfestigkeit von

5% für Stahl
13% für Kupfer
26% für Messing

erzielt werden kann. Diese Ergebnisse gewinnen an Anschaulichkeit, wenn man bedenkt, daß die Konzentration der Sauerstoffmoleküle bei $10^{-3}$ mm Hg noch etwa $7 \cdot 10^{12}/\text{cm}^3$ beträgt.

In der zitierten Arbeit beschreibt Gough die Versuche anderer For- scher (Binnie und Lehmann); Binnie spritzte während des Dauer- versuches durch umlaufende Biegung in Luft eine Kochsalzlösung auf die Probe und erhielt dabei bei Stahl eine beträchtliche Herabsetzung der Ermüdungsfestigkeit. Bei Verwendung von handelsüblichem Wasser- stoff statt Luft, ebenfalls mit Kochsalzlösung, ergab sich eine geringe Erhöhung der Festigkeit gegenüber dem Wert in Luft. Die Verwendung von besonders gereinigtem Wasserstoff ergab schließlich eine größere Erhöhung der Festigkeit gegenüber dem Wert in Luft.

Lehmann erhielt in warmer ($+96°$ C) Kochsalzlösung ($25^0/_0$) eine Er- müdungsfestigkeit, die gleich groß oder sogar größer ist als die in ge- wöhnlicher Luft ($+17°$C) und deutlich größer ist ($6^0/_0$) als die in warmem destilliertem Wasser ($+96°$C).

Graham und Maddin [5] untersuchten die Rekristallisationseigen- schaften von Al-Einkristallen nach erfolgter Streckung und Glühung. Sobald zwischen Streckung und Glühung die Oberfläche durch Ätzen abgetragen wurde, unterblieb die Rekristallisation. Es erwies sich so- mit, daß die Oberflächenschicht ein erhöhtes Keimbildungsvermögen besitzt, dessen Reichweite aus weiteren Abtragungsversuchen zu 0,04 mm in den Werkstoff hinein bestimmt wurde. Die Rekristallisation beginnt an Gitterstörstellen, d. h. in diesem Fall in Bereichen von erhöhter Fehl- stellendichte. Die während des Streckens sich anhäufenden Fehlstellen werden durch die Einwirkung von Sauerstoff in der Oberflächenschicht blockiert und bilden die für die Rekristallisation erforderlichen Keimstellen. Wenn also ein der Luft ausgesetzter Al-Einkristall gestreckt wird, ist die Verteilung der Fehlstellen in der Oberfläche nicht die gleiche wie im Innern des Kristalles.

Bei Versuchen mit sogenannten iron-whiskers, d. h. fehlerfreien kleinen Eiseneinkristallen, die entlang einer axialen Schraubenversetzung gewachsen sind, konnten Sears, Gatti und Fullman [6] die für perfekte Kristalle zu erwartenden hohen elastischen Eigenschaften feststellen. Diese Eigenschaften gingen jedoch verloren, sobald die Kristalle einige Tage ohne Bildung einer sichtbaren Oxydhaut der Luft ausgesetzt waren.

Offensichtlich haben die bisher angeführten Versuche alle miteinander gemein, daß das Vorhandensein von Sauerstoff bzw. Luft in Berührung mit der Probenoberfläche in engem Zusammenhang mit den Festigkeitseigenschaften der Oberflächenschicht des Werkstoffes steht.

Man definiert nun den Grad der Reaktionsfähigkeit einer Oberfläche mit dem umgebenden Medium als Aktivität. Diese Aktivität ist jedoch nicht gleichförmig verteilt, sondern besitzt Verteilungsmaxima an den sogenannten aktiven Stellen. Diese aktiven Stellen besitzen starke Bindungskräfte, bilden z. B. Keimstellen bei der Kristallisation, sind die Urheber katalytischer Wirkungen und nehmen auch bei der Adsorption eine Sonderstellung ein. Sie befinden sich an den Ecken und Kanten der Kristalle, an Gitterstörstellen, an frisch gebildeten Gleitlinien sowie auf frischen Spaltflächen.

Die Anzahl der aktiven Stellen an der Oberfläche einer Dauerfestigkeitsprobe wird beim Einsetzen der ersten Lastwechsel, d. h. mit dem Auftreten der ersten Gleitungen stetig ansteigen, und es ist sogar gelungen, den Grad der durch Wechselbeanspruchung erhöhten Aktivität in Form erhöhter Reaktionsbereitschaft mit dem umgebenden Medium zu messen.

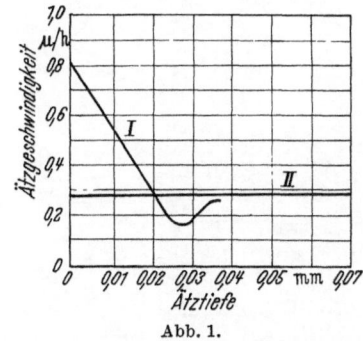

Abb. 1.

Vitovec [7] verglich die Auflösungsgeschwindigkeiten beim Ätzen zweier Proben, von denen die eine I mit 10% Überlast bis etwa zur Hälfte ihrer Lebenslänge wechselbeansprucht war, während die andere II aus dem gleichen, jedoch unbeanspruchten Material vorlag (Abb. 1).

Die Aktivierung reicht bis zu einer Tiefe von 0,02 mm, und wie Gough und Sopwith [8] in anderem Zusammenhang mikroskopisch feststellen konnten, findet der chemische Angriff bevorzugt an den Gleitlinien statt. Darunter befindet sich eine Zone verminderter Lösungsgeschwindigkeit, für deren Aufkommen der Verfasser als Ursache die Trainierwirkung annimmt.

Es ist in diesem Zusammenhang bemerkenswert, daß sowohl diese Ätzversuche als auch die vorhin angeführten Rekristallisationsuntersuchungen und die Arbeiten bezüglich der beständigen Gleitlinien größenordnungsmäßig übereinstimmende Angaben über die Tiefenwirkung in das Material hinein enthalten.

Die Erhöhung der Aktivität der Oberflächenschicht bei plastischer Verformung wird bedingt durch die durch Gleitung entstandenen neuen, d. h. von Fremdatomen unbelegten Oberflächenelemente. Die somit entstandenen freien Bindungskräfte werden auf dem Wege über Adsorption und Chemosorption von Atomen oder Molekülresten aus dem umgebenden Medium wieder abgesättigt werden. Da nun das umgebende Medium in der Regel aus Luft, d. h. abgesehen vom Stickstoff aus molekularem Sauerstoff mit einem gewissen Prozentsatz Wasserdampf besteht, wird der Chemosorption eine Aufspaltung der Sauerstoffmoleküle in Atome vorausgehen müssen, wobei ein Teil des Sauerstoffes mit dem Wasserdampf der Luft zur Bildung von $H_2O_2$ führt.

Daß die oben geschilderte Reaktion tatsächlich diesen Verlauf nimmt, konnte von Schaub und Liedtke [9] unter Ausnutzung des sogenannten Russell-Effektes gezeigt werden. Der Russell-Effekt besagt, daß photographische Platten unter der Einwirkung von $H_2O_2$ geschwärzt werden, und daß etwa durch Schmirgeln hergestellte frische metallische Oberflächen auf Grund der eben geschilderten Reaktion ebenfalls zur Schwärzung von photographischen Schichten Anlaß geben. Diese photographische Methode gestattet, einen eindeutigen Beweis von der Wirksamkeit der Aktivität bei plastischer Deformation zu liefern, wie die folgenden Aufnahmen zeigen (Abb. 2). Eine Probe aus handelsüblichem Aluminiumblech wurde auf Biegewechselfestigkeit geprüft und dabei einer Belastung ausgesetzt, die nach etwa 3.000 Biegungen zum Bruch führte. Die Be-

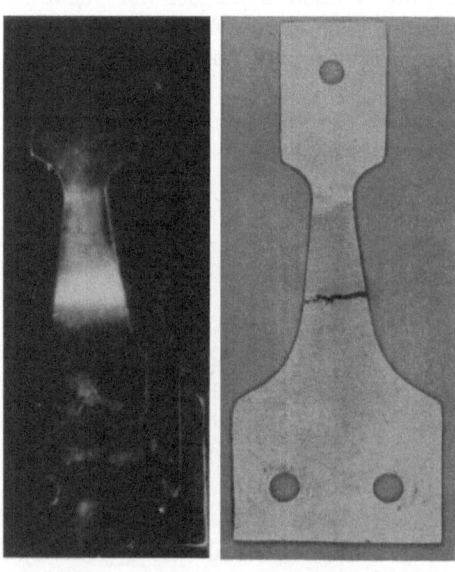

a          Abb. 2.          b

lastung lag somit weit oberhalb der Dauerfestigkeit des Materials, und die Prüflänge der Probe war einer starken plastischen Deformation ausgesetzt. Nach 1.500 Belastungswechseln wurde der Versuch unterbrochen, und die Probe für 24 Stunden auf die Emulsionsschicht einer photographischen Platte gelegt. Entwickeln und nachfolgendes Behandeln der Platte mit Uranverstärker ergab das Bild der Abb. 2a. Abb. 2b zeigt die Probe nach erfolgtem Bruch bei insgesamt 3.300 Belastungswechseln.

Die Probe ist so beschaffen, daß sie entlang der gesamten Prüflänge einen „Träger gleicher Festigkeit" darstellt und somit auch einer zumindest am Anfang über die ganze Länge gleichmäßig verteilten Deformation ausgesetzt ist. Die durch diese Deformation erfolgte Aktivierung erkennt man auf Abb. 2a an der gleichmäßig „belichtenden" Prüflänge. Infolge der hohen Belastung hat sich ein „Ermüdungsbereich" ausgebildet, in dem gemäß Abb. 2a ein erhöhtes Fließen stattgefunden hat und in dem dann gemäß Abb. 2b der eigentliche Ermüdungsbruch eingetreten ist. Die geringe Empfindlichkeit des photographischen Verfahrens macht es unmöglich, derartige Effekte bei niederen Belastungen aufzuzeigen. Vereinzelte Gleitlinien sind verglichen mit dem Auflösungsvermögen der photographischen Emulsion zu klein, zum anderen reicht die Menge des gebildeten $H_2O_2$ nicht aus, um eine sichtbare Schwärzung zu ergeben. Diese experimentelle Schwierigkeit besagt jedoch keinesfalls, daß in einem Versuch mit obigen Bedingungen etwas anderes geschehen ist als es bei Belastungen bzw. Deformationen, die normalen Dauerbrüchen vorangehen der Fall ist. Die Wechselbeanspruchung hat in der Probenoberfläche zu einer Reaktion Anlaß gegeben, die 24 Stunden nach erfolgtem Abschalten noch nicht zum Abschluß gekommen ist und in deren örtlichem Maximum der spätere Bruch erfolgt.

## Schlußfolgerungen

Es konnte somit bestätigt werden, daß man der Oberfläche von metallischen Werkstoffen in ihrer Eigenschaft als Grenzfläche zweier Medien sowohl festigkeitsmäßig als auch reaktionskinetisch ganz besondere Bedeutung beimessen muß. Diese Bedeutung wirkt sich jedoch erst dann aus, wenn der Oberfläche die andauernde Möglichkeit zur Bildung von aktiven Stellen, d. h. Elementargleitungen, gegeben ist, wie dies bei Wechselbeanspruchung der Fall ist. Denn die Wahrscheinlichkeit für den Übergang einer solchen Elementargleitung in eine beständige Gleitlinie und schließlich in den Anriß ist umso größer, je größer die Anzahl entstandener Elementargleitungen ist. Eine derart ausgebildete Gleitlinie stellt einen Bereich erhöhter Aktivität dar, dessen Ausdehnung sich entlang der Oberfläche lamellen- oder terrassenartig über mehrere hundert Gitterebenen erstreckt und das außerdem entlang den Gitterebenen eine gewisse Tiefe in das Material hinein besitzt. Die Reaktion dieser aktivierten Oberflächenelemente mit dem umgebenden Medium wird augenblicklich beginnen, und es wird sich entlang den Gleitebenen in das Material hinein ebenfalls eine chemische Reaktion erstrecken. Dabei kann die metallische Bindung auf Kosten dieser Reaktionen mit Fremdatomen (z. B. Sauerstoff) verlorengehen.

Unserer Ansicht nach ist das Vorhandensein einer Wechselbeanspruchung notwendig, jedoch nicht hinreichend, um den entscheidenden Übergang der Gleitlinien über das Zwischenstadium beständiger Gleitlinien in Anrisse erfolgen zu lassen. Erst das Hinzutreten der eben aufgezählten Reaktionen kann im Zusammenwirken mit plastischen Deformationen zur Entstehung von Anrissen führen. Erst im weiteren Verlauf der Lastwechsel und mit dem Weiterwachsen dieses Anrisses wird die mechanische Kerbwirkung und somit die auferlegte Belastung zum dominierenden Teile und ist schließlich nahezu alleinwirkend beim Eintreten des Restbruches.

Die bisher auf diesem Gebiet geleistete Arbeit konnte nur zu vorläufigen Resultaten führen, und weitere Arbeit in der gleichen Richtung ist geplant, um die Kenntnisse von den Vorgängen beim Dauerbruch zu vervollständigen.

### Literaturverzeichnis
[1] Ström, B.: Jernkontor. Ann. 138, 17 (1954).
[2] Thompson, N.: Engineering 178, Dec. 3 (1954).
[3] Lissner, O., in W. Weibull und F. K. G. Odqvist (Edit.): Proc. Coll. Fatigue, Stockholm 1955, Berlin 1956, 148.
[4] Gough, H. J. und D. G. Sopwith: J. Iron St. Inst. 126, 651—652 (1932, II).
[5] Graham Jr, C. D. und R. Maddin: J. Inst. Metals 83, 169—172 (1955).
[6] Sears, G. W., A. Gatti und R. L. Fullmann: Acta Metallurgica 2, 727 (1954).
[7] Vitovec, F.: Berg- u. Hüttenm. Mh. 97.
[8] Gough, H. J. und D. G. Sopwith: Proc. Roy. Soc. (A) 135, 392 (1932).
[9] Schaub, C. und W. Liedtke: Z. Metallk. 44, 570—572 (1953).

# A proposed mechanism of fatigue failure

By

## F. R. Shanley

With 1 figure

## 1. Introduction

Some years ago the author suggested the possibility of a phenomenon which, if it exists at all, would explain the formation of fatigue cracks [16]. In this paper the proposed mechanism will be described and compared with some of the available experimental evidence.

## 2. Unbonding as a result of slip

Fig. 1 a shows an idealized model of atoms near the surface of a crystal. Under zero load the atoms will be separated by an equilibrium distance $L_1$. In fig. 1 b the crystal is assumed to have slipped along a diagonal slip plane, under the action of the shear stress caused by tensile loading. For simplicity only three atoms are shown; the actual number may of course be very large.

If the distance $L_2$ should exceed the interatomic spacing corresponding to the cohesive stress, the original bond would be broken. This suggests how unbonding could occur at nominally low values of the tensile stress.

For purposes of illustration, all three atoms shown in fig. 1 b will be considered unbonded and are therefore indicated by hollow circles.

It is possible that the localized stress between the atoms being unbonded might reach a very high value. In unidirectional loading this would suggest that there is a "skin effect", in which a very thin layer of atoms at the surface tends to operate at a high local stress level, after plastic slip of the interior atoms has begun. Such skin effects have long been suspected; for example WEIBULL [1] demonstrated that the volume and surface effects on porcelain rods may be separated by statistical methods. He also made the following significant statement: "It is a well-known fact that surface condition plays an important role in fatigue. The existence of surface effects such as found in cast iron is very plausible. A closer examination of the problem is of fundamental importance . . ."

The idea of surface unbonding originally occurred to the author as a possible explanation of the abnormally high tensile strength of very

fine wires. In an unpublished paper a simple equation was developed
from this viewpoint, using an "effective width" concept similar to that
originally introduced by v. KARMAN for plate buckling [2]. This equa-

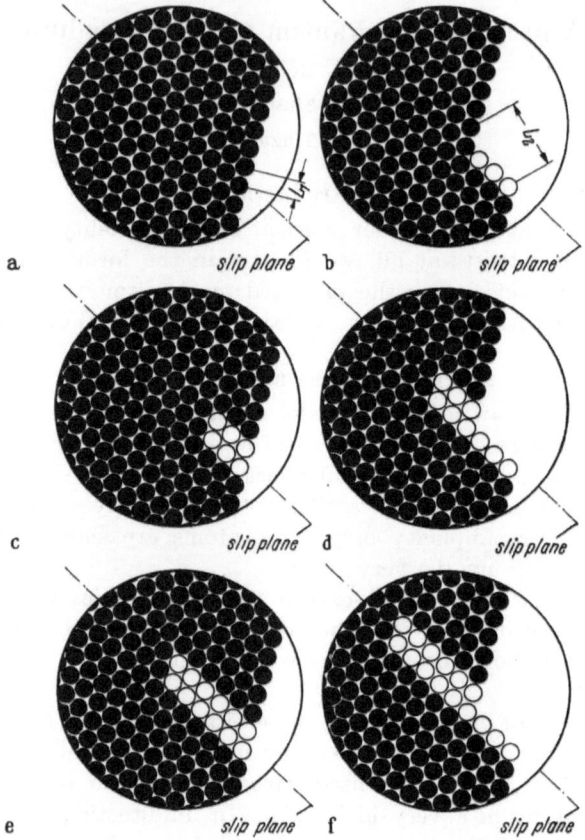

Fig. 1. Model illustrating unbonding by reversed slip.

tion agreed exactly with the empirical expression found by KARMARSCH
in 1858, from tests of fine metal wires, and accurately fitted GRIFFITH's
test results for glass fibers. (See [3], page 182.)

### 3. Development of a fatigue crack

*It will be assumed that a crystal, having slipped in one direction along
a certain plane, at a free surface, will slip in the opposite direction, along
the same plane, when the loading is reversed.* This assumption may appear
to be contrary to some of the concepts of strain hardening. Never-

theless, let us examine the possible results of making such an assumption.

In fig. 1c the slip has been reversed and the unbonded atoms are assumed to have returned to their original positions in the crystal. Will all of these atoms regain their original bonds ? To do so would probably require very high local compressive stresses, or thermal agitation, or both. *It will be assumed that some fraction of the unbonded atoms will not rebond.* In sketch 1c it is indicated, for simplicity, that all three of the atoms remained unbonded. This breaks the original bond which existed with their previous partners; the latter have therefore been designated by hollow circles.

The operation is now repeated, in 1d. It seems reasonable to assume that some of the unbonded atoms above the slip plane will not rebond with those which move into place below them, especially since there will be a tensile stress across the slip plane. The atoms immediately below are therefore indicated by hollow circles. If this process is repeated over and over again *a progressive unbonding will take place.* This will cause a "crack" to grow along the slip plane.

Before proceeding further it would appear desirable to discuss what is meant by the word "crack", in fatigue. In fig. 1, imagine that the surface shown in sketch 1f were to be examined under the most powerful microscope available. It would no doubt appear to be a slip plane. When the specimen is unloaded there is no reason why there should be an open crack. Such a crack would probably become visible only after unbonding had proceeded to such an extent that local permanent deformation or attrition had occurred. Any crack revealed by available methods of inspection might therefore represent a rather advanced stage of unbonding. In this connection, an interesting experiment was reported by BULLEN, HEAD and WOOD [4]. They stopped the cyclic stressing of a specimen at an early stage (about half the nominal life) and took photomicrographs ($\times 200$) which revealed typical intensified lines representing slip planes. They then loaded the specimen in tension to produce a permanent strain of about 5 per cent. The microscope now revealed relatively large cracks on some of the slip planes. It would seem reasonable to suppose that there had been some unbonding prior to the application of the static load and that the cracks merely opened up or became larger.

## 4. Essential features of the mechanism

Several features of the proposed mechanism of unbonding during reversed slip will now be noted. (a) *There must be a free surface.* This might occur at internal voids, as well as on the boundary of the material. (b) *Unbonding is caused by slip.* This associates fatigue with *plastic strain.* (c) *Cracks will tend to form along the "weak" shear planes in crystals.*

Fatigue cracks nearly always start at the surface of a specimen. The few exceptions to this generally show that the crack started at an internal void.

The surface effect is strongly supported by the well-known influence of shot-peening, which causes a residual compressive stress in a thin layer of material at the surface. The internal tensile stresses are not thereby reduced (in fact they are increased slightly), yet a shot-peened specimen will withstand considerably higher repeated stresses than a normal specimen (for the same life).

Item (b) indicates that fatigue is not associated with some critical value of tensile stress at which a crack will occur, but is governed by the amount of plastic strain involved. This is supported experimentally by the fact that fatigue cracks have been produced in specimens which were loaded entirely within the compression range.

Item (c) agrees with observations that fatigue cracks actually follow a zig-zag path in which the straight portions coincide with the slip planes of the individual crystals.

Another phenomenon which fits perfectly into the proposed mechanism is that of *corrosion fatigue*. A specimen may suffer a large loss of fatigue strength if the corrosive medium is permitted to attack the surface while the test is going on. It seems possible that the degree of unbonding per cycle would be increased by chemical attack.

It will now be shown that the proposed mechanism offers a basis for a mathematical theory which will explain observed relationships between fatigue life and magnitude of applied stress.

## 5. Influence of stress amplitude on fatigue life

It will be arbitrarily assumed that the number of atoms unbonded during each cycle is controlled by the amount of reversed slip that takes place. This will be controlled, in general, by the plastic deformation of the *entire specimen* (excluding notch effects). This is represented, in repeated loading, by the width of the hysteresis loop (See fig. 1 of [5]). If there is no such loop the action will be purely elastic. If all crystals behave elastically there will be no slip and therefore no fatigue failure. For some materials this appears to be confirmed experimentally by the existence of an *endurance limit*. Furthermore, it is known that, for other materials, cyclic loading will cause a gradual narrowing of the hysteresis loop, resulting eventually in virtually elastic behavior. This may explain why small fatigue cracks sometimes stop growing after a certain period of cycling at low stress levels. (See GENSAMER's discussion, based on the work of GOUGH [5], pp. 1—3.)

In a tension test the plastic strain varies with stress in a highly non-linear manner. A power function has long been used to express this relationship for many materials. (See NADAI's equation in [6].) This function will now be adopted for the plastic strain which occurs in repeated loading.

Let
$$\varepsilon_P = C\,\sigma^x \tag{1}$$

where  $\varepsilon_P$ = plastic strain
  $\sigma$  = maximum stress reached in a completely reversed cycle
  $C$  = constant and $x$ = exponent, to be determined experimentally.

(Note: The same type of function is used in the OROWAN theory of fatigue [7], but for an entirely different purpose.)

The simplest possible fatigue equation will be obtained when the rate of crack growth (per cycle) is assumed to be constant. Using (1),

$$h = A\sigma^x\,n \tag{2}$$

where  $h$  = depth of crack
  $A$ = constant
  $n$ = number of cycles.

To obtain an equation for fatigue failure *it will arbitrarily be assumed that failure occurs when the crack depth reaches a certain value, $h_0$.* The number of cycles at which this occurs will be designated by $N$. (It is well known that crack growth is very rapid in the period just preceding failure; hence the precise value assigned to $h_0$ will usually have little effect on $N$.)

$$h_0 = A\sigma^x\,N \tag{3}$$

From which
$$N = \frac{B}{\sigma^x} \tag{4}$$

where $B$ and $x$ are constants.

This is the well-known fatigue equation represented by a straight line on a log-log plot of $\sigma$ against $N$, since

$$\log N = \log B - x \log \sigma \tag{5}$$

In [8] another type of crack-growth function was used, in which the rate growth of the crack (at a given stress level) was assumed to be proportional to the depth of the crack itself. This type of exponential function was chosen because it tends to account for the stress-concentration effect of the crack. It also agrees well with experimental measurements of crack growth, which show a relatively low initial rate which rapidly becomes greater as failure is approached.

For the exponential crack-growth function it was assumed that

$$h = A e^{C\sigma^x\,n} \tag{6}$$

Replacing $h$ by $h_0$ and $n$ by $N$ and taking the natural logarithm of both sides gives

$$\sigma^x\,N = \frac{\log h_0 - \log A}{C} \tag{7}$$

If the term on the right is replaced by a constant, the equation becomes identical with (4).

These two examples show that the straight-line $\sigma$-$N$ plot on *log-log* paper can be interpreted simply to mean that the rate of crack growth (or "damage") varies as a power of the stress. This will be true for any assumed function for rate of crack-growth, provided that the corresponding crack-growth curves are affine.

Another possible expression for relating plastic strain to stress amplitude is the exponential function:

$$\varepsilon_P = Ae^{C\sigma} \tag{8}$$

If this is used instead of the power expression, the resulting fatigue equation becomes

$$\sigma = B - C \log N \tag{9}$$

This gives a straight line on *semi-log* paper, representing another common way to plot fatigue data. (Both of the above functions are frequently used in connection with creep, to represent strain rate.)

The *endurance limit* effect can be introduced in various ways. The original equation by NADAI for plastic strain [6] provided for a stress below which no plastic strain would occur. Equation (1) then becomes

$$\varepsilon_P = C \left( \sigma - \sigma_0 \right)^x \tag{10}$$

This changes (4) to

$$N = \frac{B}{\left( \sigma - \sigma_0 \right)^x} \tag{11}$$

The behavior of low-carbon steel suggests that there may be a "cut-off" effect such that there is no plastic strain below a certain stress value, $\sigma_0$, but that above this value the stress-strain relationship follows the original power expression (1). On the $\sigma$-$N$ diagram this would be represented by a horizontal "cut-off" line at $\sigma_0$, giving the usual two straight lines on *log-log* paper.

WEIBULL [9] has suggested a further modification of the $\sigma$-$N$ equation in which a constant is added to $N$, to provide a better fit in the low-cycle range. This can be physically interpreted by the proposed theory as follows. The rate of crack growth is assumed to depend on the amount of reversed plastic strain. The power expression (1) gives a satisfactory fit for relatively low stresses, but fails to predict enough strain at stresses near the nominal ultimate tensile stress. On the $\sigma$-$N$ diagram this can be accounted for by assuming that a stress very slightly less than the ultimate tensile stress causes a much lower strain and therefore can be applied a certain number of times without failure.

In [10] EPREMIAN and MEHL discovered that the left end of the $\sigma$-$N$ diagram could be made to coincide with the ultimate tensile stress by using a probability scale instead of a logarithmic scale for plotting stress. (WÅLLGREN's data from [11] were used.) These results suggest that, for cyclic loading at room temperature, the dependence of alternating plastic strain on stress amplitude is primarily of a statistical nature.

The proposed theory provides a realistic interpretation for the relationship between fatigue and the nominal ultimate tensile stress. For a ductile material the latter has no connection whatever with rupture; it is controlled entirely by plastic strain phenomena. It is therefore reasonable to expect the fatigue curve, at one-quarter cycle, to coincide with the ultimate tensile stress: the hysteresis loop then degenerates to the unidirectional stress-strain diagram.

## 6. Time and temperature effects

On the basis of the proposed theory it is possible to predict, at least qualitatively, the effects of time (rate of loading) and elevated temperature. These effects might enter in several ways: (a) Elevated temperature would increase the amount of plastic strain caused by a certain cyclic stress, thereby tending to reduce fatigue life; (b) slower rates of cycling would permit greater amounts of reversed strain per cycle, hence would reduce the number of cycles to failure; (c) high temperatures might tend to promote rebonding during reversed slip, thereby decreasing or eliminating crack-growth.

A theory of fatigue was proposed by MACHLIN [12] which, for constant temperature, can be reduced to the form of (9), with $N$ replaced by $t$ (time) [8]. This gives a straight-line plot on semi-log paper, with $N$ replaced by $t$; the *fatigue life is then dependent on time only* and is independent of the rate at which the cycles are repeated. This would seem to represent an extreme case, such as very high temperature, in which "instantaneous" plastic strain is entirely replaced by time-dependent plastic strain.

## 7. Concluding remarks

It has been shown [8] that the proposed mechanism of fatigue offers a rational basis for explaining many well-known fatigue phenomena. The only direct disagreement is found with those fatigue theories in which crack initiation is attributed to a localized lowering of the strength of the material.

Perhaps it will never be possible to determine, by experiment, exactly what happens in the very early stages of fatigue. However, rapid strides are being in that direction, as indicated by the work of CRAIG [13] and BULLEN, HEAD and WOOD [4]. A recent paper by HUNTER and FRICKE [14] is particularly interesting. They obtained electron micrographs of fatigue cracks along the edge of a slip band at

15,000 ×. Their observations by various methods revealed a significant fact: the more powerful the method of observation, the earlier in the fatigue life the cracks can be seen! This is supported by the work of many other investigators, as mentioned by Head [15], whose excellent review of the facts and theories concerning the mechanism of fatigue contains other information that appears to support the proposed theory.

From present evidence it would appear either that reversed slip (with unbonding) starts from the very beginning, as originally assumed [8], or is preceded by a relatively short period during which unidirectional slip occurs on alternate planes. In that case the early action leading up to slip reversal could probably be assumed to be governed by the same stress function that governs reversed slip.

The author is indebted to The RAND Corporation for supporting the studies which led to the proposed theory of fatigue. The helpful suggestions received from many of the people who read the original RAND reports are gratefully acknowledged.

### Bibliography

[1] Weibull, W.: Appl. Mech. Rev. 3, 449—451 (1952).
[2] Karman, T. von, E. E. Sechler and L. H. Donnell: Trans. ASME 54, 53 (1932).
[3] Griffith, A. A.: Trans. Roy. Soc. (A) 221, 163—198 (1921).
[4] Bullen, F. P., A. K. Head and W. A. Wood: Proc. Roy. Soc. (A) 216, 332 (1953).
[5] Murray, W. M.: (Edit.), Fatigue and Fracture of Metals, New York 1952.
[6] Ramberg, W. and W. R. Osgood: NACA TN 902 (1943).
[7] Orowan, E.: Proc. Roy. Soc. (A) 171, 79 (1939).
[8] Shanley, F. R.: RAND Corp. Rep. (U. S. A.), P-350 (1952); also: Suppl. (1953).
[9] Weibull, W.: J. appl. Mech. 19, 109 (1952).
[10] Epremian, E. and R. F. Mehl: NACA TN 2719 (1952).
[11] Wållgren, G.: FFA Medd. (Aeronaut. Res. Inst. Rep.) (Stockholm) Nr. 28 (1949).
[12] Machlin, E. S.: NACA TN 1489 (1948). also: NACA Tech. Rep. 929 (1949).
[13] Craig, W. J.: Proc. ASTM 52, 877—889 (1952).
[14] Hunter, M. S. and W. G. Fricke Jr.: Metallographic Aspects of Fatigue Behavior of Aluminum. Presented at Annual Meeting of ASTM, June 1954.
[15] Head, A. K., J. Mech. Phys. Solids 1, 134—140 (1953).
[16] Shanley, F. R.: Strength-Weight Analysis of Aircraft Structures, New York 1952, 296.

### Discussion

R. E. Peterson: The feature of Shanley's theory associated with the surface step seems rather restrictive. It is possible for slip to occur without the step — when the slip plane is perpendicular to the surface and the slip direction is parallel to the surface. A hypothesis proposed by Orowan[1] seems to me to be more general.

---

[1] Dislocations in Metals (1955). Published by Am. Inst. Mining Metallurg. Engrs (see last two pages of book).

OROWAN suggests that during cycling there occurs a lining up of edge dislocations perpendicular to the slip plane and this causes a tension perpendicular to the slip plane — the tension resulting in the breaking of bonds causing the separation which seems as the source of fatigue failure.

Another point which may be mentioned is that for certain surface hardened specimens failure starts under the case and would not involve "surface step".

F. R. SHANLEY answered PETERSON's criticism by referring to fatigue cracks started in compression.

W. N. FINDLEY confirmed Author's statement that fatigue in compression has been found in cast iron and aluminum alloys.

D. G. SOPWITH: What is meant by "yield point" in Author's sense?

F. R. SHANLEY: I am speaking about yield point in a macroscopic sense as derived from tests.

C. E. PHILLIPS: Is there experimental evidence of slip and reversed slip on the same crystal plane?

F. R. SHANLEY: This is an important question, which I am not able to answer.

On experimental evidence, I can only add that the more powerful the experimental method, the earlier the crack can be detected.

The theory that fatigue results from reversed slip associated with a free surface (or void) does not preclude an explanation in terms of dislocations. If slip is caused by dislocations it must follow, from my theory, that fatigue phenomena can ultimately be explained in terms of dislocations. However, such deeper insight is not required in order to explain many, if not all, of the observed facts concerning fatigue; the proposed theory appears to do this without further refinement.

# Recent researches on fatigue at the
# Mechanical Engineering Research Laboratory, East Kilbride

By

## D. G. Sopwith

With 6 figures

The completion in 1951 of the Strength of Materials Laboratory, the first of seven new laboratories of the Mechanical Engineering Research Laboratory at East Kilbride, enabled the various materials researches, formerly undertaken in the Engineering Division of the National Physical Laboratory, to be expanded. Research on fatigue is thus continuing in the tradition of some of the well-known pioneers in this field of fatigue research, e. g., Sir T. E. STANTON and Dr. H. J. GOUGH.

The various fatigue researches range from the purely fundamental to the severely practical, and involve the use of a wide variety of machines. Unnotched specimens of various metals up to 2 inches diameter can be tested under conditions of either rotating bending or direct stress; machines are also available for testing materials under varying degrees of combined bending and torsion stress on specimens up to $1/2$ inch diameter.

## 1. Size effect

The acquisition, a few years ago, by the Laboratory of some 60 Ton direct-stress machines enabled comprehensive investigations to be carried out to determine the effect of size of specimen on fatigue strength of materials in various forms. It was shewn [1] that whilst no intrinsic size effect in fatigue was observed with plain specimens of a mild steel and a nickel-chrome steel, a pronounced size effect was exhibited by notched specimens. Indeed, this particular work suggests that in sections of mild steel of sufficient size, it might well be the case that the full theoretical stress concentration effects due to notches might be realized. It has long been accepted that with high-strength materials strength reduction factors much more closely approach the theoretical values than is the case for softer materials. The importance of size when mild steel is used is now demonstrated. Arising from this work, it was suggested that the importance of stress distribution in relation to fatigue strength was often overlooked, and that, in fact, most so-called size effects can be explained in terms of stress gradient.

An investigation [2] carried out in parallel with the one described
above demonstrated the effect of holes on the fatigue strength of wide
thin sheets of aluminium alloy and steel. The reduction of fatigue
strength with increase in hole diameter from 1/144 to $^1/_3$ of the net

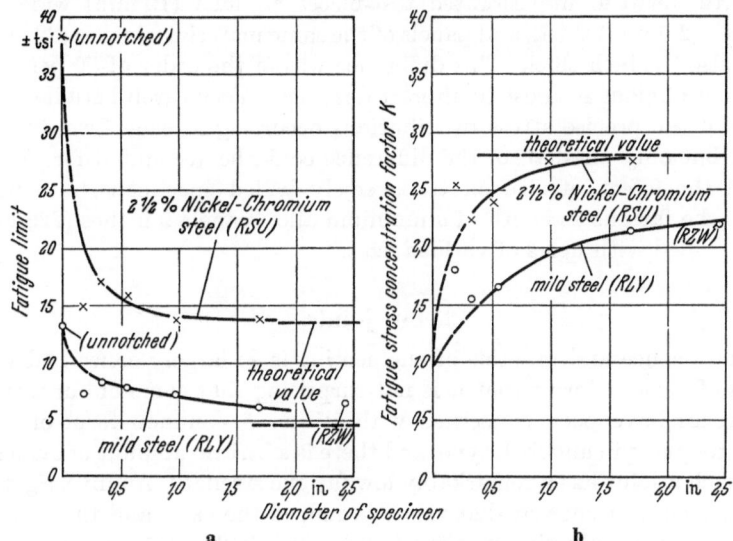

a                                        b

Fig. 1. Effect of size of transversely bored specimens
a On the fatigue limit.              b On the fatigue-strength reduction factor.

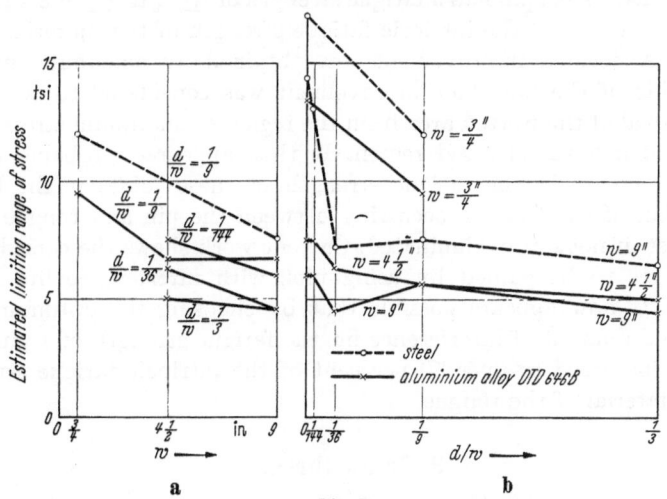

a                                        b

Fig. 2.

a Variation of fatigue limit with width of drilled test pieces ($w$)
b Variation of fatigue limit with size of hole ($d$) for test pieces of various widths ($w$)
— — ◯ — — : mild steel
——— × ····· · : aluminium alloy DTD 646 B

sheet width was over 25 per cent, but whilst, in general, the presence of a hole caused a marked reduction in fatigue strength, the smallest holes resulted in only a slight reduction, and occasionally none at all. One still unresolved anomaly in this work was the difference in fatigue strength between unperforated test-pieces $^3/_4$ inch (19 mm) wide and $^1/_{10}$ inch (2.5 mm) thick, and panels of the same material 9 inches (229 mm) wide also $^1/_{10}$ inch thick. This difference was of the order of 50 per cent, and is of obvious interest to aircraft designers. Very careful studies were made of the precise stress distributions occurring in each form of test-piece, but only one-half of the difference could be accounted for. Fig. 1 shows the effect of size on transversely-drilled specimens, and fig. 2 shows the fatigue strength of aluminium alloy panels 9 inches (229 mm) wide, drilled with holes of various sizes.

## 2. Pin joints

The science and practice of engineering is so largely concerned with joints of various forms that it is not surprising that some of our fatigue researches have been concerned with joints. A common form of joint is the tongue, pin and fork type, and there is a certain amount of evidence that such a joint has a remarkably low fatigue strength. An investigation into this subject shewed that this was indeed the case, and that a joint consisting of an aluminium alloy tongue, $2^1/_4$ inches (57 mm) wide and $^3/_4$ inch (19 mm) thick, joined to a steel fork by means of a $^3/_4$ inch (19 mm) diameter hard steel pin had a fatigue strength of $\pm^1/_2$ tsi ($\pm 0.8$ kg/mm$^2$), i. e. less than $^1/_{20}$ of the intrinsic fatigue strength of the material of the tongue. A decided improvement was obtained by machining flats on either side of the pin. The improvement was considered to be due to the removal of the fretted area from the region of maximum stress in the tongue to a lower stressed region. It thus appeared probable that a further increase in the fatigue strength of these joints might be accomplished if the fretting occurring between the pin and tongue could be almost, if not quite, eliminated. Current work shews the considerable advantages to be gained by using pins with interference fits in the tongues. It now appears possible that by choosing the optimum sizes of pin and amount of interference fit, the fatigue strength of a pin joint may be increased to over 70 per cent of the intrinsic fatigue strength of the material of the tongue.

## 3. Screw threads

The need for the unification of screw thread sizes used in American, British and Canadian practice resulted in very extensive programmes of fatigue testing of screw threads being undertaken by NPL and

continued at **MERL**. The work has included the determination of the
effect on fatigue strength of a large number of variables involved in the
production of screw threads.

Most of the work has been carried out on $^3/_4$ inch (19 mm) diameter
studs with 10 threads per inch (pitch 2.5 mm); some tests were also

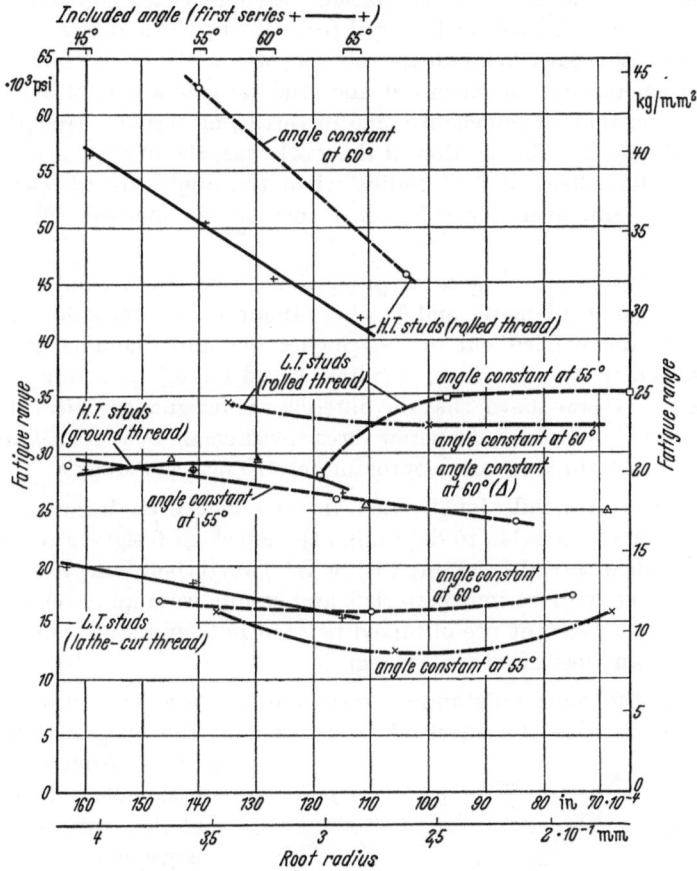

Fig. 3. Variation of fatigue strength with root radius and angle.

carried out on $^3/_8$ inch (9.5 mm) diameter and on $2^1/_2$ inches (64 mm)
diameter studs. Two stud materials and two nut materials were studied.
It was found that as far as method of production of the thread is concerned, there is little to choose between machine-cut threads and ground
threads, always provided that reasonable care in the machining operations was taken. The formation of threads from blanks by cold-rolling,
however, besides being a more rapid process, results in an increase in

fatigue strength of between 50 and 100 per cent over that of machine-cut threads.

All the screw-thread test-pieces were very accurately machined and detailed measurements taken of thread form of stud and nut of each type tested. Specimens were specially prepared so that the effect of the angle of the screw thread on the fatigue strength could be determined. The angles of thread selected ranged from 45° to 65° and covered both the British Standard Whitworth and the proposed Unified forms; the depth of engagement between nut and stud threads was kept constant. It was found that the effect of angle of thread on fatigue strength was very small (fig. 3). This section of the work was, therefore, extended to determine the effect of root radius when the angle thread was kept constant. Again, even for cold-rolled threads, no marked effect was found.

Various parts of the general programme were carried out on both $^3/_8$ inch (9.5 mm) diameter and $^3/_4$ inch (19 mm) diameter studs. A few tests were also carried out on $2^1/_2$ inches (64 mm) diameter studs of about 4 and 6 threads per inch (pitch 4 and 6 mm) to determine the effect of size. It was shewn that the difference in fatigue strength between $^3/_8$ inch and $^3/_4$ inch diameter screw threads was small, but that $2^1/_2$ inches diameter screw threads were approximately 10 per cent weaker.

After the proposals for Unified threads had been formulated, it was considered advisable to determine the effect on fatigue strength of using a Unified thread form nut with a Whitworth bolt, and vice versa. This was done with various materials and results were quite reassuring, in that the inadvertent use of mixed pairs of nuts and studs is unlikely to result in any loss of fatigue strength.

One of the most outstanding results from these tests arose from work to determine the effect of truncation on the fatigue strength. It arose from the fear occasionally expressed that loss of depth of engagement of thread between nut and bolt might result in a corresponding loss in fatigue strength. Accordingly, several series of test-pieces were prepared, in which truncation of stud thread or nut thread, or both, had been carried out to a varying degree (fig. 4). The results shewed, surprisingly enough, that reduction of depth of engagement resulted in an increase in fatigue strength; combined truncation of nut

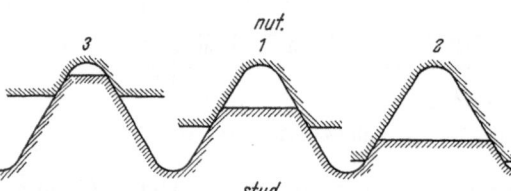

Fig. 4. Forms of truncated threads.

and stud threads giving a depth of engagement of only 25 per cent of the normal basic value, gives an overall increase in fatigue strength of 40 per cent, although the resulting product bears very little resemblance to normal screw thread practice. The strengthening effect is due to a number of causes of which the most important appears to be the more uniform load distribution due to indentation of the softer component,

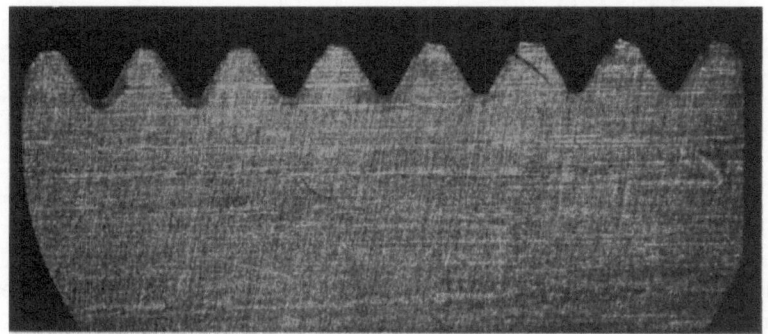

Fig. 5. Section through nut thread, tested with truncated bolt.
Note indentation of nut thread, increasing towards bearing face of nut,
and crack commencing from edge of indentation.

normally the nut. This is shewn in fig. 5, which also shews that the indentation may result in fatigue cracking; this can be avoided by rounding the crests in the bolt.

Occasionally it is necessary to use nuts which are smaller than standard, and a few tests have been carried out to determine the effect of nut height. The results indicate that failure under fatigue conditions still occurs in the stud when the nut height is reduced, even to below one-third of the standard value. The fatigue strength of the assembly decreases as the nut height is decreased, but at a much smaller rate.

## 4. Fatigue under high strain

Considerable interest has of late been shewn in the fatigue properties of materials under stresses so high that failure occurs after very short endurances. We have carried out some work in this connection, particularly in aluminium-magnesium alloy under conditions of plane bending [3]. Stress levels were chosen so that fractures were obtained at endurance ranges from less than 10 cycles to over 10 million cycles. As the specimens were subjected to constant bending moment over a parallel test section, it was possible to determine, fairly accurately, the strain applied. When the results of the tests were plotted it was found that smooth curves of strain against endurance were obtained down to the lowest endurances (fig. 6). The normal stress-endurance curve consequently shewed an initial portion almost horizontal from an

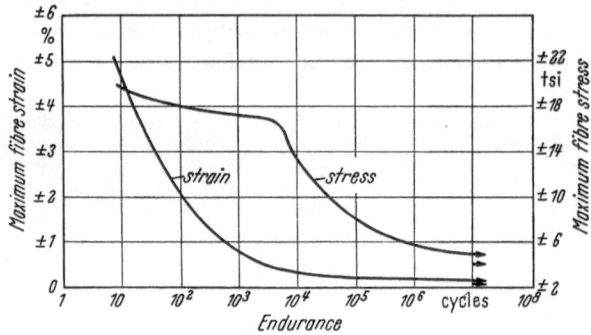

Fig. 6. Result of fatigue tests.

endurance of a few cycles up to several thousand cycles, at a stress corresponding roughly to the "yield" stress of the material.

## 5. High and medium-strength aluminium alloys

A short investigation was undertaken to explore the effect of ductility on fatigue strength of a medium-strength aluminium alloy. A large block of material was available and by selecting specimens from different parts of this block it was possible to test the material in two conditions of ductility, the tensile strength being almost the same in each case. It was found, as has been suggested by many other investigators, that there was no correlation between ductility and fatigue strength.

## 6. Crack propagation

The work on crack propagation forms the subject of a separate paper to this Conference, and therefore it will be dealt with very briefly in this resumé. The work ranges from the study of crack formation in square-section test-pieces to the fatigue strength of plain test-pieces, artificially notched by fatigue cracks. It is worth mentioning that the use of a square-section test-piece under combined tension and torsion readily permits of the study of crack initiation and propagation in relation to the directions of maximum principal tension and maximum principal shear stress.

## 7. Fatigue of surfaces in contact

Fatigue is an important factor in the life of gear teeth, not so much as causing actual breakage of teeth but as at least a contributory factor to pitting damage, which also limits the life of rolling contact bearings.

In an investigation of this type of damage, contact fatigue tests were made in which a cyclically varying load was applied between two 1 per cent carbon-chrome steel balls $1/_2$ inch and 2 inch (12.7 and 50.8 mm) in diameter; the maximum Hertzian stresses applied were three to four times those recommended in the British Standard for gear teeth, and the minimum one third the maximum.

In the hard condition (800 D.P.N.)[1] surface cracks appeared after about $6 \times 10^6$ cycles at 330 tsi (520 kg/mm$^2$); at about $10^7$ cycles an ultrasonic crack detector suggested the presence of sub-surface cracking, but in only one case was this confirmed by an electron-microscopical examination of the sectioned sphere. Spheres tempered to 350 D.P.N. shewed considerable plastic deformation, but no cracking, after $15 \times 10^6$ cycles at 250 tsi (400 kg/mm$^2$).

These results should help in the interpretation of tests on rotating discs in contact under conditions of rolling and sliding, and of back-to-back endurance tests on actual gears, both of which are in progress.

## 8. Extra-departmental researches

Arrangements are often made for researches to be sponsored by the Laboratory and carried out at a University. One such contract concerns the determination of stresses occuring in gear wheels when transmitting load. A technique has been evolved whereby photo-elastic patterns can be obtained from suitable model gears under running conditions. The work so far indicates, quite clearly, that small errors in gear manufacture may exert a profound influence on the stresses actually induced in the roots of gear teeth. Another University contract has resulted in the construction of a resonant type fatigue machine capable of testing small specimens at a speed of 60 thousand cycles per minute. Work in this machine has yielded very useful fundamental information. It has been shewn that in the case of pure copper fatigue cracks develop in areas of gross slip which occur on the surface of a specimen. Moreover, although most slip lines can be removed by electrolytic polishing, a stage during the fatigue test is eventually reached at which markings in areas of heavy slip can no longer be removed. Fatigue cracks develop from these areas of damage; the association of these areas of damage with the piling-up of dislocations which is usually associated with slip appears reasonable. It is of interest to note that in this work on pure copper, the smallest cracks detected usually extended completely across one grain; propagation of the crack from either end of this initial crack took place not necessarily in the same direction as the original crack.

---

[1] $H_v = 800$

## Bibliography

[1] PHILLIPS, C. E. and R. B. HEYWOOD: Proc. Instn mech. Engrs **165**, 113—124 (1951).
[2] PHILLIPS, C. E. and A. J. FENNER: Proc. Instn mech. Engrs **165**, 125—140 (1951).
[3] LOW, A. C.: J. Roy. aeronaut. Soc., **59**, 502—506 (1955).

## Discussion

P. E. WIENE: As quoted on page 319, [1] Burmeister & Wain has tested models of piston rods in fatigue. One of the steps to improve them was to cut down the radial height of the thread on the rod, which gave about 15% amelioration. The explanation is that bending in the thread gives stresses of the same order of magnitude as the simple tension stresses in the core. At the root of the thread those two actions add, so the crack starts here (and not at the bottom of the fillet). The single thread in the nut is subjected to higher stress and to compensate for that, the nut was made of nickel steel, the price of the nut being small as compared to the piston rod. In addition the nut was so shaped as to distribute the stresses better among the threads.

D. G. SOPWITH: I agree with WIENE's explanation of the increase in strength of his piston-rod with reduced thread height. In this case the stress in the nut would be increased but I have not found it necessary to increase the strength of the nut material; in general, I prefer the use of a nut material softer than the bolt. With regard to the improvement in stress-distribution along the nut, WIENE might be interested in the following papers:

SOPWITH, D. G.: Proc. Instn mech. Engrs **159**, 373—383 (1948)

BROWN, A. F. C. and V. M. HICKSON: Proc. Instn mech. Engrs **1 B**, 605—612 (1952—53).

# Experimental design and methods of analysis used in studying effects of metallurgical variation on fatigue

By

## R. J. Taylor

## 1. Research programme in the fatigue testing laboratory of B.I.S.R.A.

The Fatigue Section of the Metallurgy (General) Divisional Laboratory of BISRA was established at Sheffield in September 1952, but the laboratory did not commence full operation until December 1953 when the workshop facilities were completed.

It was decided that the initial research should be confined to a study of the influence of inherent metallurgical factors on the fatigue strength of alloy steels. For investigations of this nature it is desirable to subject an appreciable length of test piece to a uniform stress, thus increasing the chance for metallurgical condition to play a part in fatigue failure. Twelve testing machines of uniformly loaded rotating beam type have been installed. These machines employ a Wöhler type test which applies a uniform stress to the tested zone. Detailed descriptions of the laboratory and testing facilities are given in [1] and [2].

The performance of the machines was of primary interest and the first investigation to be completed by the laboratory was to obtain an estimate of machine variation. It was intended that the analysis of the results would also determine whether the equipment and techniques adopted by the laboratory could reproduce results within sufficiently narrow limits of variability. The material used was a mild steel to specification B. S. 970 En 4; it was thought that the results would not be obscured by the variability displayed by this material.

The planned programme was to complete six tests in each of the twelve machines; the test pieces were randomly allocated among the machines. Satisfactory results were not obtained immediately — tests were completed at two stress levels but it was found that the variability from test piece to test piece was so large that only very pronounced differences between machines could have been detected. A further 72 test pieces were prepared under closer control and the experiment was repeated at a stress level of $\pm$ 17.5 tsi. It was apparent that the variability displayed by individual test pieces had been considerably reduced.

The data were examined using the technique of analysis of variance. The variance of the complete results may be divided into two components:

1. "Between machines" variance.
2. "Within machines" variance.

The criterion used to decide whether there is a true difference between machines is the ratio of the former to the latter. This ratio is distributed as the statistic $F$ provided that the basic distribution is normal (the distribution of log life approximately fulfills this condition), and that the individual machine variances are of the same order, i. e. no machine must have produced much more or much less variable results than the others. The analysis of variance is detailed in table 1.

Table 1. *Machine comparison — Analysis of variance*
En 4. Stress Level $\pm$ 17.5 tsi

| Source of variation | Degrees of freedom | Observed variance | Expected value of variance |
|---|---|---|---|
| Between machines | 11 | 0.06481 | $\sigma_1^2 + 6\,\sigma_2^2$ |
| Within machines | 60 | 0.01997 | $\sigma_1^2$ |
| Total | 71 | — | — |

Variance ratio = 3.25 (significant, $p < 0.01$)

$\sigma_1^2$ = variance due to test pieces alone

$\sigma_2^2$ = variance due to machines alone

     = $^1/_6$ (0.06481−0.01997) = 37.4% $\sigma_1^2$

The variance ratio is 3.25, BARTLETT's significance test reveals no difference between individual machine variances, hence the probability that the ratio would be as great as or greater than 3.25 through chance may be found from tables of $F$ (degrees of freedom 11 and 60). The probability is less than 1 in 100 and it must therefore be concluded that significant differences exist between estimates of endurance obtained by different machines. The effect of machine differences is to increase the variability of results and to reduce the precision of conclusions. Table 1 shows that the variance due to the testing machines equals approximately 40% of the variance due to all other causes.

The above investigation was extended to study the differences between the BISRA and other laboratories using the Wöhler type fatigue test. The results of this investigation are more complex. The variations between laboratories are higher than that within laboratories, but it is not possible to measure the increase quantitatively. These investigations are discussed more fully in [2]. References [3] and [4] describe the statistical tests of significance mentioned in this paper.

At the present time the major project of the laboratory is an inquiry into the variations in fatigue properties, within and between ingots of the same cast. Fatigue tests have been completed for the alloy steel En 100 specification, at 60 tsi ultimate tensile strength. The alloy steel En 24 specification has been tested at 85 tsi U. T. S. and the programme is being continued for the same cast of steel but tempered to 110 tsi U. T. S. In association with the fatigue testing metallurgical examinations are being made on the steels, particular attention being paid to a study of the size, composition, distribution and shape of the inclusions.

It is too early to draw positive conclusions from the results of this investigation. For the En 100 steel, however, a small but significant difference exists between the fatigue properties of the top portion of the ingot and the remainder. There is no evidence as yet that fatigue properties vary between ingots within a cast.

The experimental procedures described above illustrate features common to many fatigue studies both in the design of the experiments and in the subsequent analysis. It is these aspects of fatigue experimentation which will be considered for the remainder of the paper.

## 2. Design of experiments

In studying the effects of metallurgical variation, many of which may be small, precautions must be taken to ensure that variation due to other factors does not mask or bias the results. This is true for all scientific inquiry but the high variability of fatigue data necessitates every effort to achieve precision.

As an example of experimental design consider the experiment comparing fatigue properties over individual casts of steel. Ten bars were selected from each of the top, middle and bottom of one ingot and from the middle portions of two other ingots. Thus five different ingot positions were to be compared and it was essential that the influence of other factors, such as testing machines, should be balanced. The experimental design is illustrated in table 2.

Table 2. *Ingot position comparison — Experimental design*
100 tests for each of five ingot positions

| Machine number | | | | |
|---|---|---|---|---|
| 10 stress levels for En 100 | (i) | (ii) | . . | (x) |
| ± 34.00 | 1.a | 2.b | . . | 10.j |
| ± 34.25 | 2.a | 3.b | . . | 1.j |
| . . | . . | . . | | . . |
| ± 36.25 | 10.a | 1.b | . . | 9.j |

Numbers 1 to 10 represent ten consecutive bars in ingot positions.
Letters a to j represent ten consecutive positions in each bar.

A test was made on material from each bar, at each of ten stress levels and in each of ten machines. The same design was used for all five ingot positions; although test pieces were cut from different bars, the ten bars were considered in rolling order and numbered in the same manner. By this means errors due to testing machines, choice of stress level and bar to bar variation, within an ingot position, were balanced. Errors due to heat treatment and to variation within bars were confounded with machine differences. The method used was to see that test lengths in the same relative position in different bars (all the b's say) were batched together for heat treatment, and then allocated to a common machine (machine (ii) for the b's). Test pieces were prepared and run to fracture in strict stress level order. Hence the effect of differences due to time factors would be indistinguishable from the effect of stress factor differences.

The particular design used in the above experiment is termed a *latin square*. The design allows errors due to machines and bars to be eliminated (along with errors due to confounded variables). Unbiassed estimates of mean endurance may be obtained at each stress level and the standard error of these estimates is a minimum. The standard statistical analysis would entail comparing estimates of endurance from each ingot position. The nature of fatigue data does not permit this at every stress level, but whatever method of analysis is used it must still estimate parameters from the collected data. For this reason it is always worth-while applying effort to find the best experimental design before commencing an investigation which will not be completed for weeks or even months. Advantages and disadvantages of alternative experimental design are discussed in [5].

## 3. Characteristics of fatigue data

The distribution of life obtained from a series of fatigue tests, at a given stress level, has two pronounced characteristics. One is the skewness of the data, the median life generally being considerably lower than the mean life. The other is the considerable scatter observed, coupled with the presence of tests yielding no failure within practicable limits. For several steels these unbroken test pieces display quite different endurance to apparently identical test pieces which do fail. It seems that at nearly every stress level there is more than one distribution of endurance. At higher stress levels a low endurance distribution is predominant, and it is characterized by skewness and high variation. As the fatigue limit is approached another distribution dominates. The form of this distribution is unknown save that each individual result lies above an arbitary value.

Little is known of the fundamentals determining these distributions but limited research on this aspect is at present being attempted by BISRA, although no results are as yet available.

## 4. Methods of analysis of results

The method of analysis used in a particular experiment will depend on the range of stress levels used. If estimates of mean endurance and associated standard error are required experimentation has to be confined to the higher stress levels. When the chosen stress is too near the fatigue limit some tests will result in a non-break and then there is no satisfactory manner to use mean endurance in the analysis. The alternative is to determine the proportion of non-breaks at a given stress level and to consider the behaviour of this parameter instead.

Standard statistical tests of significance are only applicable even at higher stress levels if no unbroken test pieces occur and if a transformation of fatigue life can be found approximating to the normal distribution. There has been a great deal of argument as to the validity of the logarithmic-normal hypothesis, be that as it may, for practical purposes the logarithmic transformation has been found adequate for many common statistical tests for several different types of steel.

Data from the experiment considering differences between ingot position, for En 100 steel, will be used to illustrate the alternative methods of analysis. At stress level $\pm$ 36.25 tsi every test resulted in a break; the analysis of variance for these fifty results is shown in table 3.

Table 3. *Ingot position comparison — Analysis of variance*
En 100.  Stress level $\pm$ 36.25 tsi

| Source of variation | Degrees of freedom | Observed variance | Variance ratio |
|---|---|---|---|
| Between ingot positions | 4 | 0.10523 | 3.29 [1] |
| Between machines | 9 | 0.02614 | 0.99 [2] |
| Residual | 36 | 0.02648 | — |
| Total | 49 | — | — |

[1] Significant $p < 0.01$
[2] Non significant

Differences between the ingot positions are found to be significant at the 1 in 100 level. The testing machines do not differ according to this analysis, but one reason for this is that the residual variance is swollen by interactions between factors involved in this study. When the mean log life is examined for each ingot position (see table 4), the top of ingot 1 is found to be chief contributor to ingot position differences.

Table 4. *Mean life at* $\pm$ 36,25 tsi

| Position ingot | Top 1 | Middle 1 | Bottom 1 | Middle 15 | Middle 31 |
|---|---|---|---|---|---|
| log $N$ | 5.74 | 5.51 | 5.49 | 5.53 | 5.54 |

In fact the "$t$ test" confirms that the remaining four ingot positions do not differ. The same analysis cannot be repeated at other stress levels as unbroken test pieces occur. The alternative technique has now to be used.

Each test must be classified as a break or non-break. The criterion used is whether the observed life exceeds some threshold value and, if it does, the test is stopped and recorded as a non-break. Otherwise the test is recorded as a break, the actual life of the test piece not now being important. The threshold value used in the present experiment was $30 \times 10^6$ cycles.

At each stress there are ten tests and of these a number $m_i$ of non-breaks. The ratio $\frac{m_i}{10}$ estimates the probability that a test will result in non-break at the $i$th stress level. The relation between these estimated probabilities and the stress levels is unknown. However if the marginal distribution of stress (or more likely log stress) is approximately normal then the probit transformation

$$\frac{m_i}{10} = p = \int_{x+5}^{\infty} \frac{1}{\sqrt{2\,\pi}}\, e^{-\frac{1}{2}\,x^2}\, dx$$

defines a variable $x$ which is linearly related to log stress [6]. The angular transformation (equivalent to replacing the ordinate of the normal curve by $\sin 2\varphi$)

$$\frac{m_i}{10} = p = \sin^2 \varphi$$

will also produce an approximate linear relation, and has the advantage of a simpler fitting procedure [7].

Another approach is of a sequential form. In this case a test is made at some convenient stress level and if a break occurs the next test is run at a stress one step lower than before. If no break occurs the next test is run at a stress raised one step. Exactly the same procedure is repeated at the new stress level. The experimental procedure and subsequent analysis are detailed in [6] and [8]. The method of analysis (which also assures the marginal distribution of log stress to be normal) is legitimate for fatigue data provided the sample is large.

These three methods are each used to estimate the fatigue limit of the material. The solution is expressed as the $x\%$ fatigue limit, which is defined as the stress level where only $(100-x)\%$ of the tests will be expected to fail before reaching the threshold value. The choice of $x$ is arbitrary as long as it is compatible with the proportion of failures observed in the stress range considered. The $50\%$ and $95\%$ fatigue limits are convenient values and it is important that the stress levels used should at least cover this range.

The main advantage of using either the probit or angular method is that a balanced experimental design may be used; this is not generally true for the staircase method. However, unlike the staircase method, the range of stress levels has to be predetermined for both probit and angular methods. In the staircase method the experiment can be stopped when the fatigue limit estimate is sufficiently precise. The precision may be determined by the size of the estimated standard error. The staircase method generally concentrates results about the 50% fatigue limit. This ensures a good estimate of the median fatigue limit but the estimate of the 95% fatigue limit, say, will not be as reliable. Two practical difficulties in the use of the staircase method are firstly the necessity of predetermining the step to be used between stress levels, and secondly the impossibility of using a multiple testing scheme with a battery of machines, as no test may be started before the result of the previous test is known.

The probit estimates of the 50% fatigue limit confirmed the results of the analysis of variance. The fatigue limit for the top of ingot 1 is expected to lie in the range 35.22—35.72 tsi, whereas the fatigue limit range for the other four ingot positions is 33.21—34.53 tsi.

Table 5 compared the estimates of fatigue limit obtained from the top of ingot 1 using all three methods of analysis. During the three analyses it is possible to check the validity of the method by means of a $\chi^2$ test of "goodness of fit". In no case was there reason to doubt the validity of the method. It is to be noted that the estimates for the 50% fatigue limit are practically identical. However at the 95% fatigue limit the estimates are not in such close agreement, particularly the large standard error of the staircase estimate of the fatigue limit.

Table 5. *Ingot position comparison — Estimates of fatigue limit*
En 100.   Top of ingot 1

| Method of analysis | 50% fatigue limit | | 95% fatigue limit | |
|---|---|---|---|---|
| | Estimate of fatigue limit | Estimate of standard error | Estimate of fatigue limit | Estimate of standard error |
| Probit . . . | 35.47 | 0.11 | 34.34 | 0.23 |
| Angular . . | 35.46 | 0.09 | 34.41 | 0.16 |
| Staircase[1] . . | 35.53 | 0.10 | 34.43 | 0.36 |

[1] Although the experiment was not conducted in the manner required by the staircase method, nevertheless the analysis is still applicable as the stress levels were equally spaced and comprehensive for this ingot position. It was assumed that the results came from only one machine but in the same order as they occurred in the actual experiment.

The estimate of the fatigue limit obtained by any of the three methods described must be dependent in part on the initial threshold value. In general as the threshold value increases the fatigue limit will decrease. The threshold value is usually determined on the basis of past experience. However if the material exhibits two endurance distributions, as observed for some steels, it may be possible to run tests to a lower threshold value. The 50% fatigue limit may be defined as the stress level at which the two endurance distributions are equally represented. Then the threshold value need be chosen only to exceed all likely values in the lower distribution. Table 6 shows that the estimate of fatigue limit remains unaltered for an appreciable range of threshold values. In this analysis, of 400 tests, a threshold value of $10 \times 10^6$ (log $N = 7.00$) could have been used instead of $30 \times 10^6$ (log $N = 7.47$). The saving in this instance would have exceeded $100 \times 10^6$ cycles.

Table 6. *Sensitivity of fatigue limit estimate*
En 100. (Excluding top of ingot 1)

| Threshold value log $N$ | Number of non-breaks | Estimate of 50% fatigue limit |
|---|---|---|
| 7.50 | 60 | 32.40 |
| 7.47[1] | 64 | 32.43 |
| 7.25 | 64 | 32.43 |
| 7.00 | 64 | 32.43 |
| 6.75 | 65 | 32.43 |
| 6.50 | 66 | 32.43 |
| 6.25 | 76 | 32.55 |
| 6.00 | 122 | 33.60 |

[1] Threshold value used in the experiment.

## 5. Conclusions

a) In planning an investigation to study the effect of metallurgical differences, the variation introduced by extraneous factors must be exactly balanced in the experimental design.

b) The influence of metallurgical factors on the endurance of steel can only be determined at stress levels well above the fatigue limit. It is then legitimate to use standard statistical techniques if the logarithmic-normal hypothesis is acceptable for the endurance distribution of the steel.

c) The fatigue limit can be estimated from balanced experiments by the use of either the probit or the angular sigmoidal transformation. The probit method has a sounder theoretical justification, but the angular method reduces the effort necessary for computation.

d) If multiple testing is not used an economic and precise estimate of the 50% fatigue limit can be obtained by use of a sequential method of experimentation.

e) Any estimate of the fatigue limit will depend on the criterion used to decide whether a test is a non-break. Owing to the nature of the endurance distribution for steels, the fatigue limit does not appear sensitive to small changes in the threshold value.

### Bibliography

[1] CLAYTON-CAVE, J. and E. INESON: Metal Treatment, **20**, 553—556 (1953).
[2] CLAYTON-CAVE, J., R.J. TAYLOR and E. INESON: J.Iron St.Inst., **180**, 161—169 (1955).
[3] TIPPETT, L. H. C.: Methods of Statistics, New York 1952.
[4] GOULDEN, C. H.: Methods of Statistical Analysis, New York 1952.
[5] FISHER, R. A.: The Design of Experiments, Edinburgh 1949.
[6] FINNEY, D. J.: Probit Analysis, Cambridge 1952.
[7] FISHER, R. A. and F. YATES: Statistical Tables for Biological, Agricultural and Medical Research, London 1948.
[8] Report submitted by the Statistical Research Group, Princeton University, to the Applied Mathematics Panel, Statistical Analysis for a New Procedure in Sensitivity Experiments, AMP Rep. Nr. 101. 1 R, SRG-P Nr. 40.

### Discussion

F. TURNER questioned the value of smooth test pieces and if it would not be possible to develop a standard notched test piece.

R. J. TAYLOR: For fundamental research work polished test pieces should be preferred, as a greater volume then will be tested.

P. KUHN: It is not easy to produce a suitable standard notch.

# A contribution to the theory of the fatigue of metals

By

## G. V. Uzhik

With 6 figures

Research into the causes of the fatigue of metals has been going on continously for many years now. However, neither X-ray analysis [1], [2], [3] nor microscopic study of the structural changes that take place during repeated loading [4], [5], [6] have permitted elucidation up to now of the origin of the limiting state at which, long before any visible effects appear, latent destruction of the metal begins that invariably leads to fracture.

At the same time, the research done has revealed some of the conditions that give rise to fatigue. Most important of these, and indisputable, are the following:

a) Fatigue fracture starts, as a rule, at points of stress concentration, i. e., at notches such as grooves, fillets, holes, scratches, cavities, slag inclusions, etc.

b) The process of fatigue is always accompanied by repeated local microplastic deformation as a shear or displacement of the grains along their boundaries.

c) Under the action of repeated microplastic deformation the shearing strength, yield stress, hardness, etc. of the metal increase with an increase in the number of cycles.

To elucidate the causes of fatigue the following highly important questions must first of all be examined.

1. How and under what conditions does initial plastic deformation develop at the points of stress concentration?

2. What happens in the concentration zone after formation of plastic strain? What will the distribution of stresses be in this zone?

3. Does any further re-distribution of stresses take place under the action of repeated plastic deformation? This question may be put in still another way. Is there any difference in the distribution of the stresses in the concentration zone, when the load is applied just once and when the same load is applied a certain number of cycles $N$?

## 1. Formation of initial plastic deformation in the zone of stress concentration

To elucidate the conditions of formation of the initial plastic deformation in the concentration zone, it is necessary to examine the state
of stress at the points of maximum stress. In most of the published
papers [7], [8], [9] it is shown that these points are to be found where
there is a change of section, i. e. at the bottom of various notches such
as grooves, holes, etc. (Points A and B in fig. 1).

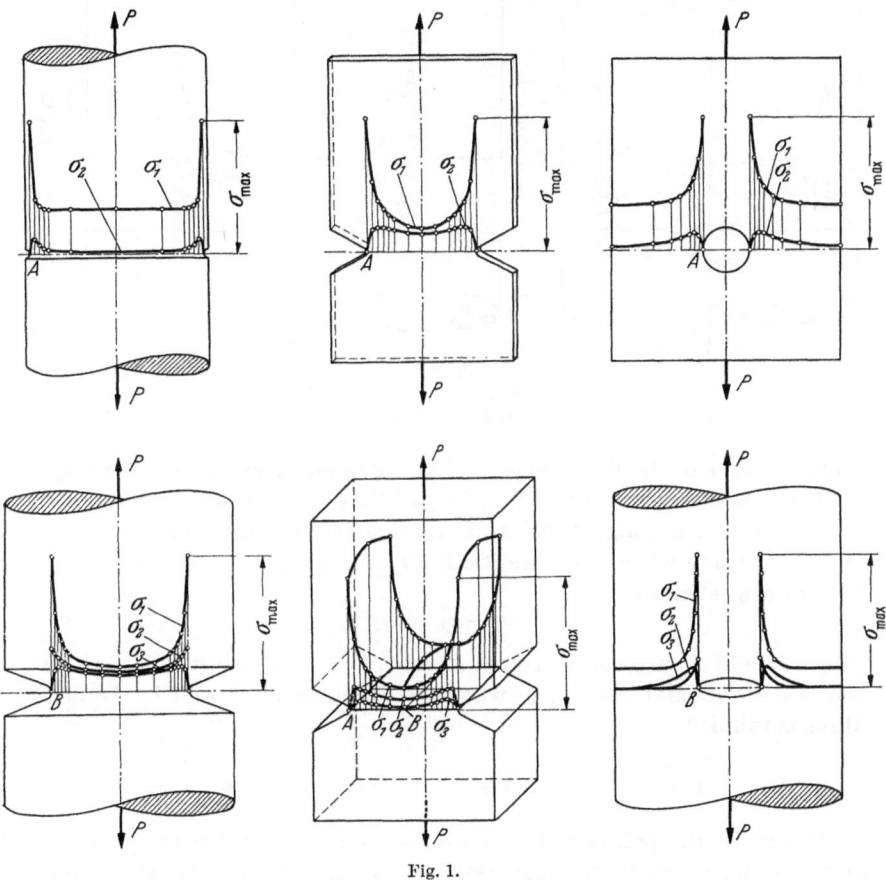

Fig. 1.

With respect to the difference in character of the state of stress at
these points, most of the known stress raisers [7], [8], [9] may be divided
into two main groups:

a) All those where the state of stress at the bottom of the notch
(points A in fig. 1) is uniaxial, and near the bottom biaxial ($\sigma_1 > \sigma_2 > 0$).

These may be regarded as uniaxial without great error, the second component $\sigma_2$ being very small;

b) All those where the state of stress at the bottom of the notch (points B in fig. 1) is biaxial, and near the bottom triaxial ($\sigma_1 > \sigma_2 > \sigma_3 > 0$).

Here we shall consider the above questions by examining how they apply to two specimens with different notches (fig. 2), each of which is

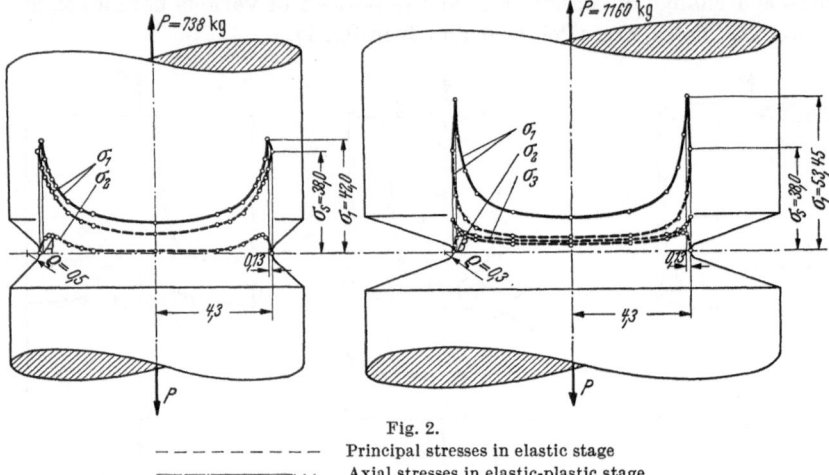

Fig. 2.
– – – – – – – – –    Principal stresses in elastic stage
————————— · · ·    Axial stresses in elastic-plastic stage

representative of the first and second group of stress raisers respectively.

It has been shown [10], [11], [12], [13] that, in the case of a combined and non-uniform state of stress, formation of the initial plastic deformation occurs, when the conditions of plasticity advanced by Saint Venant are satisfied

$$\sigma_1 - \sigma_3 = \sigma_s \tag{1}$$

where $\sigma_1$ and $\sigma_3$ are the principal stresses and $\sigma_s$ is the yield stress in the case of uniaxial tension, or when the condition advanced by Huber-Mises is fulfilled

$$\sqrt{\frac{1}{2}\left[ (\sigma_1 - \sigma_2)^2 + (\sigma_2 - \sigma_3)^2 + (\sigma_3 - \sigma_1)^2 \right]} = \sigma_s \tag{2}$$

Hence, at the points of maximum stress concentration (at points A and B in fig. 1 and 2), one may assume that, in cases of biaxial tension, and all the more so of uniaxial tension, the initial plastic deformation will form in accordance with conditions (1) or (2).

This means that under increasing load the maximum stress in the concentration zone shall stop increasing when $\sigma_1$ reaches the value of the yield stress, i. e. when

$$\sigma_{\max} = \sigma_s$$

An experimental study of the stresses in the concentration zone both at elastic and elastic-plastic deformations was made by MÖLLER and NEERFELD [14] employing the X-ray method. The data obtained, part of which are given in fig. 3, deserve special attention inasmuch as the X-ray method permits the base of the measurements to be extended

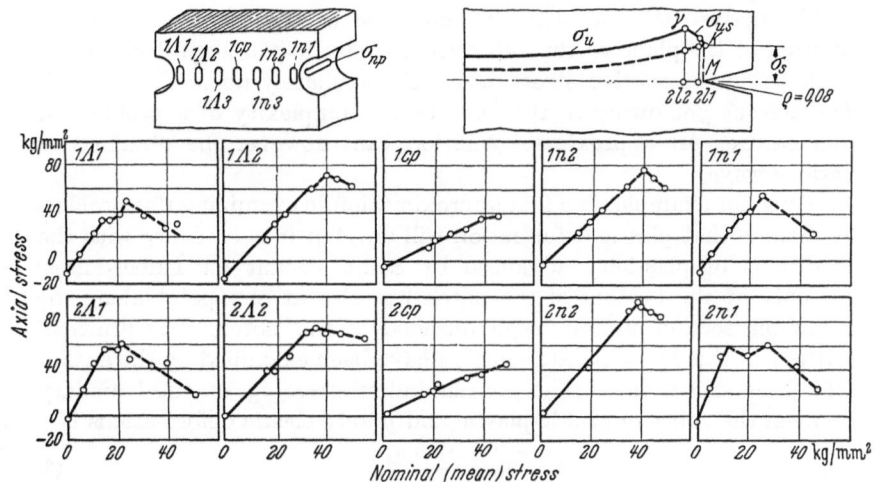

Fig. 3.

Distribution of axial stresses in elastic-plastic stage of loading according to X-ray research [14]. Distance between bottom of the notch and

point 1 Λ 1 is 0.5 mm
,,    1 Λ 2 is 2.5 mm
,,    1 c p is 40.0 mm

0.5—0.7 mm under the surface of the metal specimens, and as it is practically the only possibility of studying the stress concentrations.

In fig. 3 the graphs express the dependence of the axial stresses upon the mean (nominal) stresses along the section; the upper row refers to the front side and the lower row to the backside of the specimen. These data made it possible to establish the following:

a) A noticeable plastic deformation forms and the maximum stress $\sigma_{max}$ at the bottom of the notch (point M in fig. 3) stops increasing, when $\sigma_{max}$ has sufficiently approached $\sigma_s$. This testifies to the fact that, at the bottom of the notch the plastic deformation forms in accordance with the conditions of plasticity advanced by Saint Venant or Huber-Mises.

b) After the stresses have exceeded the yield stress at the corner of the discontinuity (point M in fig. 3), one by no means observes their equalization.

c) Plastic deformation spreads in a direction from the bottom of the notch to the central part of the section; an increase in stress occurs in the zone of plastic deformation; approximately the same character of distribution of stresses is retained in the elastically deformed zone as at the stage of purely elastic deformations along the entire section.

## 2. Redistribution of stresses in their concentration zone at the elastic-plastic stage of deformation

To analyse this problem one must be in possession of an exact solution of the plane or three-dimensional elastic-plastic problem applicable to one or another stress raiser. Unfortunately no such solution is available as yet owing to the exceptional complexity of a problem of this nature. An approximate solution can, however, be obtained in various ways.

Thus, for example, as a first approximation in examining this problem we assume that plastic deformation will develop in accordance with the conditions of plasticity advanced by Saint Venant (or Huber-Mises) not only at the bottom of the notch but also at any point along the minimum section in the neighbourhood of the notch. The principal features of this approximate solution have been examined by the author [15]. It is shown there that the maximum stress $\sigma_{1s}$ on the boundary between the zones of elastic-plastic and purely elastic deformations is

$$\sigma_{1s} = \frac{\sigma_1 \cdot \sigma_s}{\sigma_1 - \sigma_3} \tag{3}$$

where $\sigma_1$ and $\sigma_3$ are the principal stresses at any point of the minimum cross section, corresponding to the load under which the stress $\sigma_1$ has reached the value of the yield stress $\sigma_s$ in the extreme fiber (points A and B in fig. 1).

Distribution of the stresses in accordance with (3) is shown in fig. 2 and 6. As can be seen, there is a noticeable difference in the character of the stress distribution for the two groups of raisers mentioned earlier (fig. 1, points A and B). For the first group, with approximately uniaxial tension near the bottom of the notch, spread of the plastic deformations is accompanied by a relatively small increase in axial stresses (fig. 2 left). For the second group with a state of stress in the form of a triaxial unequal tension, increase in the plasticized zone is accompanied by a substantial increase in axial stresses, which is all the greater, the sharper the notch and the smaller the difference ($\sigma_1 - \sigma_3$) at the points near the bottom of the notch (fig. 2 right).

## 3. Change in stress distribution in the concentration zones during cyclic loading

The indicated approximate distribution of stresses was obtained for a single application of load. Will this stress distribution be retained and will the plasticized zone remain unchanged at repeated loading? The answer to this question was obtained indirectly by determining the change in shearing strength (yield stress) during symmetrical cycles of tension and compression of polished specimens with stress ranges equal to or greater than the yield stress. These experiments were carried out by the author [15], and also by N. N. DAVIDENKOV and G. G. NAZARENKO [16].

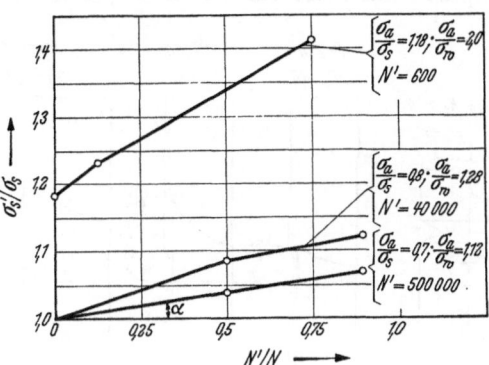

Fig. 4.

In our experiments specimens of normalized 0.45% carbon steel were tested, which had tensile strength $\sigma_B = 62.0$ kg/mm²; $\sigma_s = 38.0$ kg/mm²; $\psi = 65\%$. The tests were performed with different ratios of $\sigma_a/\sigma_s$ and $\sigma_a/\sigma_w$, where $\sigma_a$ is the stress amplitude and $\sigma_w$ the endurance limit. For a given $\sigma_a$ the number of cycles to fracture $N$ was first determined. Then at the same $\sigma_a$ specimens were run a number of cycles $N'$ less than $N$. At, for example $N' = 0.5\ N$, the specimen was unloaded and its yield stress $\sigma_s'$ determined.

The data obtained, given in fig. 4 and 5, showed that when $\sigma_a/\sigma_s = 1.0$ and especially when $\sigma_a/\sigma_s > 1.0$, there is a substantial increase in shearing strength and yield stress. In the case where $\sigma_a/\sigma_w = 1.0$, no increase whatsoever in the yield stress was observed even after $3 \cdot 10^6$ cycles.

A thorough investigation was carried out by N. N. DAVIDENKOV and G. G. NAZARENKO [16] with Steel 20 ($\sigma_s = 23.0$; $\sigma_B = 41.0\ \psi = 69\%$)

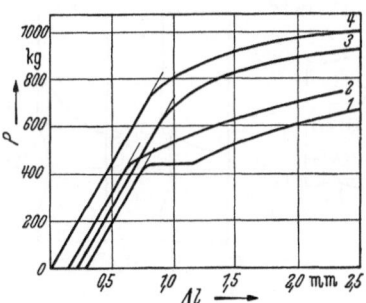

Fig. 5. Static tension curves after different number of load cycles (mild steel, [16]).

1. $\dfrac{\sigma_a}{\sigma_s} = 0.78$; $N' = 5 \cdot 10^5$

2. $\dfrac{\sigma_a}{\sigma_s} = 0.78$; $N' = 5 \cdot 10^6$

3. $\dfrac{\sigma_a}{\sigma_s} = 0.85$; $N' = 10 \cdot 10^4$

4. $\dfrac{\sigma_a}{\sigma_s} = 1.0$; $N' = 3.4 \cdot 10^4$

and with Steel 60G (0.66% C and 0.94% Mn; $\sigma_s = 37.0$; $\sigma_B = 84.0$; $\psi = 28\%$). The increase in the yield stress for Steel 20 was 45% when $\sigma_a/\sigma_s = 0.8$, and 65% when $\sigma_a/\sigma_s = 1.0$. The change in character of the tensile test diagrams after various cyclic loads is shown in fig. 5.

Naturally, in the stress concentration zone there should also be a rise in the yield stress under the action of repeated deformation, a rise that

becomes ever larger with increase in the number of cycles, which may
be even greater than that detected during the tension and compression
of smooth specimens (fig. 5 and 6).

As the yield stress increases there should be gradual and uninterrupted transition from the elastic-plastic state to the purely elastic state.

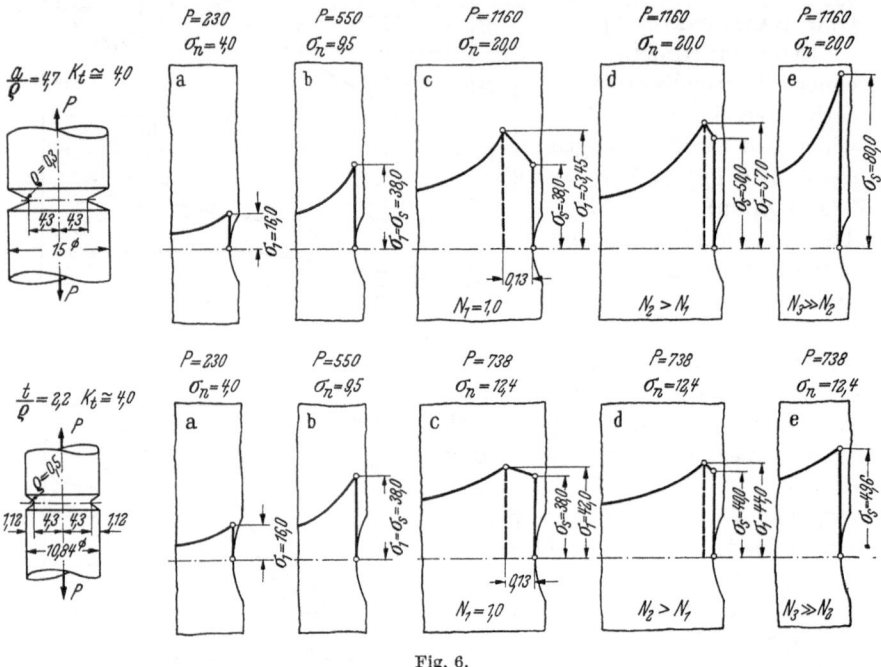

Fig. 6.

The most important feature of this transition, which is of decisive importance for elucidating one of the main causes of the fatigue of metals,
is that the continuous increase in shearing strength in the concentration
zone is accompanied by a corresponding continuous increase in stresses,
the magnitude of the applied loads being constant. The greater the
stress concentration, the larger this stress increase turns out to be
(see fig. 6). It is quite possible that this process may end up in two ways:

a) If the ever increasing stress $\sigma_{max}$ reaches a value equal to the
ultimate strength, then rupture will occur and a fatigue crack will form.

b) If, on the other hand, in the zone of maximum concentration the
transition from elastic-plastic to purely elastic deformation with a corresponding increase in $\sigma_{max}$ is completed, and $\sigma_{max}$ does not reach the value
of $R_N$, fatigue cracks can not immediately occur. However, under the
repeated action of $\sigma_{max}$ the weakening of the metal bond may continue

and, hence, the decrease in ultimate strength $R_N$ may continue until the condition of rupture $\sigma_{max} = R_N$ has been satisfied.

But there is another outcome of the completion of transition that may also be considered quite probable, namely, that the resistance to rupture proves to be greater than $\sigma_{max}$. Then the repeated action of $\sigma_{max}$ can not lead to rupture.

It is known that various metals are capable of enduring repeated plastic deformation of a certain (critical) value, whose action already does not give rise to the continuous increase in shearing strength (or yield stress) mentioned above. In this case rupture from fatigue will likewise not take place.

From the point of view of the mechanism under consideration an estimate of the ability of various metals to change their shearing strength under the action of repeated plastic deformation becomes of great importance. It is perfectly obvious that metal will resist alternating loads better, for which the angle $\alpha$ of the curve $f(N) = \sigma_s'/\sigma_s$ in fig. 4 is the smallest. Here $\sigma_s$ = yield stress without repeating and $\sigma_s'$ = yield stress efter $N$ load cycles.

Of no less importance from this point of view is a study of the change in resistance to rupture that occurs under the action of repeated loading. Available data [1], [4], [5], [6] show that under alternating loading there is a weakening of the structure, loosening of the material making up separate grains, decrease in the cohesion between separate blocks within each grain, and so forth. Of course such a process cannot but lead to a weakening of the inter- and intracrystalline bonds and to a substantial lowering in the resistance to rupture. However, exceedingly little has been done to elucidate this question, in view of the great difficulty encountered in studying it [16].

The above explanation of a number of questions in the mechanism of fatigue fracture is not in accordance with the concept of this mechanism given by AFANASYEV [4] and by OROWAN [17]. According to them, there is a continuous increase in stresses in a separate grain or group of grains when the stresses exceed the fatigue limit, until the resistance to rupture has been reached. But their hypothesis does not explain what gives rise to such an uninterrupted growth in stresses and why it should continue up to destruction. The explanation we are offering does not make stress increase up to rupture a necessary condition.

In fact, however, it would be incorrect to consider the fundamental and sole cause of fatigue to be the increase in stress, as follows from the hypothesis of AFANASYEV and OROWAN. As the data in fig. 4 to 6 show, the cause of rupture from fatigue cannot be explained by the increase in stress alone. Even when we consider this increase in the concentration zone, where it is much greater than the value given by Afanasyev and Orowan, the magnitude of the stresses still proves to be not large enough to overcome the resistance to rupture. Better grounded, it must be admitted, is the point of view of N. N. Davidenkov [16], according to which the increase in shearing strength, and accordingly in stress, should be accompanied, by a weakening in the intra- and intercrystalline bonds, loosening up the material, and a substantial lowering in resistance to destruction. Thus, *the cause of fatigue is development of these two co-operating processes: increase in shearing strength together with redistribution and increase of stresses in their concentration zone, and simultaneously decrease in resistance to rupture in the same zone during cyclic loading.*

An attempt was made to establish the character of the change (the decrease) in resistance to rupture with an increase in the number of cycles. Resistance to rupture was determined by a method devised by the author [15] for specimens with special notches at normal temperature, and also for polished smooth specimens at a temperature of $-253°$C (liquid hydrogen). The data obtained did not reveal any essential lowering in resistance to rupture under the action of cyclic loading. It is quite probable that a considerable weakening in the metal bond and a substantial lowering in resistance to rupture are localized only to exceptionally small areas. Therefore, since this resistance is determined as the mean for the whole sectional area, it is not possible to detect. To study resistance to rupture during repeated loading, new means and methods are evidently needed.

## Bibliography

[1] Gough, H. I. and W. A. Wood: Proc. Roy. Soc. (A), **154**, 510 (1936). also Proc. Instn mech. Engrs, **141**, 175 (1939).

[2] Kogan, G. and U. Terminasov: Zhur. Techn. Fiziki,' **14**, 781 and 873 (1944).

[3] Terminasov, U.: Factory Laboratory, 1952, Nr. 10, 1213.

[4] Afanasyev, N. N.: Zhur. Techn. Fiziki, **14**, 639 (1944).

[5] Bullen, F., A. K. Head and W. A. Wood: Proc. Roy. Soc. (A), **216**, 332 (1953)

[6] Head, A. K.: J. Mech. Phys. Solids, **1**, 134 (1953).

[7] Neuber, G.: Stress Concentration, Russian Ed. 1947.

[8] Timoshenko, S. P.: Theory of Elasticity, New York and London 1934.

[9] Frocht, M.: Photoelasticity, Russian Ed. 1952.

[10] Ilyushin, A. A.: Plasticity, Moscow 1948.

[11] Sokolovsky, V. V.: The Theory of Plasticity (1949).

[12] Hill, R.: The Mathematical Theory of Plasticity, Oxford 1951.

[13] Nadai, A.: Theory of Flow and Fracture of Solids, New York 1950.

[14] Möller, H. and H. Neerfeld: Jb. deutsch. Luftfahrt-Forschung, 314 (1941).

[15] Uzhik, G. V.: Resistance to Brittle Rupture and Strength of Metals, Moscow 1950.

[16] Davidenkov, N. N. and G. G. Nazarenko: Zhur. Techn. Fiziki, 23, 1953.

[17] Orowan, E.: Proc. Roy. Soc. (A), 171, 79 (1939).

## Discussion

R. Hiltscher: Als Ergänzung zu Herrn Uzhiks Vortrag möchte ich noch auf ein von mir entwickeltes spannungsoptisches Verfahren (Z. VDI, 97, 49—58, 1955) hinweisen, mit Hilfe dessen sich die von Herrn Uzhik berechnete elastisch-plastische Spannungsverteilung an Kerben studieren läßt. An Hand des Versuches von Abb. 1 sei das Prinzip dargestellt. Für das Modell-material (Polystyrol) gilt im Druckgebiet die Fließ-hypothese der maximalen Gestaltänderung. Im elasti-schen Gebiet erhält man dabei die üblichen Isochromen und Isoklinen, aus denen sich der elastische Spannungs-zustand bestimmen läßt. Bei Erreichung der Elastizi-tätsgrenze wird ein Maximum der Isochromenordnung erreicht. Als Folge des plastischen Fließens sinkt dann die Ordnung infolge eines besonderen photoplastischen Effektes wieder ab. Der Punkt der $\sigma$-$\varepsilon$-Linie, in dem Vollplastizierung erreicht ist, fällt im Isochromenbild ungefähr mit dem Wiedererreichen der Nullordnung zusammen. Die so zu gewinnende Einteilung des Spannungsfeldes in 1. elastisches Gebiet mit bekanntem Spannungszustand, 2. Übergangsgebiet und 3. voll-plastisches Gebiet mit konstantem Spannungszustand wird in den Abb. 2 und 3 auf eine Halbrund- und eine Spitzkerbe angewandt. Besonders auffallend ist für den Fall der Spitzkerbe die Teilung des Fließgebiets in zwei Äste, während auf der Symmetrieachse der Kerbe das Fließen stark behindert ist. Die Spannungsverteilung um einen Riß als Extremfall der Spitzkerbe wurde von Post (Proc. Soc. exp. Stress Anal., 12, Nr. 1, 99—113, 1954) spannungsoptisch untersucht, allerdings nur für das elastische Gebiet. Charakteristisch ist für diesen Fall, daß die Isochromenordnung auf der Symme-trieachse durch den Riß gleich Null ist. Das heißt, daß das Gebiet vor dem Riß in der Modellebene schub-spannungsfrei ist, bei dickeren Modellen praktisch auch in den beiden anderen Symmetrieebenen, so daß die Fließbehinderung im Falle des Risses noch wesentlich größer als bei der Kerbe ist. Die Frage der makroskopi-schen Spannungsverteilung an Kerbe und Riß läßt sich somit weitgehend klären. Ob damit aber ein wesent-licher Beitrag zum Studium der Ausbreitung von Dauer-brüchen erreicht ist, scheint fraglich, da die für Elasti-zitätstheorie und Spannungsoptik vorausgesetzte Ho-mogenität des Materials nicht in den mikroskopischen Dimensionen der polykristallinen Materie zutrifft.

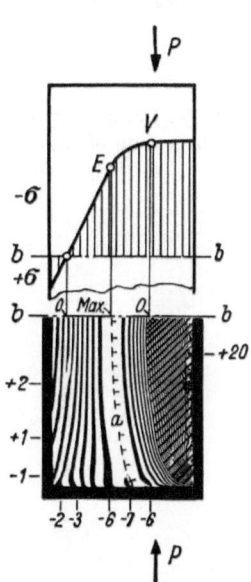

Abb. 1. Aufteilung des ela-stisch-plastischen Spannungs-feldes in einem außermittig gedrückten Prisma durch das Maximum und den Nulldurch-gang im Isochromenbild.

*Oben:* Verteilung der Span-nung $\sigma$ (über den Querschnitt b-b vom unteren Bild)

E: Elastizitätsgrenze

V: Grenze des vollplasti-schen Gebietes

*Unten:* Isochromenbild. Die Zahlen geben die Isochromen-ordnung an, der schraffierte Teil entspricht dem vollpla-stischen Gebiet.

a: Grenze des elastischen Ge-bietes.

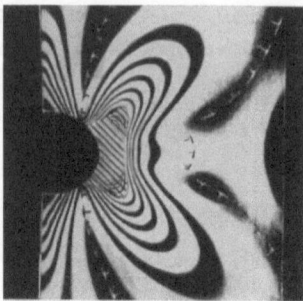

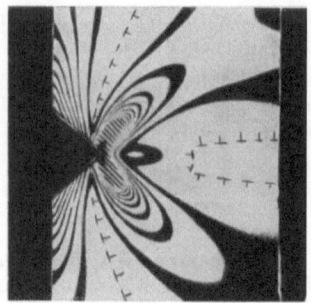

Abb. 2. Isochromenbild einer Halb-
kreiskerbe bei elastisch - plastischem
Spannungszustand

Abb. 3. Isochromenbild einer Spitzkerbe bei elastisch-plastischem Spannungszustand.

⊥ ⊥ ⊥ ⊥   Elastizitätsgrenze

/ / / / / / /   vollplastisches Gebiet

G. V. UZHIK: I wish to thank HILTSCHER for his interesting discussion and for his suggestion of experimental stress analysis at the elastic-plastic stage of deformation by a new method.

# Basic aspects of fatigue

By

## W. Weibull

With 5 figures

It is convenient to think of a specimen under repeated stresses as undergoing a progressive, accumulating damage. This concept has been applied to the total fatigue process with more or less success, in some cases leading to controversial opinions.

The purpose of this paper is to demonstrate that some of the difficulties may be eliminated, if due consideration is taken to the fact that the fatigue process consists of two stages of quite different nature: the crack *initiation* and the crack *propagation*, and if the concept of cumulative damage is applied, not to the total complex process, but to a single point of the specimen, during the first stage that point where the crack is suspected to start, and during the second stage an arbitrary point at the prospective path of the crack.

If $D$ denotes the damage, by definition equal to $100\%$ when fracture occurs, and $N$ any number of stress cycles, the damage factor $k$ may be defined by

$$D = k \cdot N \tag{1}$$

The damage factor is a function as well of the stress as of the strength of the material (and possibly also of $N$ which for the present will be neglected).

The real stress field within the specimen is composed of the smooth nominal stress, calculated according to the theory of elasticity and denoted by $\sigma$, and local stress concentrations, caused by scratches, inclusions or similar stress raisers, whereas the real strength may be that of the idealized material, weakened by dislocations and imperfections of microscopical and macroscopical nature.

In this way, we may visualize a $k$-field within the specimen with statistically distributed local maxima.

If this field does not change under the influence of the pulsating load (which in fact it sometimes does), it is obvious that the first crack starts at the point with the highest $k$-value. In most cases this point is located at the surface of the specimen.

After some time, other cracks may appear. It is not absolutely excluded that the first crack stops to grow and that someone of the later
ones will develop into the final rupture, because of the possibility that
the first crack may change the initial $k$-field.

From a phenomenological viewpoint, we may describe the $k$-field in
the vincinity of a local stress raiser at $x_0$ by the expression

$$k = f_0 \left[ \sigma, (x - x_0) \right] \tag{2}$$

where $\sigma$ is the nominal stress and $x$ a coordinate along the prospective
path of the crack (limiting us for the present to the one-dimensional

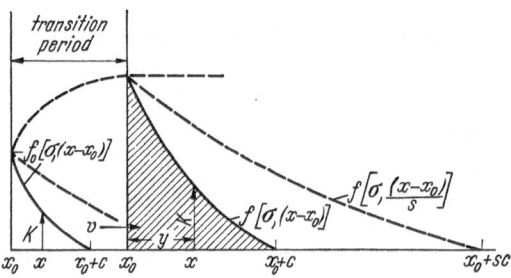

Fig. 1. Geometric distribution of the damage factor $k$.

case). This expression is
illustrated by fig. 1. The
value of $k$ falls off rapidly
from its maximum value
at $x_0$ to zero at $(x_0 + c)$,
that point where the real
stress is equal to the endurance limit. (It is tacitly
understood that there is
a one-to-one relationship
between the real and the
nominal stresses).

*The first stage* is characterized by the condition that $x_0$ is a fixed
point, for instance the bottom of an initial surface scratch. Accordingly,

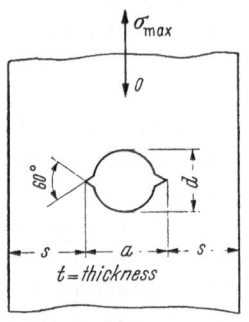

$s = 20$ mm.
$d = 4$ "
$r = 0.10$ "
$a = 5.50$ "
$t = 2$ "

Fig. 2. Test specimen.

the damage $D$ in an arbitrary point $x$ increases
in proportion to the value of $k$ under the influence of a constant stress amplitude. After a
certain number of stress cycles, denoted by $N_0$,
the damage reaches the value 100% at $x_0$ and
the crack starts moving. This is the end of the
first stage.

By (1) and (2), we have

$$N_0 = 1/f_0 (\sigma, 0) \tag{3}$$

As a consequence of the preceding considerations, two general conclusions may be drawn.
First, since $f_0 (\sigma, 0)$ depends on the surface
conditions (scratches, imperfections and the like)
the quantity $N_0$ is a random variable with large
scatter. Second, the probability of encounter-
ing heavy stress raisers increases with the surface
area. In other words, a considerable size effect is to be expected on $N_0$.

Both conclusions have been verified experimentally by means of
plate specimens as shown in fig. 2. In most of the tests, the central

hole was provided with two sharp V-notches in order to facilitate the simultaneous start of the cracks (left and right). The stress was pulsated between a maximum value $\sigma_{max}$ and zero. The quantity $N_{10}$ i.e. the number of cycles at which the crack has developed to 10% of the width, has been used as a measure of the duration of the first stage, thus including the transition period (see below). As a measure of the propagation time, the difference $(N_B - N_{10})$ has been chosen, where $N_B$ denotes the number of stress cycles at failure. The coefficients of variation $V$ computed show (see table 1) that the scatter of the crack initiation is extremely high, particularly if the extra notches are absent.

Table 1. *Scatter of* $N_{10}$, $N_B$, *and* $(N_B - N_{10})$

| Material | $\sigma_{max}$ kg/mm² | Coefficient of variation | | | Extra notches |
|---|---|---|---|---|---|
| | | of $N_{10}$ % | of $N_B$ % | of $(N_B - N_{10})$ % | |
| 24 S-T | 15.6 | 37.1 | 34.0 | 2.2 | No |
| 24 S-T | 12.0 | 31.2 | 27.6 | 3.8 | No |
| 24 S-T | 8.0 | 8.2 | 5.3 | 3.4 | Yes |
| 75 S-T | 7.0 | 19.8 | 17.0 | 10.6 | Yes |
| 75 S-T[1] | 7.0 | 24.4 | 20.5 | 8.5 | Yes |
| Cr-Mo Steel $\sigma_B = 90$ kg/mm² | 19.0 | 51.1 | 36.7 | 14.5 | Yes |
| $\sigma_B = 70$ kg/mm² | 19.0 | 2.6 | 4.1 | 9.0 | Yes |

[1] Coated with kerosene

The size effect on geometrically similar specimens is demonstrated in table 2. It may be concluded that the diameter of the hole is responsible for the large size effect. The difference between the values of the $50 \cdot 10$ and $10 \cdot 10$ mm specimens, 76 and 111 respectively, is considered to be due to the different stress concentration. The values of $K_t$

Table 2. *Size effect on* $N_{10}$
Material: 24 S-T, Alclad; $\sigma_{max} = 80$ kg/mm²

| $s$ mm | $d$ mm | $r$ mm | $N_{10}$ kc | $K_t$ | Plate marked |
|---|---|---|---|---|---|
| 10 | 2 | 0.05 | 506 | 2.64 | 1 |
| 20 | 4 | 0.10 | 99 | 2.64 | 1 |
| 30 | 6 | 0.15 | 82 | 2.64 | 1 |
| 50 | 10 | 0.25 | 76 | 2.64 | 2 |
| 10 | 10 | 0.25 | 111 | 2.27 | 2 |
| 50 | 50 | 1.25 | 54 | 2.64 | 2 |

Tabled values of $N_{10}$ are averages of 3 tests each.

give the theoretical stress concentration of holes without extra notches which are assumed to raise the stress concentration proportionally because of the geometrical similarity.

*The second stage* is characterized by the condition that $x_0$, now denoting the tip of the crack, is a moving point. The rate of crack propagation $v$ is defined by

$$v = \mathrm{d}\,x_0/\mathrm{d}\,N \tag{4}$$

At the beginning of this stage, the material just in front of the crack has suffered a certain amount of damage which is very nearly 100%. The curve of $f_0$ (but not $f$) thus represents the distribution of the damage by using a scale which makes the ordinate at $x_0$ equal to 100%. It is easily understood that a less sloped curve, as indicated by the dotted lines in fig. 1, corresponds to a larger rate of propagation.

During the crack propagation, the $k$-curve is moving with $x_0$, in the most simple case without changing its shape. This seems to happen, when the tip of the crack is well away from the initiating scratch. Thus $k$ is changing during a "transition period" from $f_0$ successively to a stable form $f$. It seems as generally $f_0\,(\sigma, 0) < f(\sigma, 0)$, but sometimes the reverse may happen, depending on the stress raising effect of the initial crack.

A fixed point $x$ is apparently subjected to a pulsating stress of increasing amplitude. When the tip of the crack is moving from $x_0$ to $x_0 + \mathrm{d}x_0$, the material at $x$ suffers an increased damage $\mathrm{d}D$ which by (1) is

$$\mathrm{d}\,D = k \cdot \mathrm{d}\,N \tag{5}$$

Considering (2) and (4), the total damage accumulated at this point, after it has been passed by the whole $k$-curve, is

$$D = \int_{x-c}^{x} \frac{f\,[\sigma, (x - x_0)]\,\mathrm{d}\,x_0}{v} \tag{6}$$

with the necessary condition that

$$D = 1 \text{ for } x = x_0 \tag{7}$$

Substituting

$$y = x - x_0 \tag{8}$$

we have

$$\int_0^c \frac{f\,(\sigma, y)\,\mathrm{d}\,y}{v} = 1 \tag{9}$$

In general, $f$ and $\sigma$ and accordingly $v$ are functions of $x_0$. If $f$ and $\sigma$ do not change with $x_0$, it follows that $v =$ constant and then from (9)

$$v = \int_0^c f\,(\sigma, y)\,\mathrm{d}\,y = A \tag{10}$$

where $A$ denotes the shaded area in fig. 1.

If we now enlarge all the dimensions $s$-fold, keeping $\sigma$ unchanged i.e. increasing the load $s$-fold, it follows from the law of similarity that the area will be $s \cdot A$ and from (10) that the rate of propagation will

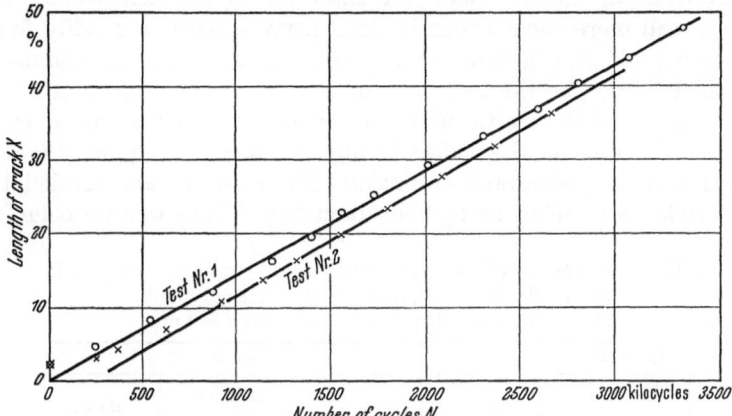

Fig. 3. Crack propagation at constant stress amplitude. Material 24 S-T.
$\sigma_{\max} = 4{,}0$ kg/mm².

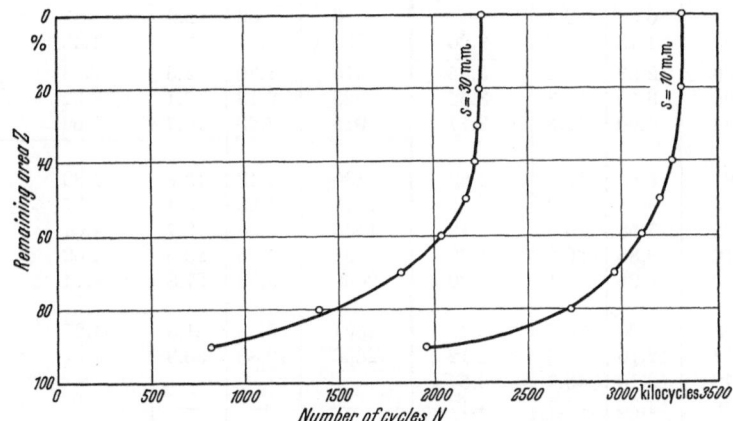

Fig. 4. Crack length vs. number of stress cycles at constant load amplitude.

also be $s$ times enlarged. This means that the propagation time is independent of the width of the specimen.

It is possible to carry out this deduction also in that case when $\sigma = f_1(x_0)$, as for instance when the load amplitude is constant and accordingly the stress amplitude increases reciprocally with the remaining cross-sectional area.

The statement that the rate of propagation after the transition period is independent of the length of the fatigue crack has been verified in the following way: The stress was pulsated between $\sigma_{max}$ and zero. By decreasing the load at intervals ($\Delta x \sim 1$ mm), given in table 3, the value of $\sigma_{max}$ was kept between 3.90 and 4.10 kg/mm². The mean velocity $\triangle x/\triangle N$ over an interval does not show any systematic trend. This result is still more conspicuous in fig. 3 from which it is readily found that the rate of propagation is constant as soon as the transition period has been passed. The theoretical conclusion that the propagation time is independent of the width of the specimen is verified by fig. 4, where the ($z$ vs $\cdot N$) curves for the widths 10 mm and 30 mm are plotted ($z$ = remaining area in percentage of initial). These curves are parallel but offset 110 kc (size effect as to hole diameter). There was no complete

Table 3. *Growth of fatigue cracks at nearly constant stress amplitude*
Material: 24 S-T; $\sigma_{max} = 3.90 - 4.10$ kg/mm²
Dimensions: $s = 30$; $d = 6$; $r = 0.15$; $t = 2$ mm

| Test Nr. 1 | | | | Test Nr. 2 | | | | |
|---|---|---|---|---|---|---|---|---|
| $N$ kc | Length of crack mm | Length of crack % | Rate of propagation $10^{-3}$ mm/kc | $N$ kc | Length of crack mm | Length of crack % | Rate of propagation $10^{-3}$ mm/kc | |
| 0 | 0.63[1] | 2.1 | — | 0 | 0.66[2] | 2.2 | — | Transition period |
| 250 | 1.43 | 4.8 | 3.20 | 259 | 1.03 | 3.4 | 1.43 | |
| 536 | 2.53 | 8.4 | 3.85 | 375 | 1.30 | 4.3 | 2.33 | |
| 866 | 3.70 | 12.3 | 3.55 | 625 | 2.13 | 7.1 | 3.32 | |
| 1184 | 4.90 | 16.3 | 3.77 | 915 | 3.20 | 10.7 | 3.69 | |
| 1387 | 5.83 | 19.4 | 4.58 | 1130 | 4.13 | 13.8 | 4.33 | |
| 1555 | 6.88 | 22.9 | 6.25 | 1313 | 4.93 | 16.4 | 4.37 | |
| 1725 | 7.58 | 25.3 | 4.12 | 1553 | 5.90 | 19.7 | 4.04 | |
| 2010 | 8.80 | 29.3 | 4.28 | 1798 | 7.05 | 23.5 | 4.69 | |
| 2300 | 9.93 | 33.1 | 3.90 | 2068 | 8.33 | 27.8 | 4.74 | |
| 2583 | 11.00 | 36.7 | 3.78 | 2361 | 9.58 | 31.9 | 4.27 | |
| 2798 | 12.10 | 40.3 | 5.12 | 2656 | 10.88 | 36.3 | 4.41 | |
| 3078 | 13.10 | 43.7 | 3.57 | — | — | — | — | |
| 3366 | 14.30 | 47.7 | 4.17 | — | — | — | — | |
| | | | M. v. 4.24 ± 0.77 | | | | M. v. 4.41 ± 0.24 | |

[1] The crack length $x = 0.63$ was obtained by applying
$\sigma_{max} = 4.5$ kg/mm² during $\triangle N = 850$ kc (crack visible)
8.0 ,, ,, 30 ,,
6.0 ,, ,, 220 ,,
4.0 ,, ,, 480 ,,
5.0 ,, ,, 100 ,,

[2] The crack length $x = 0.66$ was obtained by applying
$\sigma_{max} = 8.0$ kg/mm² during $\triangle N = 30$ kc (crack visible)
6.0 ,, ,, 117 ,,
5.0 ,, ,, 121 ,,

similarity, the diameter of the hole in the first series being 4 mm instead of 2 mm, but the diameter does apparently not play an important role as soon as the fatigue crack is fully developed. Table 4 gives the observed data of $N$, $z$, and $x$.

Table 4. *Crack propagation at different widths of specimen*

| $z$ %$_0$ | Series 80142x | | Series 80362x | | $N_1 - N_2$ kc |
|---|---|---|---|---|---|
| | $x$ mm | $N_1$ kc | $x$ mm | $N_2$ kc | |
| 90 | 1 | 196 | 3 | 82 | 114 |
| 80 | 2 | 274 | 6 | 139 | 135 |
| 70 | 3 | 297 | 9 | 182 | 115 |
| 60 | 4 | 311 | 12 | 204 | 107 |
| 50 | 5 | 320 | 15 | 217 | 103 |
| 40 | 6 | 327 | 18 | 222 | 105 |
| 30 | 7 | 330 | 21 | 223 | 107 |
| 20 | 8 | 332 | 24 | 224 | 108 |
| | $N_B = 332$ | | $N_B = 225$ | | 107 |

M. v. $= 111.2$

Values of $N_1$ and $N_2$ are averages of 6 values, viz., left- and right-hand cracks from 3 test specimens.

The second stage ends with tensile rupture, when the mean stress over the remaining area reaches a value which is very little influenced by the crack length as demonstrated in table 5. The specimens have been run in a fatigue machine. When the crack had developed to a predetermined value of $z$, the test was stopped and the ultimate tensile strength measured. The heading "100" means that the specimens were drawn without preceding fatigue. The tensile strength over the remaining area is remarkably independent of the various factors which means, among other things, that machined V-notches (bottom radius 0.05 and 0.1 mm) are just as severe stress raisers as the fatigue crack.

Tables 5. *Tensile strength in kg/mm² of remaining cross-sectional area*

| Series | Remaining cross-sectional area in percentage of initial | | | | | | |
|---|---|---|---|---|---|---|---|
| | 100 | 90 | 80 | 70 | 60 | 50 | 42 |
| 120362x | 38.3 | 38.1 | 38.1 | 37.6 | 37.8 | 37.4 | — |
| 80362x | 37.5 | — | 36.0 | — | — | 35.3 | — |
| 120262x | 39.3 | — | 38.7 | — | 38.2 | — | 38.2 |
| 120363x | 36.4 | — | 36.2 | — | 36.5 | — | 36.7 |
| 120342x | 39.2 | — | 38.1 | — | 37.8 | — | 39.2 |
| M. v. | 38.2 | 38.1 | 37.4 | 37.6 | 37.6 | 36.4 | 38.0 |

The preceding considerations have some bearing on the experimental determination of the $P$-$S$-$N$-relationship. The central part of the $P$-$S$-$N$-field may be investigated with reasonable means, but the boundaries $P = 0$ and $N = \infty$ have to be determined by extrapolation. This is an unsafe procedure even with large samples under the actual condition that the distribution function of fatigue life and the $S$-$N$ equations are not exactly known (and probably never will be). An illustration is given in fig. 5 which shows 103 test values plotted on a normal probability paper.

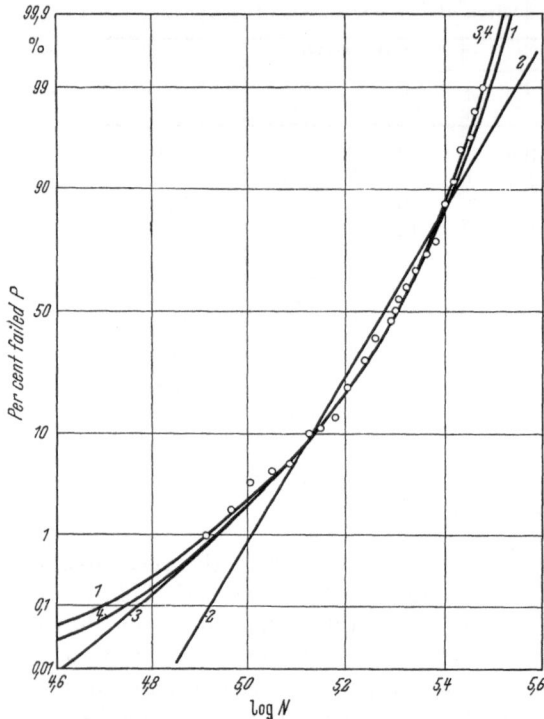

Fig. 5. Distribution of fatigue life of 24 S-T flat specimen, notched by two holes. Stress pulsating between 14 kg/mm² and zero.
1. $P = \Phi\,(N)$;   2. $P = \Phi\,(\log N)$;
3. $P = F\,(N)$;   4. $P = F\,(\log N)$.

Four different distributions have been examined and corresponding curves drawn. The normal distribution function is denoted by $\Phi$, whereas $F(x)$ denotes the function

$$F(x) = 1 - e^{-\left(\frac{x - x_u}{x_0}\right)^{1/a}} \quad (12)$$

The only obvious result is that the distribution is not log-normal (Curve 2). An experimental decision as to the three remaining functions is quite impossible without increasing the number of tests to several thousands, in spite of the fact that the functions give very different values of the lower bound $N_u$ and $(\log N)_u$, respectively, of the distribution, viz.,

Curve 1: $N_u = -\infty$
2: $(\log N)_u = -\infty$
3: $N_u = 24.9\ kc.$
4: $(\log N)_u = 2.108$

The statistical treatment of fatigue data should be very much simplified and the results safer, if it could be proved that the $S$-$N$-curve for $P = 0$ may be identified with the crack propagation time, as ascertained in a large series with flat, drilled specimens of 24 S-T, and the lower bound of the endurance limit with that stress at which a crack does not propagate.

Preliminary tests have however shown that the latter hypothesis is complicated by the fact that the non-propagating stress does not take a fixed value but depends highly on the preceding fatigue history.

The present theoretical considerations have been induced by results from extensive experimental investigations, made possible by liberal grants from the Saab Aircraft Company and carried out in close co-operation with Mr. FRED TURNER, Head of the Stress Department of that company, and Mr. GUNNAR WÅLLGREN, Head of the Structures Department of the Aeronautical Research Institute of Sweden.

## Discussion

R. B. HEYWOOD: Tests on crack propagation have been made at the Royal Aircraft Establishment on BTD 546 clad aluminium alloy sheet panels of 20 g thickness by loading in repeated tension (zero to maximum) at about 30 r/min., and giving failure in 70 to 100,000 cycles. The specimens were 72 in. by 36 in., and contained a central transverse slot 0.5 in. long by $^1/_{16}$ in. wide, with semi-circular ends.

The results were in agreement with WEIBULL's finding that considerable scatter in the initiation of cracks was obtained, but that little scatter in the propagation was found. Thus the crack from one end of the slot might be 0.2 in. long before the crack from the other end had started, but with progression of the two cracks across the panel, this difference in length became no greater.

However the results were not in accordance with WEIBULL's finding that cracks propagate themselves uniformly with cycles, for the cracks grew at a progressively faster rate as their length increased. This result was obtained even when the load was reduced during the test, so that the nominal stress across the remaining section was constant. It is suggested that the difference in behaviour of these specimens with those of WEIBULL's may have been due to the fact that the theoretical elastic stress at the extremity of a crack in an infinite sheet is proportional to the square root of the length — conditions which were approximated in the large sheets — but that the maximum stress may actually fall as the crack approaches the edges of the sheet — conditions which are more nearly approached in WEIBULL's experiments.

In other tests in which the maximum load was kept constant but was of a different value in different tests, the final catastrophic failure of the slotted panels was approximately in accordance with a relationship that has been suggested by WELLS, namely that $\sigma^2 L$ is a constant, where $\sigma$ is the nominal stress on the full area of the panel and $L$ is the overall length of cracks from one crack extremity to the other.

J. SCHIJVE: The difference between the results of WEIBULL and of HEYWOOD may probably be explained by a speed effect. In HEYWOOD's tests the stress was higher and the frequency was considerably lower (30 r/min instead of 2,000 r/min) than in the tests of WEIBULL. So in each load cycle of HEYWOOD's tests a higher peak stress was maintained for a larger time at the end of the crack. It then may be expected that a kind of creep will come into the fatigue process of the crack propagation. The speed effect at high fatigue stresses has been noted by various authors.

E. GASSNER had made the same observations as SCHIJVE on aluminum alloy 24S-T.

B. LUNDBERG: WEIBULL's statement that most of the scatter is attributed to the pre-crack period, whereas the time or number of load cycles for the propagation of the crack has little scatter, is a very interesting one. The observation seems also rather natural if one assumes that a certain "unit damage" — the greater the higher the stress or strain range is — is caused by each load cycle. This unit damage should not be confused with a crack. In the pre-crack period such a unit damage would occur at outer surfaces or at interior surfaces of cavities at weak places subjected to high stresses or strains. It seems natural to assume that these unit damages, which might have the nature of unbonding of atoms according to SHANLEY's theories, might occur at quite a large number of differently located weak spots. Sooner or later a number of unit damages occur at one and the same spot, and this implies the formation of a sub-microscopic crack. This occurrence is, quite naturally, characterized by a large scatter as the surfaces in a "submicroscopic sense" normally are widely different from each other even for nominally identical specimens, and it is thus more or less a question of probability when a number of unit damages begin to occur at one and the same spot.

After the crack has been formed, all, or at least the majority, of the subsequent unit damages will probably occur at the root of the crack, as this then has become the weakest spot and is subjected to high stresses. It seems natural that the continued propagation of the crack is of the nature of a straight-forward mechanical procedure (or rupture) which follows a certain law and would not be expected to have a large scatter between nominally identical specimens.

P. E. WIENE: As a practical confirmation of the slow propagation of cracks I can mention that some ten years ago we had at Burmeister and Wain some cases of broken piston rods (how this was cured, see ref. [1] in my paper).

We therefore controlled all piston rods by magnetic tests once a year, i. e. about every 40 million stress-cycle, and nearly always found starting cracks, but we never had a broken rod; this indicates that the sharpest cracks are not always the most dangerous.

W. WEIBULL: In most cases, the rate of propagation has been observed to increase during the "transition period" which ends, when the crack has reached a length depending on the applied stress-amplitude. Between the values 10% and 50% (which is the highest value studied), the rate of propagation is remarkably constant. If the results of HEYWOOD refer to crack lengths smaller than 10% only, there seems to be no discrepancy between his and the author's observations.

# Ausscheidungsvorgänge in Stählen
## bei ruhender und wechselnder Beanspruchung

Von

**F. Wever**

Mit 15 Abbildungen

Eine Untersuchung der physikalischen Ursachen der Ermüdung als Grundlage für eine Erklärung dieser Werkstoffeigenschaft kann nicht an der Fragestellung vorübergehen, ob nicht bei langdauernden Beanspruchungen, insbesondere bei erhöhten Temperaturen, Veränderungen im Gefügeaufbau ablaufen, die in irgendeiner Weise mit der Ermüdung zusammenhängen.

Zunächst wird man geneigt sein, einer derartigen Vermutung entgegenzuhalten, daß Stähle, die einer Dauerbeanspruchung unterworfen werden sollen, sich im allgemeinen in einem Gefügezustand befinden werden, der dem strukturellen Gleichgewicht entspricht oder ihm jedenfalls sehr nahe kommt. Es sollte daher nicht zu erwarten sein, daß sich während der Dauerbeanspruchung noch tiefergehende Änderungen im Gefügeaufbau vollziehen. Eine ganze Reihe von Arbeiten, an denen man nicht ohne weiteres vorübergehen kann, bringen Beweise für diese Auffassung.

Nun lehrt aber das Beispiel der Chromstähle, daß der Zustand des Gleichgewichtes noch lange nicht erreicht zu sein braucht, wenn das, was thermisch oder dilatometrisch gemeinhin als Umwandlung festgestellt wird, längst zu Ende abgelaufen ist. Nach den sehr eingehenden Untersuchungen des Max-Planck-Instituts für Eisenforschung wird bei diesen Stählen in der Perlitstufe zuerst ein Karbid von der Struktur des Eisenkarbides $Fe_3C$ gebildet, in dem etwa ein Viertel der Eisenatome durch Chrom ersetzt sind. Dieses Karbid besitzt die kennzeichnende Form sehr dünner Lamellen, wie sie in Abb. 1 für den Fall eines Stahles mit 0,4% C und 3,5% Cr nach einer elektronenmikroskopischen Aufnahme wiedergegeben sind. Dieses lamellare Karbid $(Fe, Cr)_3C$ entspricht jedoch noch nicht dem Gleichgewicht. Es nimmt bei genügend langem Halten auf Temperaturen von 600 bis 700° C weiter Chrom aus dem Ferrit auf, während gleichzeitig im Röntgenbild, allmählich an Intensität zunehmend, die Interferenzlinien des Chromkarbides $(Cr, Fe)_7C_3$ erscheinen. Die Bildung dieses Chromkarbides geht dabei von Keimen aus, die anscheinend bevorzugt an Stellen stärkerer Gitter-

störungen in den Lamellen gebildet werden. Abb. 2 zeigt eine Reihe
von Chromkarbidkeimen in einem frühen Zustand dieser Umwandlung. Die Keime des Chromkarbides treten perlschnurartig in Reihen
auf und scheinen gegen die Lamellen kristallographisch orientiert zu
sein; sie wachsen auf Kosten der Lamellen zu stäbchenförmigen Ge-
bilden aus. In Abb. 3 ist ein Stäbchen von Chromkarbid zu sehen, das
sich noch nicht von der Lamelle abgetrennt hat, aus der es entstanden
ist, in einem Fenster, das bei der Bildung des Stäbchens aus der La-

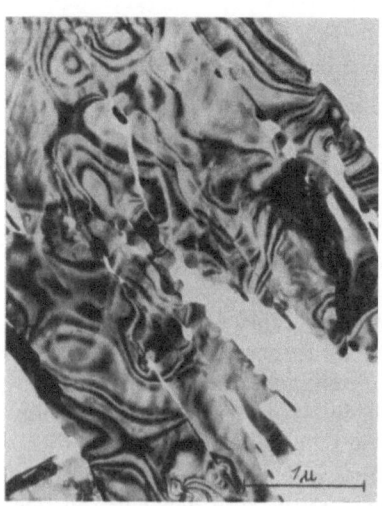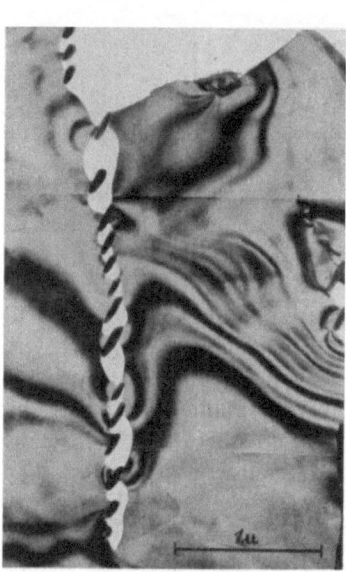

Abb. 1. Lamellen des Karbides (Fe, Cr)$_3$C aus
einem Chromstahl mit 0,4 % C und 3,5 % Cr.

Abb.2. Keime d. Chromkarbides (Cr,Fe)$_7$C$_3$
in einer Lamelle v. Eisenkarbid (Fe,Cr)$_3$C.

melle herausgelöst wurde. Abb. 4 zeigt einen fortgeschritteneren Auf-
lösungszustand; die in den Fenstern ursprünglich vorhandenen Chrom-
karbidstäbchen sind bei der Isolierung herausgefallen. Neben dem
Chromkarbid findet man auch nach sehr langen Haltezeiten langge-
streckte Reste von Eisenkarbid.

Hier liegt natürlich der Einwand nahe, daß sich bei einem Stahl
dieser Art die Einstellung des Gleichgewichtes auf einem ungewöhnlich
langen Wege vollzieht und es daher nicht verwunderlich ist, wenn sich
das Gefüge noch über sehr lange Zeiten in Richtung auf das Gleichgewicht hin verändert. Dem steht jedoch entgegen, daß sich in den
niedrig legierten Chromstählen, obwohl hier bei der Umwandlung so-
gleich das stabile Karbid (Fe, Cr)$_3$C gebildet wird, ein Einformungs-
vorgang dieses Karbides aus der lamellaren in eine körnige Form ebenfalls über sehr lange Zeiten hinzieht. Was wir aus diesen Versuchen

lernen, ist, daß sich in den Stählen, die mit karbidbildenden Elementen von geringem Diffusionsvermögen in Eisen legiert sind, die dem Gleichgewicht entsprechenden Karbidformen erst nach sehr langen Glühzeiten vollkommen ausbilden. Warum sollten dann nicht auch bei einer Dauerbeanspruchung in der Wärme ähnliche Vorgänge möglich sein ?

Hier ist auf Versuche hinzuweisen, die in dem letzten Jahre im Max-Planck-Institut für Eisenforschung an warmfesten Chrom-Nickel-Molybdänstählen mit 0,1% C, 0,7% Cr, 1,5% Ni und 0,8% Mo durchgeführt wurden, wie sie vielfach als Schraubenstähle Verwendung ge-

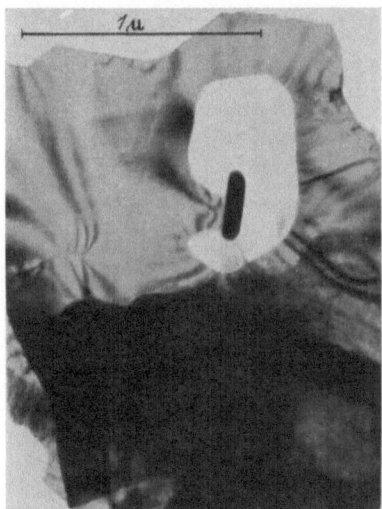 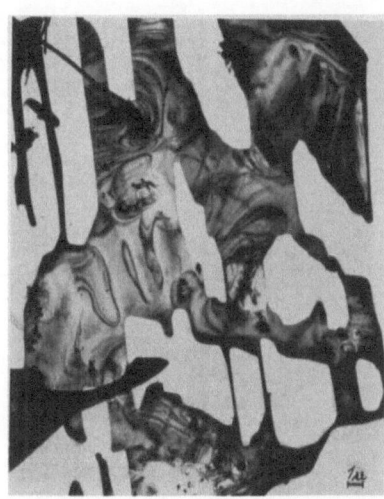

Abb. 3. Keime des Chromkarbides (Cr, Fe)₇C₃ in einem Fenster einer Lamelle von Eisenkarbid (Fe, Cr)₃C.

Abb. 4. Lamelle von Eisenkarbid (Fe, Cr)₃C im Zustande fortgeschrittener Auflösung.

funden haben. Bei diesen Stählen war die beunruhigende Erfahrung gemacht worden, daß sie nach längeren Zeiten mit sehr geringer Verformung interkristallin zu Bruch gehen können, auch wenn die Beanspruchung im Bereich der DVM-Kriechgrenze liegt.

Zu einer planmäßigen Untersuchung dieser Frage wurden Stahlreihen mit Kohlenstoffgehalten von 0,04 bis 0,3%, Chromgehalten von 0,5 bis 0,9%, Nickelgehalten von rd. 1,5% und Molybdängehalten von rd. 0,75% erschmolzen. Diese Stähle wurden teils luft- oder ölabgeschreckt auf niedrige Temperaturen von 560 bis 570° C angelassen, teils in der Zwischenstufe bei 350 bis 450° C umgewandelt, teils auch öl- oder wasserabgeschreckt auf höhere Temperaturen von 620 bis 660° C angelassen. Bei allen Stählen ergaben Proben, die bei 570° C angelassen oder bei 350 bis 450° C zwischenstufenvergütet worden waren, eine hohe DVM-Kriechgrenze in Verbindung mit einer hohen

1.000-h-Zeitstandfestigkeit. Sie brachen jedoch in diesem Zustand in allen Fällen mit geringer Verformung in den Korngrenzen. Dagegen ergaben die bei höheren Temperaturen von 620 bis 660° C angelassenen

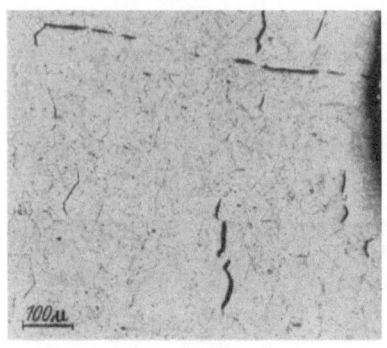
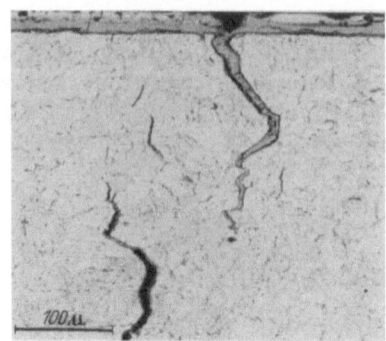

Abb. 5 a.

Abb. 6 a.
Anrisse an der Staboberfläche.

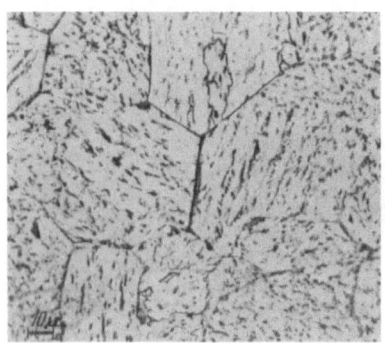
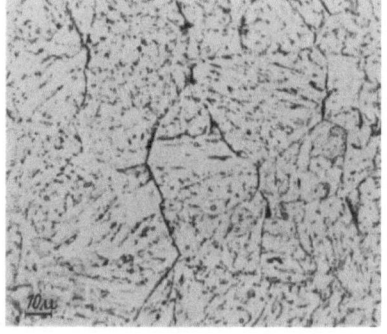

Abb. 5 b.
Abb. 5. Gefüge nahe der Bruchfläche.

Abb. 6 b.
Anrisse in etwa 20 mm Entfernung
von der Bruchfläche.

Abb. 5 und 6. Anrisse im Gefüge eines im Dauerstandversuche nach 1 314 h Belastung mit 50 kg/mm²
bei 500° C mit etwa 0,7 % Bruchdehnung und 0 % Einschnürung gebrochenen Stabes aus einem Stahl
mit 0,14 % C, 0,77 % Cr, 1,60 % Ni und 0,94 % Mo.
Behandlung: 930° C/Luft, 3 h/570° C/Ofen.

Proben je nach dem Kohlenstoffgehalt eine mehr oder weniger gesenkte DVM-Kriechgrenze und eine niedrigere 1.000-h-Zeitstandfestigkeit, sie gingen in diesem Zustand durchweg mit guter Dehnung und Einschnürung zu Bruch.

Längsschliffe senkrecht zur Bruchoberfläche der mit geringer Dehnung gebrochenen Proben der ersteren Warmbehandlungsart mit hoher DVM-Kriechgrenze ergaben, daß der Bruch bevorzugt entlang den ehemaligen Austenit-Korngrenzen eintritt. Als Beispiel ist in Abb. 5 und 6 das Gefüge einer Probe wiedergegeben, die bei 500° C mit 50 kg/mm² belastet und nach 1.314 Stunden praktisch ohne Dehnung und Einschnürung zu Bruch gegangen war. In einem ausgedehnten Bereich bis

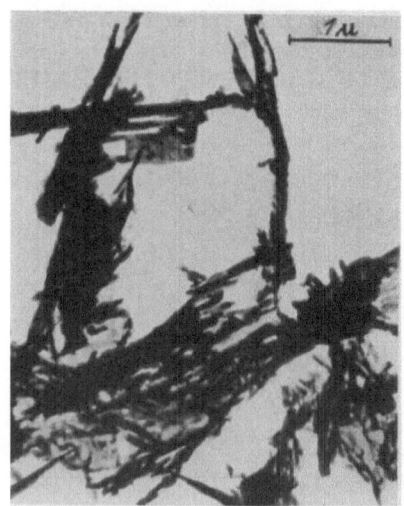 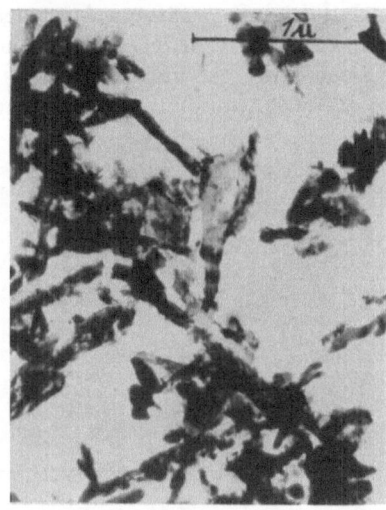

Abb. 7.                                        Abb. 8.
Elektronenmikroskopische Aufnahmen der isolierten Karbide eines Stahles mit 0,14% C, 0,77% Cr, 0,94% Mo und 1,60% Ni.

Abb. 7. Behandlung 930° C/Luft, 3 h/570° C/Ofen. Zwischenstufenform des Eisenkarbids $Fe_3C$.

Abb. 8. Behandlung 930° C/Öl, 3 h/570° C/Ofen; 2738 h bei 500° C mit 40 kg/mm² Belastung.

in beträchtliche Entfernung von der Bruchfläche sind Aufreißungen und Lockerungen in den Korngrenzen zu erkennen. Sofern diese Aufreißungen nahe der Staboberfläche liegen, sind sie ebenso wie die Bruchfläche selbst oxydiert, doch sind auch im Stabinnern ohne erkennbaren Zusammenhang mit der oxydierten Oberfläche Aufreißungen vorhanden.

Eine Erklärung für das unterschiedliche Verhalten dieser Stähle wurde wieder durch eine Isolierung und Untersuchung der Karbide gefunden. Bei beiden Anlaßarten wurde schon im Ausgangszustand eine Anreicherung des Chroms und Molybdäns in der Karbidphase festgestellt. Bei den niedrigen Anlaßtemperaturen liegt das Karbid durchweg als Eisenkarbid $Fe_3C$ vor, in dem ein Teil der Eisenatome durch Chrom und Molybdän ersetzt sind. Im Verlauf der Dauerbeanspruchung nehmen die Gehalte an Chrom und Molybdän im Isolat weiter beträchtlich zu. Nach Belastungen über 500 Stunden bei 500° C wird eine neue Phase im Isolat beobachtet, die so fein anfällt, daß sie beim Ausschleudern in der Zentrifuge kolloidal auch im Elektrolyten verteilt bleibt und erst durch besondere Maßnahmen teilweise ausgeflockt

werden kann. Dieser kolloide Anteil ergab bei der Analyse sehr hohe
Gehalte an Molybdän; bei der Röntgenanalyse erwies er sich als das
Molybdänkarbid $Mo_2C$. Abb. 7 und 8 geben elektronenmikroskopische
Aufnahmen der isolierten Karbide wieder. Man erkennt in Abb. 7,
Karbid des luftvergüteten Ausgangszustandes nach Anlassen auf 570° C,
die bekannten gedrungenen Formen des Eisenkarbides, wie sie in der
Zwischenstufe gebildet werden. Nach der Belastung über 2.738 Stunden
bei 500° C (Abb. 8) treten daneben sehr feine Nädelchen auf, die das

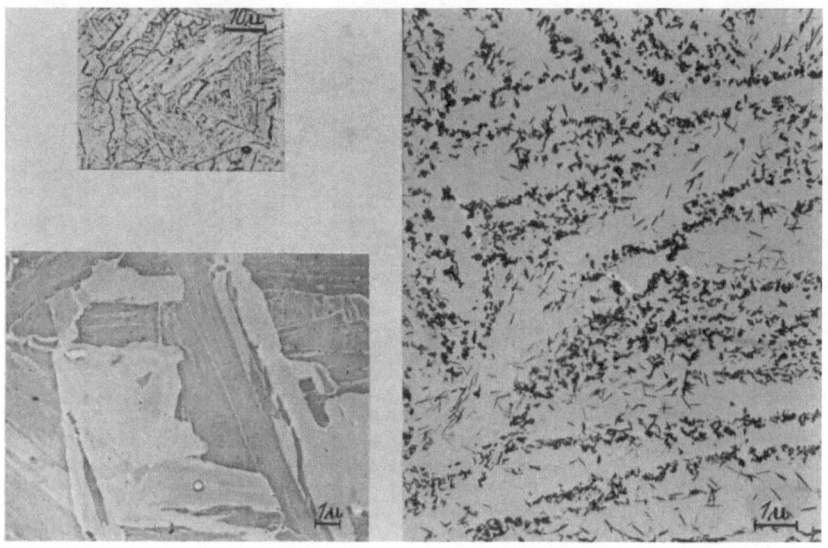

Abb. 9. Vergütungsgefüge und Ausscheidungen des Molybdän-Karbides $Mo_2C$.
Stahl mit 0,04 % C, 0,48 % Cr, 0,7 % Mo, 1,4 % Ni.
Behandlung: 930° C/Wasser, 2h/660° C/Luft.

röntgenographisch nachgewiesene Molybdänkarbid $Mo_2C$ sind. Ihre
sehr geringe Größe macht verständlich, daß sie beim Ausschleudern
des Rückstandes in der Lösung bleiben.

Völlig anders ist das Bild bei den Stählen, die vor der Dauerbeanspruchung bei höheren Temperaturen von 620 bis 660° C angelassen
worden waren. Hier ist von vornherein eine stärkere Anreicherung der
Karbidphase an Molybdän und Chrom vorhanden, die beträchtlich über
die Werte hinausgeht, die im niedriger angelassenen Zustand beobachtet worden waren. Bei der Dauerbeanspruchung nimmt diese Anreicherung weiter zu, während gleichzeitig der Molybdängehalt des
Ferrits auf sehr niedrige Werte absinkt. Nach dem Röntgenbefund
tritt schon im Ausgangszustand das Molybdänkarbid $Mo_2C$ neben
Eisenkarbid $Fe_3C$ auf. Im Elektronenmikroskop findet man neben den

derben Formen des Eisenkarbids von Anfang an die Nadeln des Molybdänkarbides, die sich während der Dauerbeanspruchung nicht erkennbar verändern.

Es gelang später auch durch einen Kunstgriff, die Ausscheidung dieses sehr feinen Molybdänkarbides elektronenmikroskopisch unmittelbar im Gefüge sichtbar zu machen. Abb. 9 zeigt das Gefüge eines Stahles dieser Versuchsreihe mit 0,04% C nach zweistündigem Anlassen auf 660° C. In dem lichtoptischen Gefügebild sind keinerlei Ausscheidungen zu erkennen. Der darunter wiedergegebene Lackabzug nach Gefügeätzung zeigt im Ferrit eine außerordentlich feine Karbidausscheidung. Eine wenig stärkere Ätzung genügt, um diese Karbidteilchen so weit freizulegen, daß sie an dem Lackhäutchen hängenbleiben (rechtes Teilbild). Es ist nun deutlich zu erkennen, daß sie feinste Körnchen und Nädelchen bilden. Eine Elektronenbeugungsaufnahme ergibt eindeutig die Interferenzringe des Molybdänkarbides $Mo_2C$.

Nach diesem Befund ist in den auf hohe Temperaturen angelassenen Proben von Anfang an ein Teil des Karbides als Molybdänkarbid $Mo_2C$ vorhanden. Bei den niedriger angelassenen Proben ist dieses Karbid im Ausgangszustand noch nicht nachweisbar; es wird erst während der Dauerbeanspruchung in äußerst feiner Form ausgeschieden.

Hier erhebt sich jetzt die Frage, ob überhaupt und gegebenenfalls in welcher Weise diese Ausscheidungen sehr fein verteilten Molybdänkarbides in Verbindung mit der dadurch hervorgerufenen Verarmung des Ferrits an Molybdän mit der Kornversprödung dieser Stähle zusammenhängen. Bei den hoch angelassenen Stählen sollte der von vornherein kleinere Kriechwiderstand des Ferrits, bedingt durch den niedrigeren Molybdängehalt, zur Folge haben, daß die Verspannungen der Korngrenzen im ganzen geringer bleiben, weil sich das Korn selbst schon bei niedrigeren Spannungen verformen kann. Das schon im Ausgangszustand ausgeschiedene Molybdänkarbid kann dabei nur in geringerem Maße eine festigkeitssteigernde Wirkung ausüben. Bei den niedriger angelassenen Proben durchläuft die erst während der Beanspruchung erfolgende Ausscheidung von Molybdänkarbid einen Zustand kritischer Dispersion mit allen bekannten Folgen auf das Verformungsvermögen. Das Ferritkorn wird dadurch verfestigt, und die Verspannungen an den Korngrenzen können solche Ausmaße annehmen, daß es zu einem Aufreißen kommt.

Man wird hier vielleicht einwerfen, daß die Chrom-Nickel-Molybdänstähle heute als Schraubenstähle überholt sind, weil sie nach den inzwischen gewonnenen Erkenntnissen nicht genügende Stabilität besitzen, und daß die soeben besprochenen Ergebnisse im Grunde nur diese Auffassung bestätigen. Hierzu können jedoch neuere Beobachtungen unseres Instituts an austenitischen Stählen auf der Grundlage Chrom-

Nickel-Molybdän-Vanadin vorgelegt werden, die mit Titan oder mit
Niob/Tantal stabilisiert worden waren. Auch hierbei erwies sich wiederum das Verfahren der Karbidisolierung als nützlich.

Als ein Beispiel aus dieser Versuchsreihe ist in Abb. 10 das Gefüge
eines Stahles mit 0,04% C, 17% Cr und 14% Ni wiedergegeben, der
mit 0,7% Nb/Ta stabilisiert worden war. Im vergüteten Ausgangszu-

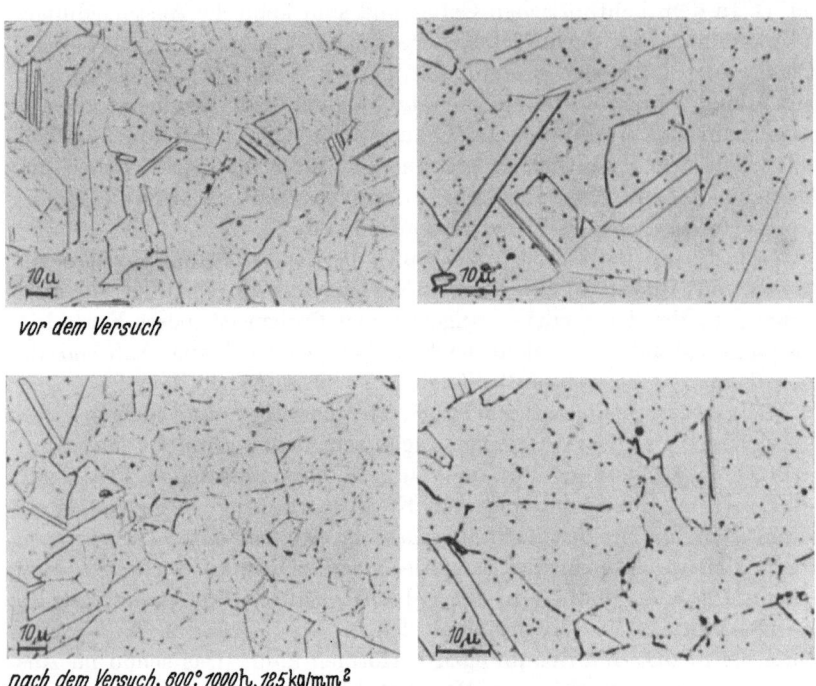

vor dem Versuch

nach dem Versuch, 600°, 1000 h, 12,5 kg/mm²

Abb. 10. Gefüge vor und nach dem Zeitstandversuch.
Stahl mit 0,04% C, 17% Cr, 14% Ni, 0,7% Nb/Ta. Behandlung: 20 min/1100° C/Luft.

stand (Abb. 10, obere Reihe) sind in der austenitischen Grundmasse
neben gröberen Nitriden und Karbiden fein verteilte Einschlüsse vorhanden, die vorwiegend innerhalb der Austenitkörper liegen. Nach einer
Belastung von über 1.000 Stunden bei 600° C treten deutlich neue Ausscheidungen auf den Korngrenzen hervor (Abb. 10, untere Reihe). Die
röntgenographische Prüfung der Isolierungsrückstände ergab bei diesen Versuchen mit Unterschieden, die durch die Zusammensetzung der
Stähle bedingt sind, im Ausgangszustand und nach kurzen Belastungen
bis zu 1.000 Stunden bei 600° C lediglich die Karbide der Stabilisierungs-
elemente TiC bzw. (Nb/Ta)C. Nach Beanspruchungen von mehr als

1.000 Stunden tritt allmählich neben diesen das Karbid $Me_{23}C_6$ hervor, das vielleicht aus dem Kohlenstoff gebildet wird, der nicht an das Stabilisierungselement gebunden ist. Nach Belastungen über 6.000 Stunden wird bei diesen Stählen die $\sigma$-Phase beobachtet, deren Linien nach 7.500 Stunden die stärksten des Röntgendiagramms werden.

Inzwischen liegen Beobachtungen vor, daß sich bei diesen Stählen die gleichen Veränderungen im Aufbau auch ohne Belastung, allein

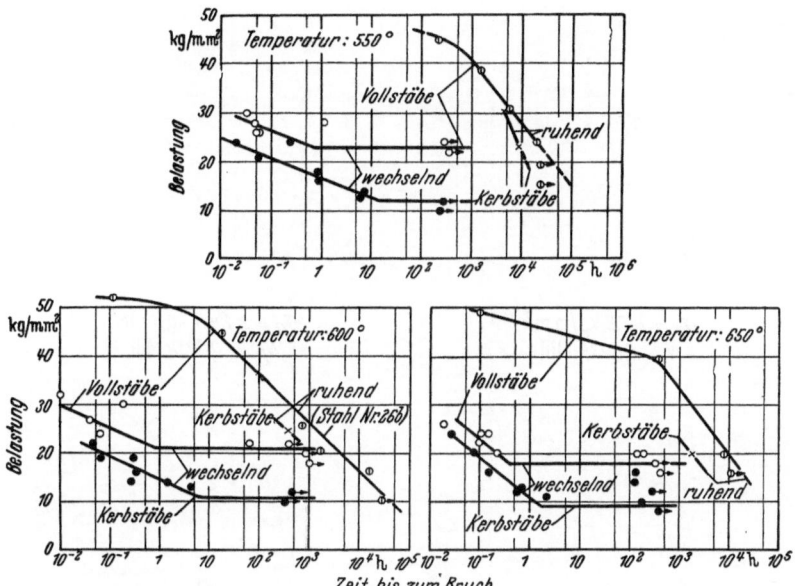

Abb. 11. Spannungs-Bruchzeit-Linien eines austenitischen Stahles mit 0,12 % C, 15,4 % Cr, 15,4 % Ni, 1,98 % Mo, 1,04 % Nb und 0,119 % N bei ruhender und wechselnder Belastung für 550°, 600° und 650° C.

durch eine Glühbehandlung von ausreichender Länge vollziehen. Es ist möglich, daß die Geschwindigkeit dieser Veränderungen ohne Belastung etwas kleiner ist als mit Belastung. Der Unterschied ist jedoch, wenn überhaupt vorhanden, nur gering. Hierzu werden noch weitere Versuche notwendig sein, bis ein endgültiges Urteil abgegeben werden kann.

Wie steht es nun mit dem Werkstoffverhalten bei schwingender Beanspruchung? Hierzu seien zunächst Versuche mit einem austenitischen Stahl mit 0,12% C, 15,4% Cr, 1,98% Mo, 15,4% Ni, 1,04% Nb/Ta und 0,119% N mitgeteilt, dessen Wöhler- und Zeitstandlinien für 550, 600 und 650° C in Abb. 11 wiedergegeben sind. Bei allen drei Temperaturen verlaufen die Wöhler-Linien der Voll- und Kerbstäbe für Wechsel-

belastung mit 1.000 Lastwechseln pro Minute weit unterhalb der Zeitstandlinien für ruhende Belastung. In Abb. 12 sind Gefügebilder dieses
Stahles wiedergegeben, die den Einfluß der Belastungshöhe und -dauer
auf die Gefügeausbildung bei 600° C kennzeichnen sollen, die Schliff-
proben wurden einmal aus dem Einspannteil und zum anderen aus der

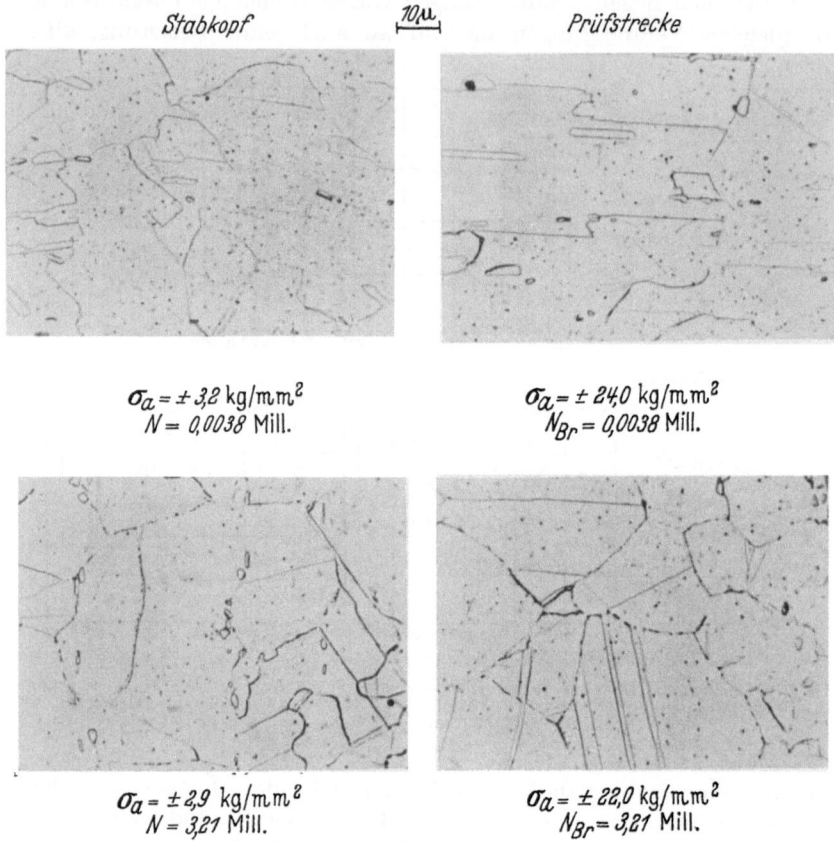

Abb. 12. Gefügezustand eines austenitischen Stahles mit 0,12% C, 15,4% Cr, 15,4% Ni, 1,98% Mo,
1,04% Nb und 0,119% N nach Wechselbeanspruchung bei 600° C.
Zug-Druck: $\sigma_m = 0$; $n = 1000$ r/min.

Prüfstrecke der Schwingungsproben entnommen. Bei den Proben der
unteren Reihe, die mit rd. 3,2 Mill. Lastspielen oder rd. 53 Stunden
beansprucht worden waren, sind schwach ausgeprägt feine Karbidausscheidungen auf den Korngrenzen vorhanden, und zwar auch in den
nur mit rd. $\pm 3$ kg/mm² belasteten Einspannenden. Eine Versuchsdauer
von 3.800 Lastspielen oder rd. 4 min bewirkt dagegen nur vereinzelte
Ausscheidungen auf den Korngrenzen (s. die obere Reihe in Abb. 12).

Wesentlich deutlicher treten die Ausscheidungen auf den Korngrenzen der bei 650° C wechselbeanspruchten Proben auf (Abb. 13). Eine sehr niedrige Beanspruchung von nur $\pm 2{,}6 \ \text{kg/mm}^2$ mit 13.400 Lastspielen oder rd. 13 min (Abb. 13, oben links) bewirkt nur geringe Änderung des Gefüges. Bei einer mit $\pm 20 \ \text{kg/mm}^2$ und der gleichen Laufzeit beanspruchten Probe (Abb. 13, oben rechts) sind schon Ausscheidungen auf den Korngrenzen zu erkennen, die bei den langzeitig mit rd. 8,5 Mill. Lastspielen oder 142 Stunden beanspruchten Proben (Abb. 13, untere Reihe) noch deutlicher werden. Von der Schliffprobe

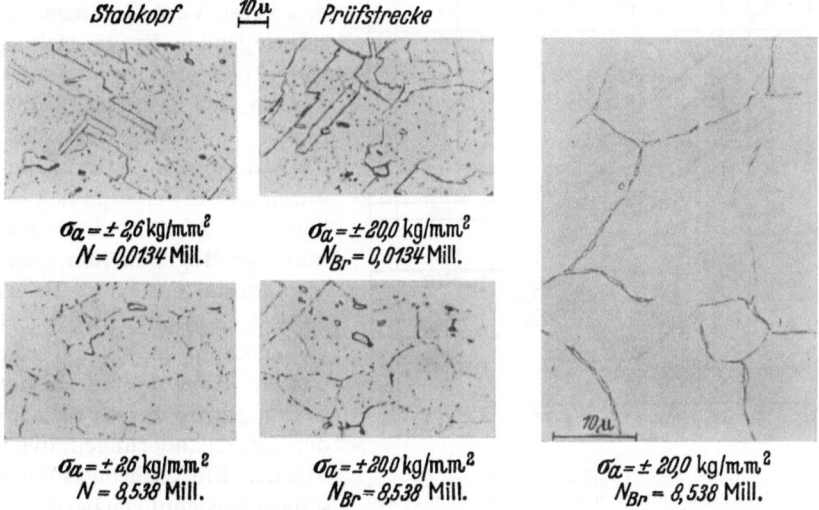

Abb. 13. Gefügezustand eines austenitischen Stahles mit 0,12 % C, 15,4 % Cr, 15,4 % Ni, 1,98 % Mo, 1,04 % Nb und 0,119 % N nach Wechselbeanspruchung bei 650° C. Zug-Druck: $\sigma_m = 0$; $n = 1000$ r/min.

dieser letzteren mit $\pm 20 \ \text{kg/mm}^2$ beanspruchten und nach 8,5 Mill. Lastspielen gebrochenen Probe (Abb. 13, unten rechts) wurde ein Lackabdruck angefertigt, der im rechten Teilbild in Abb. 13 mit 1.000-facher Vergrößerung wiedergegeben ist. Man erkennt sehr deutlich, daß die Korngrenzen mit Karbidausscheidungen erfüllt sind.

An einer Reihe von Vollstäben dieses Stahles wurden Isolierungen durchgeführt. Die Karbidrückstände aus unbelasteten oder nur bis zu verhältnismäßig niedrigen Lastspielzahlen belasteten Proben besaßen nach der Mikroanalyse angenähert die gleiche Zusammensetzung. Dagegen konnte bei einer Probe, die $53^{1}/_{2}$ Stunden bis zum Bruch belastet worden war, eine deutliche Anreicherung des Chromgehaltes festgestellt werden. Die Röntgenanalyse ergab in allen Fällen das Karbid (Nb/Ta)C neben $\gamma$-Eisen.

Das bei den Dauerstandsversuchen mit ähnlich zusammengesetzten Stählen gefundene Karbid $Me_{23}C_6$ konnte bisher bei den schwingungsbeanspruchten Proben nicht nachgewiesen werden. Ebenso wurde bisher auch die $\sigma$-Phase bei den Schwingungsversuchen in keinem Falle gefunden. Die Versuche bedürfen hier noch der weiteren Ergänzung. Auf jeden Fall ist jedoch heute schon sichergestellt, daß sich bei der Schwingungsbeanspruchung unter erhöhten Temperaturen die gleichen oder ähnliche Veränderungen in den Karbiden vollziehen wie bei ruhender Last, mit dem bemerkenswerten Unterschied, daß diese Veränderungen bei schwingender Beanspruchung wesentlich schneller ablaufen.

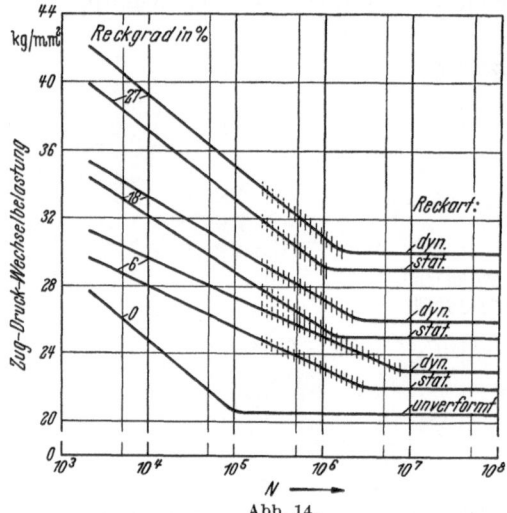

Abb. 14.

Bereich der Gefügeänderungen im Zeitfestigkeitsgebiet von Weicheisenproben nach Kaltverformung und Wechselbelastung bei Raumtemperatur,

Die verbesserten Hilfsmittel zum Nachweis dieser Veränderungen, die vor allem durch die Anwendung der Isolierung gegeben sind, eröffnen nun auch Möglichkeiten, solche Veränderungen unter Bedingungen zu untersuchen, wo sie bisher kaum erwartet worden wären. Eine weitere Untersuchungsreihe befaßt sich mit den Gefügeänderungen, die in weichem Flußstahl unter Wechselbeanspruchungen bei Raumtemperatur auftreten. Hierzu wurden Proben aus einem Stahl mit 0,02 % C um verschiedene Beträge sowohl statisch in einer Zerreißmaschine als auch dynamisch in einer eigens für diesen Zweck entwickelten Schlagvorrichtung vorgereckt und danach auf ihre Zug - Druck - Wechselfestigkeit untersucht. Die Wöhlerkurven dieser verschiedenen Zustände sind in Abb. 14 zusammengestellt. Die Wechselfestigkeit wird durch die vorhergehende bildsame Verformung beträchtlich erhöht. Nach Beanspruchungen, die *unterhalb* und *weit oberhalb* der Wechselfestigkeiten liegen, werden keine Gefügeänderungen beobachtet, dagegen werden in den Belastungsbereichen *nahe oberhalb* der Wechselfestigkeit deutliche Gefügeänderungen festgestellt. Als Beispiel ist in Abb. 15 das Gefüge einer Probe wiedergegeben, die 18 % dynamisch vorgereckt und danach bei $\pm$ 27 kg/mm² nahe oberhalb ihrer Wechselfestigkeit beansprucht worden war. Der Bruch war dabei nach 2,53 Mill. Lastspielen eingetreten. In den Ferritkristalliten haben sich dunkel erscheinende, kugelige Ausscheidungen in perlschnurähnlicher Anordnung gebildet. Nach der Fry-Ätzung ist zu erkennen, daß diese Ausscheidungen bevorzugt in den Gleitlinien liegen.

Zur Klärung der Natur dieser Ausscheidungen wurden Proben in verschiedenen Behandlungszuständen der elektrolytischen Isolierung nach KLINGER und KOCH unterworfen und die dabei erhaltenen Rückstände nach Trennung in einen magnetischen und einen unmagnetischen Anteil röntgenographisch bestimmt. Die unverformte Probe liefert neben

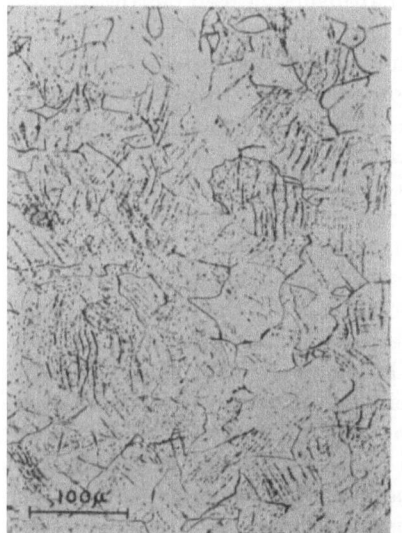 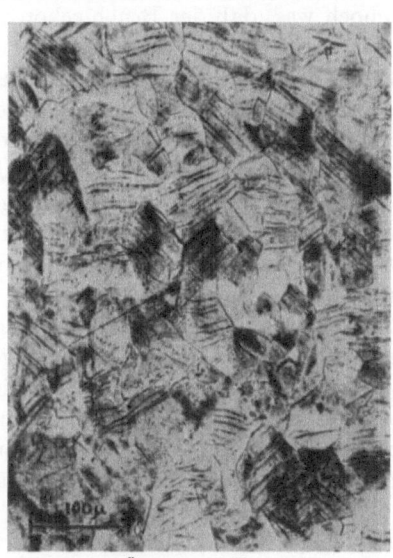

Ätzung mit Pikrinsäure.        Ätzung nach Fry.

Abb. 15. Ausbildung und Lage von Ausscheidungen in kaltverformten und wechselbeanspruchten Weicheisenproben. Behandlung: 18 % dynamisch gereckt bei + 20° C. Zug-Druck-Wechselbelastung bei + 20° C mit $\sigma_a = 27$ kg/mm² und $N = 2{,}53$ Mill. Lastspielen.

einem unmagnetischen Anteil, der durch das Röntgenbild als Mangansulfid MnS ausgewiesen wird, einen groben und einen feinen magnetischen Anteil, die beide aus $\alpha$-Eisen bestehen. Die Bildung dieser Anteile ist so zu erklären, daß einzelne Ferritkristalle bei der anodischen Auflösung aus dem Metallverband herausgetrennt werden; sie fallen dann zu Boden und werden im Rückstand gefunden. Wir haben später gelernt, die Lösungsbedingungen so abzuändern, daß diese, unter Umständen störende Erscheinung nicht mehr auftritt. In einer 18 % vorgereckten Probe finden sich die gleichen Anteile im Rückstand, eine erkennbare Veränderung gegenüber dem Ausgangszustand ist nicht eingetreten. In einer statisch vorgereckten und darauf mit 27,1 kg/mm² bis zum Bruch nach 75.500 Lastspielen beanspruchten Probe bestehen die magnetischen Anteile aus Eisenkarbid $Fe_3C$; damit ist nachgewiesen, daß es bei der Wechselbeanspruchung dieses sehr kohlenstoffarmen Stahles zur Ausscheidung von gebundenem Kohlenstoff als Zementit

$Fe_3C$ kommt. Diese Ausscheidung ist offenbar an die Bedingung geknüpft, daß die Belastung oberhalb der Wechselfestigkeit liegt, weil nur dann die notwendige Beweglichkeit des Kohlenstoffs gegeben ist. Sie erfolgt bei einer Beanspruchung unterhalb der Wechselfestigkeit, wenn überhaupt, so langsam, daß wir sie bisher nicht beobachten konnten. Sie benötigt aber auch bei einer Belastung oberhalb der Wechselfestigkeit erhebliche Zeit und ist daher nicht nachweisbar, wenn die Belastung so hoch war, daß der Bruch schon verhältnismäßig bald eintritt.

Die vorgelegten Beobachtungen sollen die Aufmerksamkeit darauf lenken, daß bei der Dauerbeanspruchung der Stähle in der Wärme Veränderungen im Gefügebau, insbesondere in der Art und Zusammensetzung der Karbide vor sich gehen. Diese Veränderungen laufen im unbelasteten Zustand und bei statischer Beanspruchung sehr langsam ab. Sie sind bei Wechselbelastungen um Größenordnungen schneller und können dann auch bei Raumtemperatur nachgewiesen werden. Diese Veränderungen sind offenbar nicht eine seltene, technisch uninteressante Ausnahmeerscheinung, es besteht vielmehr Grund zu der Annahme, daß sie bei der großen Mehrzahl der für Dauerbeanspruchungen bei erhöhten Temperaturen eingesetzten Stähle vorkommen.

Dabei muß einstweilen noch die Frage offen bleiben, welcher Zusammenhang zwischen dieser Erscheinung und dem Bruchverhalten, insbesondere dem verformungsarmen Bruch besteht. Es kann aber wohl keinem Zweifel unterliegen, daß die beobachteten Änderungen im Aufbau der Karbidphase und die damit verbundene Verarmung der ferritischen oder austenitischen Mischkristallphase an Legierungselementen nicht ohne Einfluß auf die Festigkeitseigenschaften sein kann.

## Diskussion

I. ODING fragte, ob tatsächlich irreversible Ausscheidung von Karbiden bei Wechselbeanspruchung beobachtet worden ist (wird vom Verfasser bejaht). In der Sowjet-Union hat man solche Ausscheidungen zwar bei statischen Versuchen, jedoch nicht bei Wechselbeanspruchung beobachtet.

A. JOHANSSON called attention to the irreversible precipitation of carbide in non-stabilized austenitic chromium-nickel steels, fatigued at 500°C, as revealed by fig. 9 in his own paper, see p. 120.

L. HIMMEL: Evidence that accelerated local precipitation may occur under the action of fatigue stresses has also been obtained recently by P. J. E. FORSYTH, the Royal Aircraft Establishment. Working with Al + 4% Cu-solid alloys this investigator found that the material within the slip band region was actually extruded above the surface of the specimen when fatigued at room temperature. It is thought that the material extruded from the surface may be a depleted solid solution formed as the result of accelerated over-ageing during the test.

P. LAURENT: L'Auteur a observé une précipitation de $Fe_3C$ dans un acier doux écroui, donc instable; comme nous le rapportons dans une autre communication de ce Colloque, le Dr. HENDUS a observé dans un fer Armco recuit au voisinage de certaines fissures de fatigue une précipitation en plaques parallèles à (110) que nous pensons être le carbure $\varepsilon$, voir p. 144.

# Bending fatigue of large welded test pieces with regard to velocity of crack propagation

By

## P. E. Wiene

With 6 figures

The present series of experiments forms part of the investigations constantly being untertaken by Burmeister & Wain with a view to increasing the safety of diesel engines [1]. In this case the main object was to decide on the often discussed problem of the justification of annealing frames and bed plates after welding; and as the experiment shows an increase in fatigue strength of 20 per cent by annealing at 650° C, it is concluded that such annealing is expedient for components exposed to heavy varying stresses, the most important of which are situated at the surface of the material — at least when operating temperatures are not so high that annealing may be expected to take place during service.

The *experimental arrangement* is shown in fig. 1. In the main experiment, a 28 mm plate had been welded in $T$ for a length of 1 m to an 80 mm plate. The material was semi-killed S. M. steel from the Danish Rolling Mills with Lloyd's certificate, C = 0.17%, Si = 0.14% and Mn = 0.75%. 8 test pieces of this type were made, 4 of which were tested in the as welded condition, and the other 4 after 4 hours annealing at 650° C followed by slow cooling in furnace for 20 hours. For the welding low hydrogen electrode was used, hand-welding, no pre-heating, no peening. After the welding were allowed to elapse about two months before fatigue tests were started, whereby a natural ageing similar to that in practice was obtained.

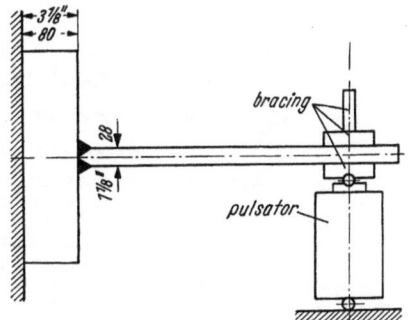

Fig. 1. Experimental arrangement. Length of weld-seams perpendicular to paper's plane is 1 m.

The fatigue test was carried out by the Structural Research Laboratory at The Technical University of Copenhagen, by means of an

Amsler pulsator (250 r/min), for one-sided bending stresses, the force
acting in one point on the middle of the length and immediately below
the bracing (fig. 1), the load thus being distributed fairly evenly throughout the length of the welding. However, the stress calculated at the

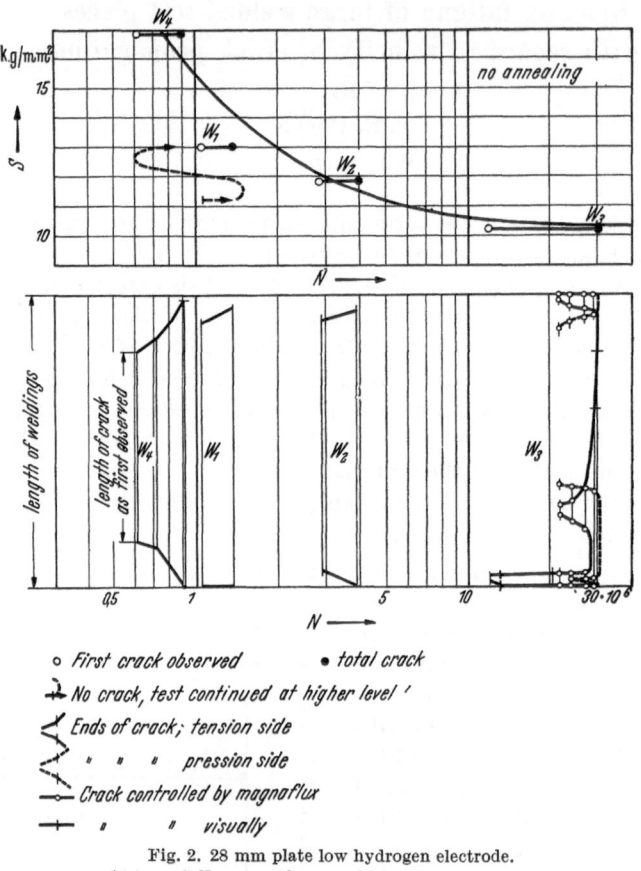

Fig. 2. 28 mm plate low hydrogen electrode.
At top: $S$-$N$-curves ($S$ = nominal stress)
At bottom: cracks as function of number of cycles $N$.

centre was about 3 per cent higher, and at the ends about 4 per cent
lower, than the nominal stress (fig. 4). The calculation of this was
checked by strain gauge measurements, both statically and dynamically.
A check was also made to ensure that no vibrations of significance
occurred (natural frequency 250 Hz, frequency of pulsator 4.17 Hz). The
stress was measured by means of manometers on the pulsator, and was
checked by dial gauge and partly also by strain gauge.

*The results* of the main experiment are shown in fig. 2 and 3 giving

$0-10.3 \text{ kg/mm}^2$ as endurance limit after welding, increasing to $0-12.4 \text{ kg/mm}^2$ after annealing.

The reasons for the *improvement in the fatigue strength by annealing* may be: a) the welding stresses are relieved; and b) the hardened

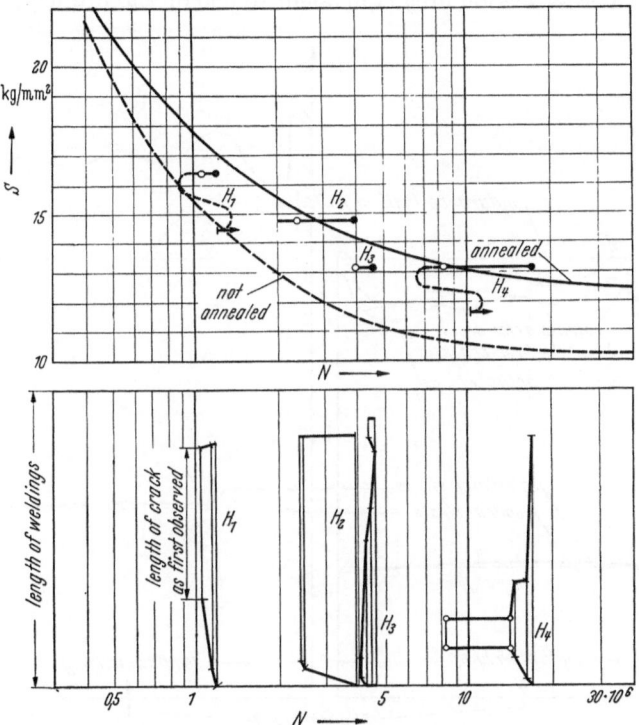

Fig. 3.  28 mm plate, low hydrogen electrode.  Same as fig. 2, but annealed at 650° C.  In dotted line the curve from fig. 2.

areas in the transition zone are tempered. A closer study of the welding stresses has not been made; but there is no doubt that these are at least of the order of the yield point.

In drawing the fatigue curves *Weibull's formula* was used [2]:

$$\frac{S - E}{T - E} = e^{-k \, (\log N)^m}$$

where $T =$ (about) tensile strength, $E =$ endurance limit, $S =$ endurance strength at $N$ cycles of stress. Though less correct and more difficult to apply than later formulas [3] it has the advantage of a single function covering the whole curve from $N = 1$ to $N = \infty$.

The maximum deviation from the fatigue curves, fig. 2 and 3, is about 6 per cent, which is surprisingly little considering the scatter to be expected with welding. Probably if a larger number of test-pieces were employed, some would be found to give a greater deviation. On the other hand, it must be borne in mind that each of these test-pieces has a cross-section area equivalent to 650 of the ordinary 7.5 mm

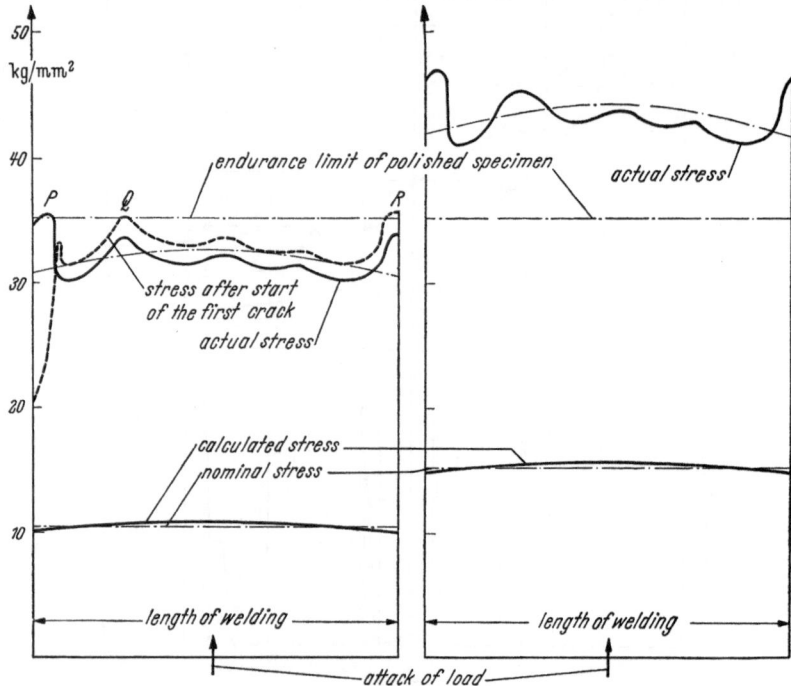

Fig. 4. Left: estimated stresses in tension side of weld W 3 (Fig. 2).
Right: same weld exposed to a higher load.

rotating beam test-pieces. Thus it is highly probable that a large number of "chance" flaws are present in all the big test-pieces.

The beginning of the *fracture* was generally ascertained by visual inspection; it appeared, however, that local heating could be felt some time before the crack became visible. At some points of W 3 (fig. 2) and H 4 (fig. 3) magneto-flux testing was used.

As could be expected, the *fracture started* in most cases near the centre of the weld length where the maximum stress occured. An exception is W 3, fig. 2, where the crack P started, after 11 million cycles, at the tension side near one end of the welding, where the termination had probably not been very well carried out.

It is noteworthy that, after this crack had developed to about 5 percent of the length of the weld, it stopped, and it was not till after about 10 million further cycles that new cracks $Q$ and $R$ were observed, while a further crack was found extending over about 60 per cent on the *compression side*. Nevertheless, another 10 million cycles had to take place before the plate broke.[1] The stresses indicated (in this case 10.2 kg/mm$^2$) are calculated without regard to the areas getting reduced by cracks; but as *the force* was kept constant during each experiment, the real stress in the cross-section of the fracture increased as the latter was weakened by the cracks. This also showed in the deflection increasing

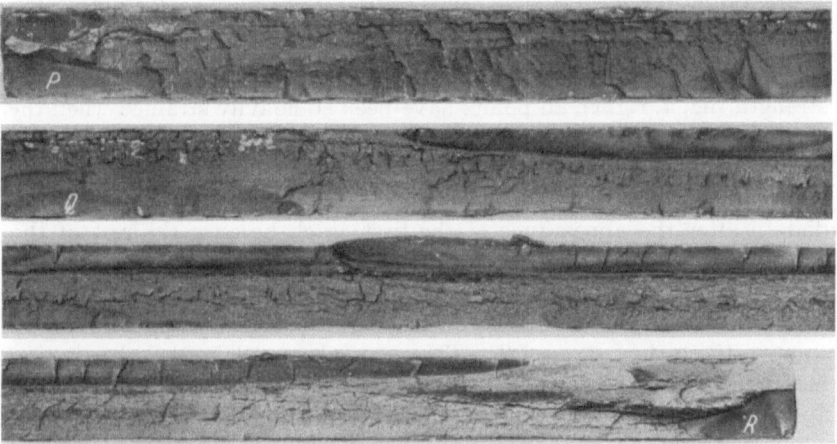

Fig. 5. Crack in W 3, photographed in 4 consecutive pictures. Tension side down. Letters P, Q and R correspond to fig. 4.

as the cracks extended. The stresses will often increase like this in practice (though not for statically indeterminate structures, and not for thermal stresses).

The actual tension along the welding may possibly take the course sketched in fig. 4, which shows, left, the tension under a load just about the fatigue strength. As mentioned above, the tension is a little greater in the middle. The transition between welding and plate gives a geometrical and metallurgical notch effect, which may be estimated to about 3; but in addition to this there are local notch effects arising from occasional flaws — for example, at the terminations of the welding. We thus get a single tension peek $P$ above the fatigue strength for material in polished condition, with the fracture beginning after, say, 11,000,000 cycles. As some of the surrounding material is also stressed

---

[1] The crack $P$ thus is what PHILLIPS has called non-propagating.

near the fatigue strength, the fracture quickly spreads through this material — in the fig. 4 to the left-hand edge of the plate, after which the course of the tension is as shown by dotted line. At the two other tension peeks $Q$ and $R$ the tension thus exceeds the fatigue strength; but as up to then it has been appreciably below, some 10,000,000 more cycles are needed before these tensions lead to cracks. When this occurs, the whole assembly is so much weakened that large sections of the material are loaded above the fatigue strength and the fracture now proceeds somewhat more rapidly.

The course of fig. 4 corresponds to $W3$ (fig. 2). A crack taking a similar course is seen in $H4$ (fig. 3). These prolonged stops are indicated in the fracture by clear "annual rings" (see fig. 5). Possibly also slag inclusions work as crack arrestors for a while.

If, however, the plate is loaded appreciably above the fatigue strength (fig. 4, right), all points have been so heavily strained when the first fracture occurs that the course of the crack will be more rapid and more continuous.

In highly uniform material the fracture will occur almost immediately after the appearance of the first crack because the rest of the material will also have been damaged. Heavily notched rods, on the other hand, will give a slowly proceeding fracture, since the fissure will continue to meet new material on its way which has been subjected to comparatively low stress [4]. This may also explain the observation mentioned by WEIBULL that in rotating beam test-pieces, stressed just above the fatigue limit, a crack starts from one point of the periphery whereas at higher load cracks develop so quickly that they seem to start at many points approximately at same time.

In actual machine-construction the tension will usually vary considerably more along a welding seam than in the present test. For this reason there is some chance of stopping a crack before serious injury occurs by control with magnetic tests, for example.

Similar experience has been gained about ten years ago with screw threads [1], where cracks likewise appear to develop comparatively slowly. The tension in the bulk of this material is appreciably less than at the thread root, where the bending tension in the thread itself is added to the simple tensile stress, while the notch effect doubles or trebles the tension.

That cracks also develop intermittently in practice is clearly shown by the "annual rings" in the fatigue fractures.

Finally, a test was made with three plates of *aluminium-killed*, probably oxygen-blown converter steel of Austrian origin. In this test the construction was annealed at 650° C (as in fig. 3); but, as

indicated by fig. 6, this material at any rate shows no better fatigue
strength than the normal Siemens Martin steel, which is appreciably
cheaper, despite the fact that the aluminium-killed steel was strained in
the rolling direction whereas the normal steel was strained perpendicular

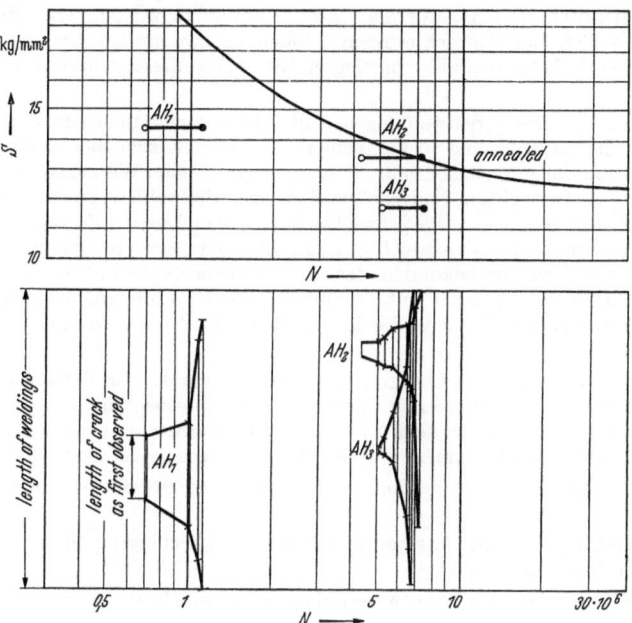

Fig. 6. 28 mm Al-killed plate, low hydrogen electrode, the curve from fig. 3,
drawn in.

to the rolling direction. The transition temperatures as obtained in
impact tests are appreciably more favourable for aluminium-killed
steel than for normal steel; yet this is not reflected in a corresponding
improvement in the fatigue strength of the welded and annealed construction.

## Bibliography

[1] WIENE, P. E.: Rev. gén. Mécan. 39, 51—57 (1955).
also: Ingeniøren 63, Nr. 29 (1954).
also to be published in Trans. Inst. Mar. Engrs. (Paper read Nov. 1955)

[2] WEIBULL, W. in W. M. MURRAY (Edit.): Fatigue and Fracture of Metals,
New York 1952, 182—196.
also: Tekn. Tidskr. 80, 1059—1064 (1950).

[3] WEIBULL, W.: Saab Aircr. Comp. TN 30 (Linköping, Sweden), 1954.

[4] Battelle Memorial Institute, Prevention of the Failure of Metals under Repeated Stress, New York 1949, 229—230.

## Discussion

M. HEMPEL: Sind die Proben röntgenographisch auf Schweißfehler geprüft worden?

Im Max-Planck-Institut für Eisenforschung, Düsseldorf, wurden 12 bis 16 mm dicke Blechproben aus St 37 geschweißt und die Proben röntgenographisch geprüft und nach Einteilung in bestimmte Fehlergruppen in Zugschwellversuchen untersucht (M. HEMPEL und H. MÖLLER: Arch. Eisenhüttenw. **20**, 375—383, 1949) Dabei ergab sich bei den fehlerfreien Proben ein wesentlich höherer Schwellfestigkeits-Wert als bei den hier vorgelegten Biegeschwellfestigkeiten von T-Schweißungen.

P. E. WIENE: Die T-Schweißungen sind schwer zugänglich für Röntgen und werden bei der B. u. W. nie so kontrolliert. Es handelt sich hier nicht etwa um Laboratorienausführung, sondern um in einer gewöhnlichen Werkstatt ohne irgendwelche spezielle Instruktion und von gewöhnlichen Schweißern ganz routinemäßig ausgeführte Schweißungen. Die Schweißer haben aber Lloyd's Zertifikat. Leichter zugängliche, auf Zug beanspruchte Schweißungen werden regelmäßig durch Röntgen kontrolliert und bekommen fast immer die beste oder nächstbeste Zensur. Der Unterschied beruht daher wahrscheinlich in erster Linie auf der viel größeren Kraftkonzentration bei T-Schweißungen in Biegung als bei Stumpfschweißungen in Zug.

I. ODING: Wir haben bei 60 mm Rundstäben, woran vier Platten radiell angeschweißt waren, in rotierender Biegung Ermüdungsfestigkeiten von $\pm$ 2 bis $\pm$ 3 kg/mm² gefunden; nach dem Ausglühen bekamen wir $\pm$ 4 bis $\pm$ 5, aber nach dem Bearbeiten $\pm$ 18 kg/mm². Sind Ihre Proben mechanisch bearbeitet worden?

P. E. WIENE: Nein, weder durch Hämmern noch durch spanabhebende Bearbeitung.

N. G. LEIDE: War die Analyse des Aluminium-beruhigten Stahls derjenigen des anderen Stahls ähnlich?

P. E. WIENE: Die Analysen waren einander ziemlich ähnlich:

|               | C    | Si   | Mn   | P     | S     | N      |
|---------------|------|------|------|-------|-------|--------|
| Hauptversuch: | 0.17 | 0.14 | 0.77 | 0.023 | 0.042 | 0.005  |
| Al-beruhigt:  | 0.12 | 0.25 | 0.50 | 0.010 | 0.016 | 0.0088 |

# Cumulative damage in fatigue

By

## E. W. C. Wilkins

With 9 figures

## 1. Introduction

Cumulative damage in fatigue is a problem which in recent years has become of interest to designers in almost all branches of structural engineering. To the aircraft designer however — especially under present-day conditions of operation — it is of paramount importance. During its lifetime, an aeroplane is subjected to repetitions of loads of various magnitudes and frequencies, and operating conditions involve take-off and landing at high loads, and flying at high speeds, aircraft which are large and flexible and which, in the attempt to achieve high structural efficiency, have been designed to an absolute practical minimum of weight. The aircraft designer today therefore is faced with the necessity of estimating not only the strength of a structure, but also its life — a task with which he was not confronted before.

Considerable work in this field has been done already [*10*], [*13*], [*19*], [*27*], [*28*], [*33*], [*34*], [*39*]. Most of this however has been of an ad hoc nature, and it is virtually impossible from it alone to propound any general hypothesis which would help a designer to predict the life of a particular structural assembly of new design. The fact is of course that there are too many variables, and if the situation is to be remedied, it is essential that much work of a more fundamental kind must be done.

The purpose of this paper is to describe a programme of basic research on the problem — along different lines from those normally adopted — initiated by the author, under the auspices of the Royal Aeronautical Society, about two years ago, and now being carried out at the Battersea College of Technology in London.

## 2. Method of investigation

It is well known that the relationship, generally attributed to MINER [*9*], but actually first proposed by PALMGREN [*1*], viz., $\Sigma n/N = 1$, does not hold generally, although it is thought that it may not be far wrong for the range of repetitions corresponding to maximum fatigue damage [*27*], [*39*]. Most of the work done up to now has been to test the validity

of this relationship, but the results have been far from conclusive. One
of the difficulties of course is that there are so many variables. Another
is that the situation is considerably masked by the large scatter that
fatigue test results always show.

In the present investigation, the PALMGREN-MINER hypothesis is
not assumed; on the contrary, the aim is to determine what the relationship is. An attempt has been made also to minimize the difficulties
arising from the large number of variables involved and from scatter.
In the first place, all the specimens for the tests have been made from
a single melt of material and the tests are being done under carefully
controlled conditions; in the second place, the work is being planned
so that the results can be interpreted statistically.

The main feature of this investigation is then to find a relationship
between the numbers of repetitions at various levels of stress when the
specimen being tested is failed at one of them.

Consider first the case of only two stress levels. Let $N_1$ be the number
of cycles necessary to produce failure at one level and $N_2$ the number

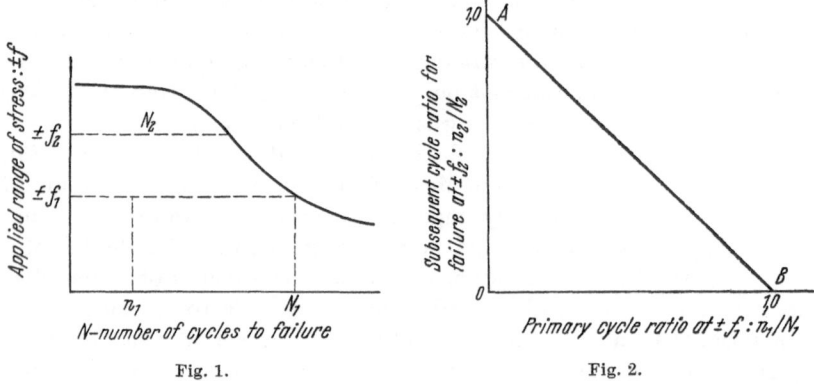

Fig. 1.                                Fig. 2.

to produce failure at the second level. Because of scatter, the actual
values of $N_1$ and $N_2$ adopted would be those corresponding to a specified
degree of probability.

Suppose now that we subject a specimen to $n_1$ cycles at the first level
of stress, $n_1$ being less than $N_1$ (fig. 1), and then fail this specimen at the
second level of stress. If the relationship $\Sigma n/N = 1$ held generally we
would have $n_2 = N_2 (1 - n_1/N_1)$, a relationship in which, for any given
values of $N_1$ and $N_2$ — and therefore for any given two levels of stress,
$n_2$ varies linearly with $n_1$, and if we plotted the ratio $n_1/N_1$ horizontally
against $n_2/N_2$ vertically (fig. 2), we should get the straight line $AB$.

In fact however, the evidence of test suggests that the relationship is not linear and, further, that its form is different for different values of the stress levels. In this case the general relationship would take the form

$$\Sigma n/N = \Phi$$

where $\Phi$ is a non-linear function of two levels of stress and of the number of cycles to which the specimen is subjected at the first level. The object of this investigation is then in effect to determine the form of the function $\Phi$.

In the case of two levels of stress it is well known that if the specimen is pre-stressed at the lower level and failed at the higher one, then, generally, $\Sigma n/N > 1$, while if the stressing is done in the reverse order it is less than 1, see ref. [3], [4], [8], [14]. The former case would be represented by a curve such as $ACB$ in fig. 3, for which, it will be seen, $\Sigma n/N > 1$, and the latter by a curve such as $ADB$, for which $\Sigma n/N < 1$. In either case $n_2/N_2$ is some function of $n_1/N_1$ and, therefore, since $\Sigma n/N = n_2/N_2 + n_1/N_1$, we should have

$$\Sigma n/N = \Phi(n_1/N_1)$$

It is clear from fig. 3 that the function $\Phi$ will only be numerically equal to unity, for all values of $n_1/N_1$, if the plotting of $n_2/N_2$ against $n_1/N_1$ should result in a straight line.

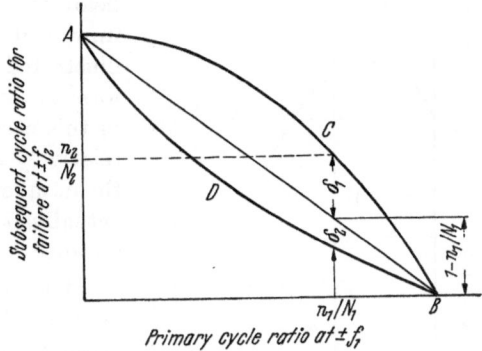

Fig. 3.

Curve ACB:
$$n_2/N_2 = 1 - n_1/N_1 + \delta_1$$
$$\therefore \quad \Sigma n/N = n_1/N_1 + n_2/N_2 = 1 + \delta_1 = \Phi(n_1/N_1)$$

Similarly for curve ADB:
$$\Sigma n/N = 1 - \delta_2 = \Phi'(n_1/N_1)$$

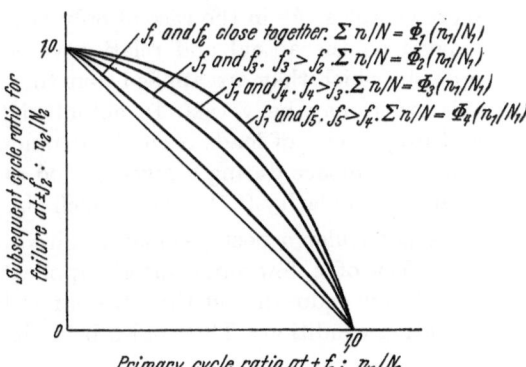

Fig. 4. Possible relationship between $n_1$ and $n_2$ for different stress levels.

Otherwise, $\Phi$ will be greater or less than unity, for $0 < n_1/N_1 < 1$, depending on whether the curve is convex upwards, as $ACB$, or concave upwards, as $ADB$. In either case of course $\Phi$ must be equal to 1 at the extremities.

21*

The actual form of the curve will be expected to vary with the relative values of the stresses. The closer together the two levels of stress, the more nearly one might expect the curve to approach linearity. This is illustrated in fig. 4. One might expect that the form of the curve would vary also with the actual values of the stresses. It is for example well known that if a specimen is subjected to a number of cycles at a low stress — particularly, in the case of ferrous alloys, at stresses just below the fatigue limit — the material is improved rather than damaged. This is illustrated in fig. 5, which represents the form of curve one could perhaps expect in this case. This curve shows that for relatively small values of pre-cycling $n_1$, the number of cycles to failure $n_2$ would actually be greater than the normal endurance $N_2$ at the higher stress.

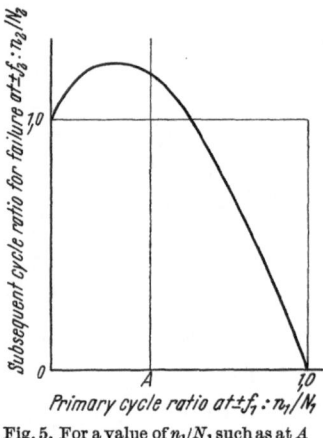

Fig. 5. For a value of $n_1/N_1$ such as at $A$
$n_2/N_2 > 1,0$ so that $n_2 > N_2$

It is also known that the results are affected if one of the stress levels is greater than the elastic limit of the material. In this case it is conceivable that the curve of $n_2/N_2$ against $n_1/N_1$ might be convex for one part and concave for the other.

If more than two stress levels are involved, the problem is much more complex. As in the case of only two levels of stress, the result will depend on the actual and relative values of the stresses, and on the order in which they are applied, but there are now more ways in which this order may be varied. In actual flight conditions the magnitudes and frequencies of loads occur in a somewhat random manner, but the general sequence during a given period of reasonable length is repeated with fair regularity [21], a fact which simplifies the problem somewhat.

A particular aspect peculiar to aircraft operation is the problem of the effect of a few intermittent applications of a high stress on the cumulative endurance at the lower stress levels corresponding to normal operating conditions. This is also being investigated.

## 3. Outline of programme

The object in this investigation is to find the relationship between the numbers of repetitions at various levels of stress when the specimen being tested is failed at one level.

To begin with, two levels of stress only are being considered. In this part of the investigation specimens are being subjected first of all to selected numbers of repetitions at one level and then failed at a higher level. The number of repetitions at the lower level of stress is varied, and so are the magnitudes of both levels of stress. The order of testing is then being reversed, the specimen being subjected first to various numbers of cycles at the higher stress and then failed at the lower stress.

The work will then be extended to the case of three levels of stress; afterwards, depending on the results obtained here, it may be further extended to the determination of complete endurance curves.

To give this work some practical design value, the tests are being done with material specifications which are actually used in aircraft construction and, in one part of the investigation, under representative loading conditions as well.

To begin with, the tests are being done in 4-point loading rotating bending machines, but it is intended later to repeat them in axial-load machines.

## 4. Details of tests

**a) Material.** The material for the rotating bending tests is L. 65 (formerly D.T.D. 364) and for the axial-load tests L. 71, which is the sheet version of L. 65.

To minimize scatter, the specimens for the entire programme have been prepared from a single melt.

This material was chosen for the following reasons:

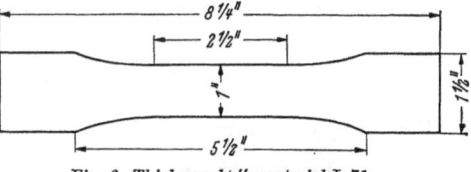

Fig. 6. Thickness $1/_8''$, material L 71. Sinusoidal transition fillets.

1. It is expected that the scatter will be less than it would probably be with other light alloy specifications, quite apart from the fact that the specimens have been produced from a single melt.

2. These materials are quite extensively used in aircraft construction.

3. Both materials are being used in a number of other investigations and it is hoped that it may be possible to correlate the results [37], [38].

**b) The test specimen.** The test specimen, for both the rotating bending tests and the axial tests, have long parallel centre portions, merging into the enlarged ends by means of transition fillets of special form. The design for the sheet specimen — for the axial tests — is shown in fig. 6. The round specimen — for the rotating bending tests — is similar. The object of the long parallel part is to increase the amount of material subjected to the test stress and the special fillets have been

designed to reduce the stress concentration at the points where the
fillets join the ends of the test portion, in order to reduce the likelihood
of failure inside the fillets. In fact, for all practical purposes the stress
concentration here is zero. The design of these specimens was the result
of a photo-elastic investigation carried out specially for the purpose
[36], [38].

c) **Range of investigation.** The general investigation will cover a range
of cycles from $10^4$ to $10^7$, with a more detailed investigation of the region
from about $5 \cdot 10^5$ to $2 \cdot 10^6$ — corresponding approximately to the
region of maximum aircraft fatigue damage.

d) **Number of tests at each point.** Twenty specimens are being tested
at each point on any curve. This was considered to be a reasonable
compromise between the need for economy and the requirements for a
statistical interpretation of the results.

e) **Testing machines.** The fatigue laboratory was specially equipped
at the Battersea College of Technology for doing this work. The machines are 4-point loading rotating bending Schenck machines; they run
at approximately 3,000 r/min.

It is intended to do the axial-load tests in a new type of testing
machine, now being designed, which will be capable of performing both
the cumulative cycle tests and the special tests involving the application
of intermittent loads during the cyclic testing of the specimen.

## 5. Preliminary tests

Certain preliminary tests have been carried out as follows:

a) To determine the mechanical properties of the materials.

b) To determine a suitable surface finish for the test specimens.

c) Endurance-probability curves for the basic material.

## 6. Part 1. Two levels of stress

a) A selected number of repetitions $n_1$, at one level of stress $\pm f_1$,
followed by repetitions to failure $n_2$, at a higher level of stress $\pm f_2$
(fig. 1).

These tests are being done for three intermediate values of the ratio
$n_1/N_1$, viz., $^1/_4$, $^1/_2$ and $^3/_4$. With the end values, this will furnish 5 points
through which a curve can be drawn to show the relationship between
the number of cycles and the two ranges of stress. This is illustrated in
fig. 7, where the points 2, 3 and 4 correspond to the three intermediate
values of $n_1/N_1$. Point 1, for which $n_1 = 0$, corresponds to the case of

a specimen failed entirely at the higher stress level $\pm f_2$, for which $n_2$ is equal, as it should be, to $N_2$. Similarly, point 5 corresponds to failure entirely at the lower stress level $\pm f_1$.

The cumulative cycle relationship for this case may be expressed as

$$\Sigma \, n/N = \Phi \, (n_1/N_1)$$

b) The tests described in 6 a) will be repeated, starting however with the larger stress range $\pm f_2$, followed by repetitions to failure at the smaller range $\pm f_1$. Now we shall have

$$\Sigma \, n/N = \Phi' \, (n_1/N_1)$$

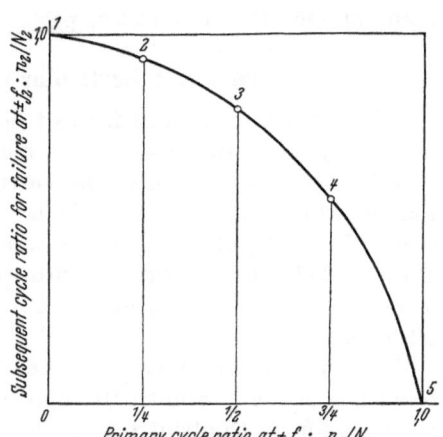

The object of these tests will be to compare the two functions $\Phi$ and $\Phi'$.

Fig. 7.   $n_1 =$ repetitions of stress at $\pm f_1$
$n_2 =$ repetitions of stress at $\pm f_2$
required to fail the specimen already subjected to $n_1$ repetitions at $\pm f_1$
$N_1 =$ endurance at $\pm f_1$
$N_2 =$ endurance at $\pm f_2$
$\Sigma n/N = \Phi \, (n_1/N_1)$

c) The tests in 6 a) and 6 b) will be repeated, starting with the same range of stress $\pm f_1$ as in 6 a), but failing at a third range $\pm f_3$, $f_3$ being greater than $f_2$, and then, as in 6 b), vice versa.

These tests will then be repeated for two further ranges of stress, $\pm f_1$ and $\pm f_4$, and again for two ranges $\pm f_1$ and $\pm f_5$.

d) All the tests are to be repeated for different values of the starting range, viz., $\pm f_2$, $\pm f_3$ and $\pm f_4$.

## 7. Part 2. Extension to three stress levels

a) In this part of the investigation the specimen will be subjected to repetitions $n_1$ at one range of stress $\pm f_1$, followed by repetitions $n_2$ at a higher range of stress $\pm f_2$, and then by repetitions to failure $n_3$ at a still higher range of stress $\pm f_3$.

In order to see whether it is possible to superimpose the results obtained for separate pairs of stress levels, the actual numerical values chosen for $f_1$, $f_2$ and $f_3$ will be those used in Part 1.

b) These tests will be repeated, if considered necessary in the light of the information obtained from the tests under 6 b), starting with the higher stress $f_3$ or even with $f_2$.

c) The tests in 7 a) and if necessary those in 7 b), will be repeated for different levels of stress.

## 8. Part 3. Extension to more than three levels

The details for this part of the work are being left until results have been obtained for the first two parts.

## 9. Part 4. A particular aircraft investigation

The problem of special interest here is to determine the effect of a few intermittent applications of a high stress on the cumulative endurance at lower stress levels. The particular case to be done first will be that in which the specimen will be subjected to continuous cycles of stress of $\pm 10\%$ of the ultimate strength of the material about a mean stress of $25\%$ of the ultimate, with, superimposed upon this, a number of regularly spaced applications of a stress of about 50 to $60\%$ of the ultimate.

The two important variables here are a) the magnitude and b) the frequency of the intermittently applied high stress. It is proposed to do the tests for up to about ten applications of each of four values of the intermittent stress, viz., 50, 55, 60 and $65\%$ of the ultimate strength. It is hoped that this will give some idea of what happens under such conditions and indicate lines along which the investigation might profitably be extended.

## 10. Some preliminary experimental results

The results of some preliminary tests of a purely exploratory nature are given in tab. 1 and 2 and in fig. 8 and 9.

Table 1. *Results of endurance tests on L. 65 plain specimens in rotating bending*

| Stress range in tsi $S$ | Specimen No. | No. of cycles to fracture $N$ |
|---|---|---|
| $\pm 12.0$ | 1 | 67,000 |
|  | 2 | 30,000 |
|  | 3 | 18,000 |
|  | 4 | 85,000 |
|  | 5 | 46,000 |
| $\pm 15.0$ | 1 | 90,000 |
|  | 2 | 156,000 |
|  | 3 | 317,000 |
|  | 4 | 285,000 |
|  | 5 | 212,000 |
| $\pm 19.0$ | 1 | 620,000 |
|  | 2 | 3,214,000 |
|  | 3 | 954,000 |
|  | 4 | 1,217,000 |
|  | 5 | 2,560,000 |

Table 2. *Results of some cumulative damage preliminary tests on plain specimens in L. 65 tested at two stress levels in rotating bending*

| Cycles at 28,000 psi | | Specimen No. | Cycles to fracture at 36,000 psi | | Average cycles to fracture of 5 specimens | | $\Sigma\, n/N$ | $\Sigma\, n/N$ Calculated from expression $1 + n_1/N_1 - (n_1/N_1)^2$ |
|---|---|---|---|---|---|---|---|---|
| $n_1$ | $n_1/N_1$ | | $n_2$ | $n_2/N_2$ | $n_2$ | $n_2/N_2$ | | |
| 190,000 | 0.2 | 1 | 94,000 | 0.90 | | | | |
| | | 2 | 106,000 | 1.01 | | | | |
| | | 3 | 101,000 | 0.96 | 95,400 | 0.91 | 1.11 | 1.16 |
| | | 4 | 72,000 | 0.69 | | | | |
| | | 5 | 104,000 | 0.99 | | | | |
| 380,000 | 0.4 | 1 | 84,000 | 0.80 | | | | |
| | | 2 | 101,000 | 0.96 | | | | |
| | | 3 | 97,000 | 0.92 | 92,200 | 0.88 | 1.28 | 1.24 |
| | | 4 | 92,000 | 0.88 | | | | |
| | | 5 | 87,000 | 0.83 | | | | |
| 570,000 | 0.6 | 1 | 73,000 | 0.70 | | | | |
| | | 2 | 68,000 | 0.65 | | | | |
| | | 3 | 80,000 | 0.76 | 72,800 | 0.69 | 1.29 | 1.24 |
| | | 4 | 67,000 | 0.64 | | | | |
| | | 5 | 76,000 | 0.72 | | | | |
| 760,000 | 0.8 | 1 | 43,000 | 0.41 | | | | |
| | | 2 | 47,000 | 0.45 | | | | |
| | | 3 | 44,000 | 0.42 | 42,000 | 0.40 | 1.20 | 1.16 |
| | | 4 | 37,000 | 0.35 | | | | |
| | | 5 | 39,000 | 0.37 | | | | |

Note:

$N_1$ = Average cycles to fracture of five specimens at $\pm$ 28,000 psi = 950,000
$N_2$ = Average cycles to fracture of five specimens at $\pm$ 36,000 psi = 105,000
$n_1$ = Number of cycles applied to specimens at 28,000 psi without fracture
$n_2$ = Number of cycles to fracture at 36,000 psi for specimens first subjected to $n_1$ cycles.

In these tests, five specimens only were used for each point on the curve. These were failed, in rotating bending, at each of three levels of stress, viz., $\pm$ 12, $\pm$ 15 and $\pm$ 19 tsi. The results are given in tab. 1. These results are plotted in fig. 8 and a smooth curve drawn through them. This provides the basic endurance curve for use in the second stage of the tests.

Five specimens were then tested, for each of four different values of the primary cycle ratio, at a stress of $\pm$ 28,000 psi, and then failed at a second level, viz., $\pm$ 36,000 psi. These results, with relevant calculations, are given in tab. 2.

The values of the failing cycle ratio $n_2/N_2$ so obtained are then plotted against the corresponding values of the primary ratio $n_1/N_1$ (fig. 9), and a smooth curve drawn through them. This curve is represented very closely by the expression

$$n_2/N_2 = 1 - (n_1/N_1)^2$$

giving, in these particular tests,

$$\Sigma\, n/N = 1 + n_1/N_1 - (n_1/N_1)^2$$

The numerical values of $\Sigma\, n/N$ calculated from this expression are given in the last column in tab. 2, for comparison with the experimental values in the previous column. The differences are quite small.

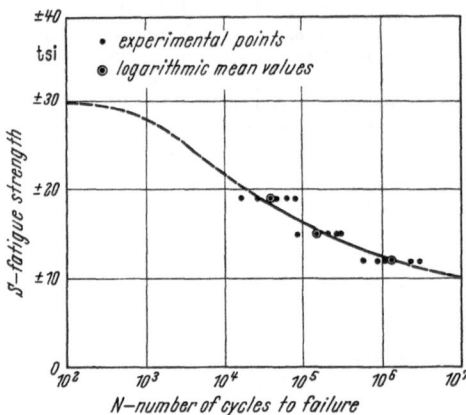

Fig. 8. Endurance curve for L.65 plain specimens used in cumulative damage preliminary tests. Five specimens tested at each of three levels in rotating bending.

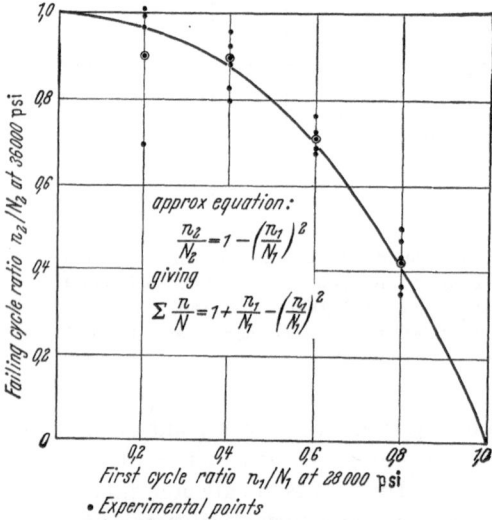

Fig. 9. Results of some cumulative damage preliminary tests on plain specimens in L. 65 tested at two stress levels in rotating bending.

## 11. Future work

It is intended to carry out a similar programme of work using copper specimens, and a start has been made in connection with a joint experimental mathematical investigation of the problem.

When the new fatigue testing machine has been built, it is proposed to carry out cumulative damage tests in which the specimens will be subjected to selected load spectra.

To conclude this paper, I would like to express my grateful appreciation to all who have made it possible for me to write it: to the Royal Aeronautical Society and to my colleagues on the staff there, and in particular to Miss PARISH for the painstaking way in which she produced the drawings for me; to the Battersea College of Technology and to my colleagues there for making available to me the facilities for doing the experimental work; and to the Aluminium Development Association for providing the material for the test specimens and for their general support for the investigation.

## Bibliography

[1] PALMGREN, A.: Z. VDI 68, 339—341 (1924).
[2] LANGER, B. F.: Trans. ASME 59, A 160—A 162 (1937).
[3] KOMMERS, J. B.: Engineering 143, 620 and 676 (1937).
[4] KOMMERS, J. B.: Proc. ASTM 38 Part 2, 249—268 (1938).
[5] KOMMERS, J. B.: J. appl. Mech. 5, 180 (1938).
[6] THUM, A. and W. BAUTZ: J. appl. Mech. 5, A 180—A 182 (1938).
[7] STICKLEY, G. W.: NACA TN 792 (1941).
[8] KOMMERS, J. B.: Proc. ASTM 43, 749 (1943).
[9] MINER, M. A.: J. appl. Mech. 12, A 159—A 164 (1945).
[10] JACKSON, L. R. and H. J. GROVER: NACA Adv. restr. Rep. 5 H 27 (1945).
[11] KOMMERS, J. B.: Proc. ASTM 45, 532—543 (1945).
[12] PUGSLEY, A. G.: Symp. Failure of Metals by Fatigue, Melbourne 1946.
[13] BENNETT, J. A.: Proc. ASTM 46, 693—711 (1946).
[14] KOMMERS, J. B.: Proc. Soc. exp. Stress Anal. 3, Nr. 2, 137—141 (1946).
[15] PUGSLEY, A. G.: J. Roy. aeronaut. Soc. 51, 715—720 (1947).
[16] RICHART JR, F. E. and N. M. NEWMARK: Proc. ASTM 48, 767—800 (1948).
[17] LUTHANDER, S. and G. WÅLLGREN: FFA Medd. (Aeronaut. Res. Inst. Rep.), (Stockholm), Nr. 18 (1949).
[18] WÅLLGREN, G.: FFA Medd. (Aeronaut. Res. Inst. Rep.) (Stockholm), Nr. 28, (1949).
[19] WALKER, P. B.: J. Roy. aeronaut. Soc. 53 (1949, Aug.).
[20] DOLAN, T. J., F. E. RICHART JR and C. E. WORK: Proc. ASTM 49, 646—682 (1949).
[21] WILLIAMS, D.: Aeronaut. Quart. 1, 291—304 (1950).
[22] NEWMARK, N. M. in W. M. MURRAY (Edit.): Fatigue and Fracture of Metals, New York 1952.
[23] ROŠ, M. and A. EICHINGER: Eidg. Mater. Prüf. Anst. Ber., Nr. 173 (1950).
[24] HARDRATH, H. F. and E. C. UTLEY: NACA TN 2798 (1952).
[25] HEMPEL, M.: Z. VDI 94, 882—887 (1952).
[26] DOLAN, T. J. and H. F. Brown: Proc. ASTM 52, 733 (1952).
[27] WILLIAMS, J. K.: J. Roy. aeronaut. Soc. 56, 842 (1952).
[28] WALKER, P. B.: J. Roy. aeronaut. Soc 57, 12 (1953).
[29] HARTMAN, A.: NLL (Nat. aeronaut. Res. Lab.) Rep. (Amsterdam) M. 1923 (1953).
[30] ERKER, A.: Schweißen u. Schneiden 5, 400 (1953).
[31] FREUDENTHAL, A. M.: Proc. ASTM 53, 896—909 (1953).
[32] MARCO, S. M. and W. L. STARKEY: Trans. ASME 76, 627—632 (1954).
[33] KENNEDY, A. P.: J. Roy. aeronaut. Soc. 58, 361 (1954).
[34] CHILVER, A. H.: J. Roy. aeronaut. Soc. 58, 396 (1954).
[35] CORTEN, H. T., G. M. SINCLAIR and T. J. DOLAN: ASTM Preprint Nr. 70 (1954).
[36] WILKINS, E. W. C. and H. T. JESSOP: J. Roy. aeronaut. Soc. 58, 435—438 (1954).
[37] SMITH, D. C.: Research Programmes under the Auspices of the Roy. aeronaut. Soc., Internat. Comm. aeronaut. Fatigue (1955) (Restricted).

[*38*] WILKINS, E. W. C.: A Summary of some current Fatigue Problems now under Investigation, Internat. Comm. aeronaut. Fatigue (1955) (*Restricted*).
[*39*] TYE, W.: J. Roy. aeronaut. Soc. **59**, 340—345 (1955).

## Discussion

E. GASSNER bemerkte, daß während des Krieges ähnliche Untersuchungen wie die vom Verfasser vorgeschlagenen an einer Reihe von Werkstoffen bei der DVL, Adlershof, ausgeführt wurden, und so verwirrende Ergebnisse ergaben, daß überhaupt keine Schlüsse gezogen werden konnten. Daher ist man zu Betriebsfestigkeitsversuchen mit vorgegebenem Programm übergegangen.

C. BRÖNN erwiderte hierzu, daß eine Schwierigkeit vorliegt ein Belastungsprogramm vorauszusehen, das den Anforderungen der Praxis genügt.

A. M. FREUDENTHAL confirmed that according to his experience rearranging the stress levels within a program cycle influences the results of program tests.

E. W. C. WILKINS appreciated GASSNER's interest and replied to BRÖNN, saying that it was essential to try to meet the practical conditions as far as possible in arranging any load programme, and he thought this could be done.

Replying to FREUDENTHAL, he noted with interest his experiance on the effect on the results, of re-arranging the stress levels within a programme cycle. This made it the more necessary to try to simulate practical conditions of loading.

# Subject index

# Table des matières

# Sachverzeichnis